"*A Step-by-Step Guide to Socio-Emotional Relationship Therapy* is a game changer. Thoughtful and well-researched, it strikes a great balance between the theoretical and the practical. It opened my eyes to power dynamics in relationships and gave me practical intervention strategies that I am already using. You will want to read it cover to cover, and then refer back to it regularly! *Everyone* can learn something from this book!"

—**Ryan B. Seedall**, *PhD, Associate Professor at Utah State University, Associate Co-Editor of* The Handbook of Systemic Family Therapy, *and Co-Author of* Deliberate Practice in Systemic Family Therapy

"This must-read book reveals how common societal discourses and interrelated 'isms' result in the individual, couple, and family relationship problems seen in therapy. This seminal book's illustrative case examples, reflective questions, specific competencies, and other core tools help novice and seasoned therapists and researchers to empower couples, families, and individuals to reject harmful societal discourses and improve their relationships according to their own values."

—**Shalonda Kelly**, *PhD, Graduate School of Applied and Professional Psychology, Rutgers, The State University of New Jersey; author of* Diversity in Couple and Family Therapy: Ethnicities, Sexualities, and Socioeconomics

"Knudson-Martin's pedagogical and clinical brilliance makes SERT principles of mutuality and equity accessible and practical. Readers will find clearly articulated definitions and clinical examples of how to engage and embody the humble contextual relationality the model offers us and our clients."

—**Jessica ChenFeng**, *PhD, Fuller Theological Seminary, co-author of* Finding Your Voice as a Beginning Marriage and Family Therapist

"In this wonderful, beautifully written book, Carmen Knudson-Martin presents her cutting-edge approach to relational therapy, the product of a lifetime of experience as a therapist, scholar, teacher, researcher, and supervisor, Knudson-Martin provides a compelling, clear theoretical framework for socio-emotional relationship therapy, offers a guide to the specific steps in its practice, and supplies numerous evocative clinical examples. This is a book that illuminates essential aspects of relational therapies that are often ignored by others: the implicit values underlying treatment. Feminist, egalitarian, but ultimately human, this book raises the consciousness of practitioners about vital aspects of relational therapy, having to do with power, social class, and other aspects of intersectionality. Valuable either as a comprehensive approach to treatment or as a source for those of various specific therapy orientations about how to incorporate issues about gender, culture, and intersectionality into relational therapy, this is *the* book about relational therapy you should read this year."

—**Jay Lebow**, *PhD, ABPP, Clinical Professor, Family Institute*
at Northwestern and Northwestern University

A Step-by-Step Guide to Socio-Emotional Relationship Therapy

Writing to the practicing clinician, this book offers a step-by-step practical guide to Socio-Emotional Relationship Therapy (SERT) when working with individuals, couples, and families.

Most therapists know sociocultural systems influence their clients' lives, but few know how to connect the dots between what happens in the wider society, interpersonal neurobiology, relational processes, and client well-being. Written by a founder of SERT, Carmen Knudson-Martin draws on knowledge from multiple disciplines to innovatively weave together a practical step-by-step guide that demystifies the connections between micro and macro processes and relational/self-development. Divided into four parts, chapters cover how to conceptualize clinical issues through a socio-emotional lens, the therapist's role in assessment, goal-setting, clinical decision-making, the "how-to" of each of the three phases of the SERT clinical sequence, and self-of-the-therapist work and clinical research that inform the model. The clear writing style and detailed examples make complex social processes accessible, demonstrating how good practice is—and must be—equitable and socially responsible.

This practical guide is essential reading for all mental health professionals, such as seasoned family therapists, counselors, psychologists, social workers, and students in training in these fields.

Carmen Knudson-Martin, PhD, LMFT, Professor Emerita, Lewis & Clark College, is a developer of Socio-Emotional Relationship Therapy. She has published widely on the political and ethical implications of therapist practices.

A Step-by-Step Guide to Socio-Emotional Relationship Therapy

A Socially Responsible Approach to Clinical Practice

Carmen Knudson-Martin

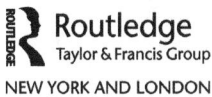

Routledge
Taylor & Francis Group

NEW YORK AND LONDON

Designed cover image: © Getty Images

First published 2024
by Routledge
605 Third Avenue, New York, NY 10158

and by Routledge
4 Park Square, Milton Park, Abingdon, Oxon, OX14 4RN

Routledge is an imprint of the Taylor & Francis Group, an informa business

© 2024 Carmen Knudson-Martin

ISBN: 978-1-032-21833-5 (hbk)
ISBN: 978-1-032-21832-8 (pbk)
ISBN: 978-1-003-27023-2 (ebk)

DOI: 10.4324/9781003270232

Typeset in Adobe Caslon Pro
by Apex CoVantage, LLC

I dedicate this book to Douglas Huenergardt and the SERT research team.

I hear your voices as I write, teach, and practice.

CONTENTS

FOREWORD

Lana Kim

As a family therapy educator, scholar, supervisor, and practitioner, there are key experiences that influenced my graduate education and training as a marriage, couple, and family therapist. Among these, was the privilege to participate as a doctoral student member of the Socio-Emotional Relationship Therapy (SERT) research team that Carmen Knudson-Martin and Douglas Huenergardt led at Loma Linda University. As a doctoral student, my clinical work had shifted from predominantly seeing parents and children to mostly working with couples, so I was invested in advancing my couple therapy skills. Therefore, the timing of this research was opportune.

What drew me to Carmen and Doug's research were the assumptions of SERT. I was inspired by the ideas that Carmen and her colleague, Anne Mahoney, had already been studying on the impact of sociocultural construction of gender and power on couple processes and how partners engage in the *Circle of Care*. I resonated with the idea that humans tend to inadvertently replicate inequitable patterns from the larger social context in their intimate relationships, that this is often invisible and unnoticed, and that this creates many of the relational problems that bring people to therapy. I connected with this premise because I saw it play out in the relationships of the couples who I worked with in therapy. I believed that learning to intervene in couple relational processes through the lens of

larger societal power processes held great potential for facilitating therapeutic change. However, I had no idea then just how significantly SERT
would shift my clinical work in the long run.

Being a part of this early research was challenging and inspiring. As
one of the research members who conducted the live couple therapy,
I remember fumbling more than not while learning to translate the theoretical concepts into practice and feeling uncertain if I was implementing
the ideas in therapeutic ways. However, the participatory action research
method allowed for Carmen, Doug, and the team to offer suggestions
and feedback on the spot during live sessions, and as the study progressed
and the team started to operationalize the ideas in practice, we witnessed
instances of what McDowell et al. (2019) have referred to as "third order
change" happen for our client couples. Motivated by seeing this change,
I started to apply the ideas with my clients outside of the research study,
and unsurprisingly, I noticed similar results.

A compelling case that validated the usefulness of this approach happened one year after I had terminated therapy with a White, early-40s,
cisgender, heterosexual client couple who had sought therapy after the
wife in the relationship had ended a year-long romantic affair with her
work supervisor. Midway through this couple's therapy, I shifted to using
the concepts I had been learning from the SERT research team, and
this transformed how I viewed the therapeutic problem as well as how
I facilitated the couple repair process. In short, the couple left therapy
reporting significant change in the way they viewed their role as partners
and how they did their relationship. The husband in this relationship left
a voicemail message to simply thank me for the work I did with them a
year ago, citing improved relational skills, active partnership, and feeling
like their relationship was stronger than it had ever felt before. This unso-
licited feedback was unexpected, but direct evidence to me that SERT
was a game changer for promoting a felt change in relational function.
In my work, using a SERT lens has served as the lynchpin to facilitating
fundamentally transformative couple therapy.

Couple and family therapy approaches do not inherently address the
societal inequities that play out in relationships, and SERT asserts that
when therapy does not attend to these power processes, it can inadvertently reinforce societal power differences that underlie client issues.

Furthermore, family therapy training programs and therapy models do not provide specific guidelines for how to work with the moment-by-moment power processes that show up in the microcosm of intimate partner relationships from a non-neutral stance. Because these conceptual ideas are difficult to operationalize and are not articulated in models, therapists often struggle to translate these into practice. Consequently, they often address power without sociocultural attunement to emotion, which leaves clients feeling invalidated, blamed, and defensive. Or they address power using language that is too conceptually abstract and can feel alienating. SERT recognizes that socio-emotional attunement and transforming power are related, so it is key to engage with sociocultural emotion and the flow of power in a relational way to promote greater shared relational responsibility between partners.

Since my first participation in SERT research 15 years ago, I have continued to collaborate with Carmen to study and articulate SERT processes, develop coding tools, explicate clinical sequences, and articulate clinical competencies, specifically around the idea of sociocultural attunement. I have continued to use SERT foundationally in my therapy, too, and to teach and train students in my graduate classes and supervision contexts about this approach. SERT is the only therapy framework I know that specifically helps partners move toward shared relational responsibility, and it positions the therapy "to counteract sociocultural forces that work against health and relationality." SERT privileges the idea of sociocultural attunement and requires the therapist to assess the relational power structure in a way that leaves clients feeling felt, understood, and seen. It reads the relational intent in clients' ways of living out partnership, while helping them recognize the ways they are practicing partnership that counters what they value. SERT provides therapists with an alternative blueprint for relationship therapy, producing meaningful, experiential change.

Whenever I teach students and other therapists about this work, the buy-in to the ideas is often immediate. Then, their first question is always: *How do I learn more? Is there a book, video, guide that can teach me how to do SERT?* I hear my former graduate student self in these questions, as I would have found such instructive resources to be invaluable in learning to practice SERT. *A Step-by-Step Guide to Socio-Emotional*

Relationship Therapy: A Socially Responsible Approach to Clinical Practice is exactly that ground-breaking text that everyone who wants to learn how to *do* SERT has been looking for. Written with the therapist in mind, it demystifies the doing of socially responsible couple therapy practice and addresses everything from contextual self-of-the-therapist development and therapist positioning and role to learning how to assess the sociocultural context of emotion, center the Circle of Care, build the therapeutic alliance, and develop treatment plans in tangible ways. It raises reflective questions for therapists, offers illustrative case examples to demonstrate higher-order concepts, provides operationalized definitions of clinical competencies, and outlines the clinical sequence. It also includes additional resources such as a SERT coding tool for research and practice as well as explaining how clinicians can study their own work as a facet of their learning. SERT is an important contribution to the field of family therapy, and this guide is a landmark text that enables readers to take SERT into the therapy room more directly than ever before. These practical ideas will revolutionize how therapists think about couple therapy, do couple therapy, and facilitate new relational realities.

Lana Kim, PhD, LMFT
Director, Marriage, Couple & Family Therapy Program
Lewis & Clark Graduate School of Education & Counseling
Portland, Oregon

ACKNOWLEDGMENTS

The development of Socio-Emotional Relationship Therapy (SERT) was, and continues to be, a shared endeavor. It is the result of many who are gifts in my life. My research with Anne Mahoney and numerous doctoral students on how gender organizes couple relationships across life stages and social contexts set the stage. Thank you, Anne, for your insightful and persistent questions, mentorship, and friendship that began when I was just starting this journey and continue to this day. Meeting and working with Douglas Huenergardt, who demonstrated commitment to relational equity not only in clinical practice but in how we worked together and with students, is the context that made SERT possible. What an unexpected gift that we joined the Loma Linda faculty at the same time!

Since the meeting of our first clinical research team in fall 2008, over 60 students have volunteered their time, hearts, and dedication to learning. I carry each of you within me. Many of your contributions, but not nearly all, are described in this book. Our team meetings have always been the highlight of my week. SERT is evolving through the impact each of you has on so many others through your practice, teaching, research, and/or supervision. Lana Kim, who joined the Lewis & Clark faculty and our SERT research teams in Oregon, has persistently and ever so gently pushed me to expand how I think about the meaning of power and how it intersects with culture. Lana, I am so honored by your preface to this book that captures the essence of SERT in so few words. Jessica ChenFeng, Elisabeth Esmiol Wilson, and Lindsey Nice also continued to work with Lana and me on several projects that expanded my understanding of the sociocultural nature of emotion.

A final unexpected gift was working with Teresa McDowell and Maria Bermudez to develop *Socioculturally Attuned Family Therapy*, now in its second edition. These overarching clinical practices and our generative back-and-forth conversations are indelibly woven throughout the SERT guidelines in this book. Your openness to building from our different vantage points is testimony to the value of a relational way of working. Of course, none of this would be possible without clients who trust us with the most precious aspects of their lives. Your stories and experiences are represented in this guide with gratitude and deep respect. Our clinical work together has always been a two-way street. I am grateful for what each of you has given me.

John, my life partner; my son Chris; daughter Kyara; and their partners, Melanie and Jerome, and grandsons, Ethan and Kai, keep me real. I am grateful for your patience with my time and professional commitments. You are with me in all that I do. Thank you for your love and the promise your lives bring.

AUTHOR BIOGRAPHY

Carmen Knudson-Martin, PhD, LMFT, is Professor Emerita of the Marital, Couple, and Family Therapy Program at Lewis & Clark College, Portland, Oregon, USA, and a founder of Socio-Emotional Relationship Therapy. Carmen has published numerous articles and book chapters on the influence of the larger sociocultural context in couple and family relationships and the political and ethical implications of therapist actions on marital equality, relational development, and couple therapy. She is editor and author of five books, including *Socioculturally Attuned Family Therapy: Guidelines for Equitable Theory and Practice, 2nd Ed.* (Routledge, 2023). Carmen was the 2017 recipient of the Distinguished Contribution to Family Therapy Theory and Practice award from the American Family Therapy Academy.

INTRODUCTION

1

AN INTRODUCTION TO SOCIO-EMOTIONAL RELATIONSHIP THERAPY

Everyone wants to be loved, to feel valued, heard, and respected. This is at the heart of my work as a systems-oriented family therapist. Whatever the initial client problems or symptoms, these relational issues are present. Moreover, these deeply personal core concerns are directly related to larger sociocultural contexts and carry implicit statements about one's worth and place in the world.

My colleagues and I developed Socio-Emotional Relationship Therapy (SERT) based on awareness that the nature of our relationship to larger societal contexts is a clinical issue foundational to other therapeutic goals. Larger contexts are like the air we breathe; they tend to be invisible to us and seem so natural that we don't question them. But unless we recognize and address them, they can make us sick or impede our development.

Most psychotherapists know sociocultural systems influence their clients' lives, but few actually connect the dots between what happens in the wider society, interpersonal neurobiology, relational processes, and client well-being. As a result, it is easy to inadvertently reinforce societal-based power differences, with detrimental effects. Seeing how larger contexts are part of the moment-by-moment of clinical processes and knowing how to respond require an intentional lens.

DOI: 10.4324/9781003270232-1

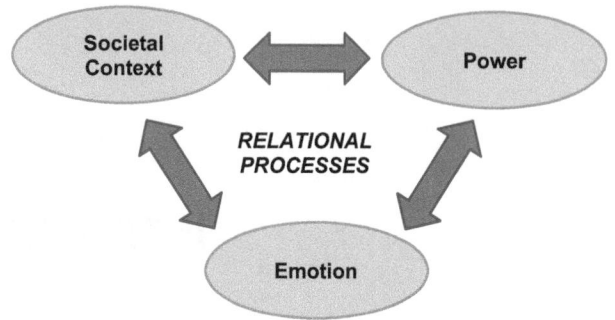

Figure 1.1 SERT Conceptual Overview

Source: Arici-Sahin, F., & Knudson-Martin, C. (2023). Socio-emotional relationship therapy in Turkey: Navigating equity and sociocultural change. *International Journal of Systemic Therapy*, p. 9 (used with permission)

SERT provides this framework. It integrates readily with other approaches or may be applied as a primary model. SERT centers the idea that healthy, just relationships provide mutual support and positions therapy to counteract sociocultural forces that work against health and relationality. As illustrated in Figure 1.1, practice focuses on what happens as societal context, power, and emotion converge in our closest relationships and social interactions.

Conceptual Overview

SERT begins with the recognition that people are fundamentally relational and need each other to thrive. How we understand ourselves, the world, and what is valued are not inherent or essential to us; they are constructed through social interactions (Gergen, 1997, 2021). The ability to define what matters is related to the flow of social power and the material conditions of life and distribution of resources that maintain the status quo (McDowell, 2015). The influence people have on one another is thus often not equitable or mutually supportive. Like contextual therapy (Boszormenyi-Nagy & Krasner, 1986; van der Meiden et al., 2020), SERT focuses on justice in the giving and receiving of care as an ethical contract between people. Distress and symptoms arise when this foundational contract is violated.

SERT draws on enduring concepts from multiple family therapy models and stands on the shoulders of many prior feminist, critical, and social constructionist scholar-practitioners. It incorporates advances in interpersonal neurobiology. SERT therapists use affective engagement and neurobiological infrastructure to promote health-affirming reciprocal care through a socioculturally attuned interpersonal process that validates, and often expands, the felt identity of each person. Therapists help clients evolve mutually supportive relationships that enable them to reflectively navigate larger societal contexts and the problems they face.

What Distinguishes SERT?

SERT therapists are intentional about our impact on social construction processes (Combs & Freedman, 2016; Murphy & Hecker, 2020). They provide leadership that interrupts societal power dynamics and orients therapy toward relationality, while maintaining a collaborative stance. Change happens as new experience based on equity and shared relational responsibility is embodied and ways of knowing oneself and others are expanded.

This book is a step-by-step guide to SERT practice, which involves:

- An engaged therapist socioculturally attuned to the felt identities of each person
- Development of relational safety through attention to interconnections between societal power and vulnerability
- Clinical dialogue/interventions that take into account varying power positions of participants
- A model of equity based on mutual vulnerability, attunement, influence, and relational responsibility
- Clinical work that invites alternatives beyond the limits of the dominant social system
- Clients able to address challenging issues from a position of mutual support
- Therapists accountable for the social impact of their work and the values it promotes

Development of SERT

One of the most important lessons SERT takes from feminist and social constructionist thought is that all perspectives come from somewhere; it is not possible to be neutral, and objectivity is an illusion. To understand and helpfully respond to a standpoint, we must know where the idea or person is coming from—what experiences and ways of knowing inform them. We also need to reflexively examine ourselves. This enables us to make responsible choices regarding our work and the values we support and to be accountable for our impact on others—on our clients and those whose lives are touched by our work, as well as to the larger community overall. This is our starting point.

Before focusing on the "how and why" of SERT practices outlined in the chapters that follow, you need to know something about me and how SERT was developed. While it will not be possible in a practice-oriented book like this to reference all whose work informs SERT, subsequent chapters will highlight many from a variety of disciplines. Beyond academic theory and research, however, is always the personal. As with any approach, SERT grew out of the confluence of personal relationships and experiences in specific contexts.

Carmen's Context

It was hard to write this heading. It seems too self-focused, too individual. In addition to a strong rule in my Lutheran, Scandinavian-heritage family of origin to never make yourself "big," I increasingly understand more clearly Bateson's (1972) concept that you cannot separate mind from environment. They are inextricably connected. This foundational family therapy idea can seem very abstract. I have come to take it very practically. It means that what I think and feel—as well as my physiological person, are not so much "mine" as a reflection of my relationships to what is around me. My story of how SERT came to be is filtered through my unique social location. Each of my colleagues would tell it somewhat differently, and while they are indelibly a part of SERT, each will evolve it in their unique ways—as will you.

I write this as a White, cisgender, heterosexual wife, mother, and grandmother who has taught, practiced, researched, and supervised family therapy for over 30 years. It has been my experience, both personally and with my students, that those of us who are White have the most difficulty recognizing the impact of larger contexts on what we think and do. It's usually easier to see these connections in areas where we hold less privilege. It's not surprising that much of my earlier work centered around gender. Becoming an adult during the women's movement made the salience of gender visible to me. The relevance of social contexts such as race, class, sexuality, nationality, abilities, etc., has taken more time and intention for me to see, and my conception of gender has become more fluid and non-binary.

Like all of us, my social locations intersect in unique ways—what Celia Falicov (1995) called a "cultural niche." Apprehending our own or another's sociocultural experience means seeking complexity beyond stereotypes. For example, I grew up on a farm in North Dakota. If you think of North Dakota at all, you probably think of it as a conservative place. But my parents belonged to a "liberal" farm organization. In this circle, my mentors were among the first Peace Corps volunteers and persons who marched for civil rights in the United States. We learned about cooperative markets and role-played perspectives of various countries in the United Nations. I read lots of books and watched television—became an observer of sorts. I knew people in the rest of the world had very different lives than mine. And people close to me were being drafted to fight in Vietnam.

Other aspects of my social location were nuanced as well. My father did not graduate from high school, and we lived frugally, but he and my mother were highly regarded in the community. In this rural setting, the Knudson name carried social capital that I inherited at birth. Everyone in the family worked on the farm; my mother's contributions always seemed every bit as important as my father's. We knew the ideology of "father knows best," but it wasn't my lived experience. In my first marriage, my husband and I shared egalitarian values; living them was not so easy. And for nearly ten years while raising young children, we lived as expatriates in Iran, Senegal, Jordan, and Costa Rica. My decision to go to graduate school followed this international experience, through which I became acutely aware that social norms and people's perspectives vary considerably. I also experienced generosity and warmth as people in each of these countries welcomed our family into theirs.

Foundation for a Socially Responsible Lens

I knew I wanted to study family therapy. That my Commission on Accreditation for Marriage and Family Therapy Education (COAMFTE)–accredited program at the University of Southern California also required me to earn a PhD in sociology was pure luck. A key sociological take-away is that human behavior cannot be reduced solely to the individual level. For example, Emile Durkheim's (1897/2005) study linked suicide rates to social factors; it showed that this most personal of acts is not purely personal (and helped establish sociology as a field). In the course of my doctoral research, I also came across Ivan Boszormenyi-Nagy's clinical focus on relational ethics (Knudson-Martin, 1992). This approach emphasizes responsibility toward one another as an ethical human contract directly related to health and healing. Nagy's work (e.g., Boszormenyi-Nagy & Krasner, 1986) said to me that we can't change the irrefutable connections to our families and social contexts, but we can change how we respond to them. It was also the only model I saw that emphasized accountability to others and to posterity as part of the clinical process. Together, the ideas that the personal is contextual and of accountability for our impact on others formed a scaffold for my evolving sense of social responsibility as it relates to the therapist role.

Once you learn to think systemically, you see patterns and connections you did not see before. I began to notice patterns among the heterosexual couples I was seeing. They (oversimplistically) seemed to boil down to that she wanted more connection and he wanted more autonomy. I was also reading about female development, including scholars such as Carol Gilligan (1982), who found that females approached moral dilemmas from a relational "voice" while males tended to take a principles-based position, and Mary Belenky and colleagues (1986), who wrote about women's ways of knowing and how these relate to the social construction of gender and power. As my students (Montana State) and I discussed how women and men tend to orient differently to relationships, we saw that these differences perpetuated and re-created patterns of power, with the more relationally oriented partner (virtually always female) carrying the relational load but unable to get the reciprocal connection they sought from a partner. Therapy "as usual" tended to perpetuate this pattern, prompting me to study the role of the therapist in gender construction (Knudson-Martin, 1994, 1995, 1997).

I met Anne Rankin Mahoney (University of Denver) at a conference. She is a sociologist, not a therapist, but she was fascinated with the gender issues I was seeing in my clinical work. We began qualitative research on how nonclinical heterosexual couples in varying life stages managed the gendered aspect of power. We discovered the "myth of equality" was prominent. Couples talked as though their relationships were equal, saying things like "we decided" or "we both," but when they described the details of how they managed their lives, these same couples repeatedly reported that, without really thinking about it, she accommodated him and took his needs into account in "her" decisions, while he functioned more autonomously and was largely unaware of the accommodations his partner was making (Knudson-Martin & Mahoney, 1996, 1998, 1999, 2005). Our work documented "invisible" ways gendered power structured heterosexual couple life not only in the division of labor but in communication and problem-solving patterns and in their disappointments regarding intimacy. Only couples who discussed gender patterns and consciously "undid" them described moving toward equality in whose needs organized their relationships and who attended to and accommodated the other.

In the meantime, I moved to Georgia and then to Loma Linda University in Southern California, where I directed the PhD in Marital and Family Therapy Program. In these contexts, I worked with more diverse students and clientele. I'll never forget when I asked a Black student in Georgia to present an overview of an assigned reading on gender. She said, "I'll do the report, but I don't know anyone like the women in this article!" At Loma Linda, my classes were seldom majority White. Many of these highly diverse students joined our research team. Due to their ability to reach out to a range of communities, participants in our studies were racially and ethnically diverse. We studied newlyweds, new parents, long-term couples with children, middle-class Black couples, immigrant couples, and retired couples and used the same interview guide with couples in Singapore and Iran.

We studied same-sex couples in long-term relationships and learned that most of them demonstrated relatively equal power, not because they set out to be equal, but because they sought to be attuned to each other and fair (Jonathan, 2009). Mutual interest in the other, rather than gender differences, tended to structure their relationships. Through our research, we were beginning to understand the relational processes involved in creating mutually supportive relationships. Anne and I compiled these studies in an edited volume, *Couples, Gender, and Power: Creating Change in Intimate Relationships* (Knudson-Martin & Mahoney, 2009). Each chapter included clinical implications and recommendations.

Action Research on Our Practices

Douglas Huenergardt and I started teaching at Loma Linda University in the same year. Our approaches to therapy had a lot in common—including having had Irv Borstein as a clinical supervisor early in our careers, at different times and in different states. Irv passed on to us a keen interest in working with in-the-moment clinical process and attending to structured relationship patterns. While I was learning from the writings of feminist family therapists such as Rachel Hare-Mustin (1978), Virginia Goldner (1985), and so many others (e.g., Goodrich, 1991; McGoldrick et al., 1989), Doug traveled regularly from Florida to Washington, DC, for a feminist supervision group with Marianne Walters, one of the founders of the Women's Project in Family Therapy (Walters et al., 1991). Doug and I began to do co-therapy and invited students to observe. As we discussed our work, new questions arose.

In fall 2008, we formed an action research project to identify the competencies involved in working with societal processes such as gender, culture, and power in therapy. Our research team took on some of the most challenging cases at our training clinic—mostly couples, but also families and individuals. Some of us watched behind the mirror while others were in session. Based on our prior research, we began with a relatively well-developed theoretical framework for how mutually supportive relationships work and why they are important to personal and relational well-being. In other words, we had an idea of the desired outcome of therapy that research showed to be so elusive. However, we did not know the clinical processes involved in getting there. How did we join with and support each partner/family member while challenging societal-based power differences in their relationships? How could we avoid imposing our own perspective, while also resisting and undoing the effects of social forces that perpetuate damaging inequities?

As will be discussed in more detail in Chapter 13, we used qualitative techniques to describe and analyze what we observed in session. We noted when societal factors appeared to be present, how therapists and clients responded, and how these clinical actions worked. As we analyzed these findings, we began to iteratively formulate a practice model that would improve our own work and provide guidance to others. We found we were working primarily with the links between three factors: societal discourse, emotion, and interaction, with societal power dynamics connected to each. We called the emergent model Socio-Emotional Relationship Therapy (SERT) (Knudson-Martin & Huenergardt, 2010; Knudson-Martin et al., 2015). Sociocultural attunement was foundational (Pandit et al., 2014).

In 2014, I joined the marriage, couple, and family therapy faculty at Lewis & Clark College in Portland, Oregon. Lana Kim, who had also been part of the research team developing SERT at Loma Linda, became an important faculty collaborator. Each year a team of graduate students joined Lana and me to further detail SERT as we grappled with the complexities of practice across cultures and contexts (Knudson-Martin & Kim, 2023) and to capture the clinical implications of the connections between vulnerability and power (Knudson-Martin et al., 2021). We also studied the students' own process of learning to integrate these issues into their practice (Morrison et al., 2022).

Third Order Thinking

While at Lewis & Clark, I also collaborated with Teresa McDowell and Maria Bermudez (University of Georgia) to develop a guide to the practice of socioculturally attuned family therapy across clinical models (McDowell et al., 2018, 2023). Teresa introduced us to third order thinking, a paradigm shift that helps us see current actions, ideas, and patterns embedded in systems of systems and makes imagining alternatives outside the dominant system possible (McDowell, 2015). This meta-perspective, along with Teresa's and Maria's insights (and those of many others) on working with race, gender and sexual minorities, socioeconomic status, nationality, legal and immigration statuses, and other ways people are marginalized and devalued, helped expand SERT to the exemplar of socially responsible, third order practice illustrated in this book.

How to Use This Book

Whatever your level of clinical experience and/or prior interest in equitable, socially just practice, this book is for you. As the title suggests, this step-by-step guide focuses on the "how to." Each chapter has numerous case examples that show what a therapist might say and do. These illustrations are based on actual cases, with identifying material and some aspects changed to protect confidentiality. Some are composites that reflect common patterns and/or more than one case. My goal is to help readers develop an overarching SERT-informed lens to guide what you think, see, and do as a clinician. If you are new to the field, the examples will offer a vision of the therapist's role in facilitating possibilities for personal and relational change and will help you critique, organize, and apply what you are learning. If you are more experienced, you will find it interesting to consider how you would typically approach similar cases. I invite you to adapt the guidance and illustrations to fit your own evolving clinical approach. Some of the concepts and examples may offer a new way to frame or address a familiar clinical issue or stimulate new ideas and questions beyond what I address.

The book is divided into four parts. It moves from case conceptualization to assessment and interventions. The chapters in Part I detail four practices that will enable you to conceptualize clinical issues through a socio-emotional lens. They describe how to expand your lens to recognize societal power processes related to emotion and vulnerability and how these affect personal and relational well-being. You will be introduced to the Circle of Care, four orienting principles that support well-being through relationships based on equity and mutual support. Part II addresses the therapist role from a socioculturally attuned perspective and leads you through SERT assessment, goal-setting, and clinical decision-making and treatment planning based on third order ethics. Part III walks you through competencies and strategies for each of the three phases of the SERT clinical sequence. We conclude with Part IV, which discusses how to contextually develop one's self-of-the therapist and the processes of studying our own practices. We conclude with a call to co-create the future.

As you go through this book and contemplate what from it you wish to make your own, consider the words of the legendary Salvador Minuchin (2017), founder of structural family therapy and social justice advocate, who called on therapists to use themselves as instruments of change:

> [A]s I got more experience it became clear that the techniques by themselves weren't all that useful. It was therapists themselves who were the instruments of change, and to be effective, they had to recognize the way they were part of the system and the process in the therapy room, not just a neutral observer.
>
> (p. 37)

My hope is that this book will help you examine your therapeutic role in the context of systems of systems. I encourage you to reflect on how to be intentional about the role you choose to play. Look for ways to collaboratively stay "with" your clients, while helping recognize, resist, and transform the effects of destructive societal inequities and dominant discourses in their lives. Reflexively examine your own contexts and responses to the difficult and unfair issues that arise in the therapeutic venture, and consider what you need to do to maintain a vision of possibility and be a keeper of hope. Though challenging, it is hard for me to imagine any work more engaging or satisfying.

PART I

SOCIO-EMOTIONAL CASE CONCEPTUALIZATION

2

EXPAND THE LENS

Practitioners are increasingly aware that our position in society is connected to our fundamental well-being and the quality of our most intimate relationships (McDowell et al., 2023; Watson et al., 2020). The implications of persistent societal inequities were foregrounded in the early 2020s as people struggled to deal with the global pandemic. Awareness of harm based on racial, gender, sexual, and legal inequities expanded through highly publicized movements such as Black Lives Matter and #MeToo (Kelly et al., 2020). The impacts of political and environmental contexts on day-to-day life—typically otherwise hidden from the consciousness of those of us in more privileged situations—are now brought to view through personalized and immediate media coverage of the effects of government policies, war, migration, climate change and environmental injustice, economic disparities, and social division.

Our challenge as therapists is to connect these broad social issues to clients' lived experience and our day-to-day work. There is a need for equitable, inclusive, and health-affirming relationships at all systemic levels—societal, community, and family (Kelly et al., 2020; Priest et al., 2019; Watson et al., 2020). We are called to use clinical practices sensitive to sociopolitical and moral issues and to challenge oppression (e.g., Piercy, 2020; Watson et al., 2020). In a key *Family Process* article, Marlene

Watson and colleagues advocated for an "ethics of care" that counters the tendency of dominant non-Latinx White Western culture to individualize problems by emphasizing our interdependence and the power of relationships. Fred Piercy, a former editor of the *Journal of Marital and Family Therapy*, appealed to the field to "be more aware, just, and affirming in our clinical work" (p. 757).

This chapter will help you expand your clinical lens to promote greater social awareness and just practice. We will review a bit of the history of what was called cultural competence, and which I now think of as sociocultural attunement and third order thinking, and use a case example to walk through five questions that will help you apply an expanded lens from the beginning of a clinical encounter.

From Cultural Competence to Socioculturally Attuned Practice

The rise of interest in cultural competence in the mid-to-latter 20th century raised awareness that therapeutic practice should be responsive to social and cultural differences. Though this mindset could result in a propensity to categorize and stereotype "others" and has been widely critiqued, it inspired questions regarding how the field determines what is normal and raised concerns that practitioners may pathologize differences without attention to sociopolitical contexts and power (Hardy, 1989; McGoldrick, 1998). Feminist and critical multicultural scholars drew attention to the dynamics of power, privilege, and marginalization and our influence as therapists to maintain or challenge inequities (e.g., Goodrich, 1991; Hare-Mustin, 1978; McGoldrick et al., 1989; Walters et al., 1991).

Social constructionists added to our understanding of culture, context, and diversity by helping us see identities and culture as fluid, changing, and differentially enacted (Laird, 1999; Paré, 1996) and by challenging the idea that we can be detached, objective observers. They showed that how characteristics of a group are described or what is considered real and good depends on who has the power to make these determinations (Gergen, 1997). Likewise, queer theorists stretched our thinking by "unmasking the social practices that construct normality" and opening space to consider a range of potentials regarding sex, gender, relationships, and family (Oswald et al., 2009, p. 43). Since therapists regularly assess behavior and make judgments about what is healthy, these perspectives raised awareness of ethical aspects of the meaning-making process inherent in therapy (Mazanec & Duck, 1999; Winslade, 2009): that what we pay attention to affects everything we say and the actions we take.

Over time, recognizing people in the context of multiple embedded systems and cultural niches within society has become foundational to systemic practice (Falicov, 1995; Imber-Black, 1992; Kelly, 2017). The notion of cultural competence has been evolving to what my colleagues and I called socioculturally attuned practice (McDowell et al., 2018, 2023) —a relational process "of seeking to know and be 'with' the experience of all clients . . . that recognizes and seeks to discover how culture and societal contexts are connected to every aspect of life, and discerns our role in it" (Knudson-Martin et al., 2020, p. 621). This means therapists must apprehend, organize, and make sense of large amounts of information in a way that captures the nuance and complexity of sociocultural context and helps our clients move toward health-affirming relationships and change (Falicov, 2014; Scher & Kozowska, 2012).

Third Order Thinking

Third order thinking enables us to connect the dots between client concerns and larger societal contexts (McDowell et al., 2019). It is based on Bateson's (1972) levels of learning and was brought to the attention of therapists by Teresa McDowell (2015). According to McDowell, third order thinking is similar to the notion of critical consciousness in which people become empowered or liberated when they become aware of the fundamental ideas and patterns that maintain the systems in which they are embedded. They begin to see alternatives within systems of systems.

Systemic therapists previously distinguished first and second order change. In first order change, the proposed solutions do not shift the basic "rules" by which a system operates; for example, people learn to manage their emotions or practice communication skills. In second order change, people recognize patterns and reorganize how their system works; instead of dealing with conflict by detouring it in arguments about the children, partners communicate their fears directly to each other. Third order thinking expands to take a meta-perspective on the systems we are in, to see them as part of larger systems of systems (e.g., economic, political, social) and to envision other possibilities. Third order change is based on this awareness; for example, recognizing emotional distress as related to social systems that emphasize productivity at the expense of relationship and taking intentional steps to reprioritize relational engagement.

When applying third order thinking, you automatically expand the lens to link intimate and family patterns to larger societal systems. In the example cited earlier, many therapists may recognize that gender roles might contribute to arguments about children. Third order thinking would also consider how other interlocking systems may operate together in a case. For instance, you would wonder how emotion and relational patterns are connected to economic structures and societal reward systems that sustain them; how dominant culture assumptions connect to multiple intersecting identities (race, class, sexuality, gender, nationality, abilities, etc.) and, in turn, are reflected in the give and take between partners; and how your own social location affects how you perceive your clients' experience and your role as therapist. Third order thinking provides a framework to connect these pieces and envision transformative third order change.

Responsibility Toward Equity

Clients generally do not see the connections between their problems and larger systems; you will need to actively facilitate this awareness. This means being both "knowing and not-knowing" (Falicov, 2014, p. 42). You must be knowledgeable enough about societal processes to know what you need to learn about or consider and how to explore alternative possibilities. At the same time, you need to engage collaboratively to understand each person's unique experience and the many intersecting factors likely to be involved. What we often think of as family and cultural processes are also inherently sociopolitical. According to Celia Falicov (2014):

> Without a lens that includes social inequities, cultural preferences may be used as explanations for economic failure, domestic violence, or poor school performance, whereas the larger negative effects of poverty and social discrimination are downplayed.
>
> (pp. 45–46)

In SERT, you begin to facilitate third order change by taking into account how these sociocultural power processes are present in the moment-by-moment of clinical work. This will enable you to position therapy so clients apprehend and experience relational possibilities beyond those defined by dominant social systems.

Socio-Contextual Questions That Expand the Lens

SERT expands case conceptualization through a socio-contextual lens that informs your internal dialogue as you meet clients and begin to know them. It shapes what you are curious about, what you ask, and the kinds of responses you make. For most of us, a socio-contextual lens does not come naturally. We experience our worlds personally, and if we are living in the West or studied concepts imported from the West, we are trained to see individual actions and identities. Expanding the lens brings otherwise invisible sociocultural processes into view.

The following five questions will help you bring an initial socio-contextual lens to client experience and your role as therapist:

- What societal power processes are part of this case?
- What societal discourses and values are at play?
- How are the client's identity and well-being connected to social power?
- How may societal power inequities affect the client's relationships?
- How is my clinical role in this case connected to societal context?

These questions challenge typically taken-for-granted power contexts and illuminate why attention to sociocultural context is at the heart of good clinical practice. Apply them to every case, not just when working with "minorities" or someone obviously culturally different from you.

Let's use an example to illustrate how to apply each of these questions as you engage with clients. Imagine you are meeting Jonah, a White, cisgender, heterosexual man, aged 38. He has been partnered with Joy (White, aged 39) for 17 years, and they have a 16-year-old daughter, Aimee, and a 12-year-old son, Nathan. Jonah is seeking therapy because he is "low energy" and "tense." Last week he had a panic attack at work and was referred to you through his employee assistance program.

What Societal Power Processes Are Part of This Case?

The philosopher Miranda Fricker referred to social power as "the capacity we have as social agents to influence how things go in the world" (2007, p. 9). She emphasized that sometimes people actively employ power to make another do something. For example, teachers can fail students if they do not complete an assignment as prescribed. But power often operates more passively—the teacher does not actually need to fail a student; the simple fact that they can do so has influence over what students do and how they perceive themselves. Moreover, the academic standards by which both teachers and students judge success reflect the priorities of dominant social groups. The interests of those in positions of power tend to define "shared" understandings and what is prized and valued in a society. Not only are these standards applied to all, according to Fricker (2007), the workings of social power processes result in epistemic injustice; that is, inequities in what constitutes the shared meanings that shape what we know and whose experience is viewed as credible. This happens in the larger society and is replicated in families and close relationships.

As you sit down to meet with Jonah, you are conscious that how Jonah has come to know himself, the actions he takes, and how he plays his part in relationships at home, at work, and in the community are connected to these generally taken-for-granted power contexts. As you get to know Jonah and hear his story, you will be noticing whose interests and needs are centered and how aware he is of the experiences of others. This attention to the flow of power is important because it affects the issues so central to clinical work—issues such as self-esteem, trust, intimacy, vulnerability, control and influence, conflict resolution, and communication (Knudson-Martin, 2013; Morrison et al., 2022).

You know that as a White, cisgender, heterosexual man, Jonah inherently brings power associated with each of these social locations into his personal world—whether he wants to or not. This does not mean that Jonah experiences himself as powerful. In fact, one of the hallmarks of being in a powerful position is that it tends to obscure awareness of one's impact on others. Others tend to accommodate to the power structured into the situation, even if those accumulating more power do not consciously intend it. And being in a powerful position tends to work against desired relational goals, such as closeness, connection, and mutual engagement (Jonathan & Knudson-Martin, 2012; Knudson-Martin & Mahoney, 1998, 1999, 2005, 2009).

◊ *Connect client concerns to power positions*

When you ask Jonah how "low energy" and "tension" are affecting his life, Jonah describes feeling "worn out and on edge." He says nothing is fun anymore; that he's fed up with all the [explicative] he has to deal with at work. You wonder how societal power processes are part of these experiences. It is clear that Jonah does not *feel* powerful, that he is not experiencing much personal agency at this point in his life. You reflect Jonah's feelings of powerlessness:

Therapist: It's hard to make your life go the way to want it to go these days—like it's out of your control?
Jonah: (sighs) Yeah. I feel like a bump on a log; like I'm not going any-where. [looks down]

Education and Socioeconomic Status

You know Jonah manages a crew that services maintenance vehicles. On his intake form he indicated his education level as a GED, a high school equivalency diploma that affords less social power than a college degree. You expand the therapeutic lens by wondering aloud about the power context of his work environment:

Therapist: (slowly, thoughtfully) You're a bump on the log . . . in the middle of . . . what? You manage a crew—what does that mean? You're in charge?
Jonah: In charge! Hah! Responsible is more like it. Those guys upstairs have no idea! They expect us to take care of everything—just like that! They don't give us the support we need. [Expletive], they don't even know what we do!

◊ *Explore social power contexts*

You begin to take in the hierarchical nature of Jonah's work situation. Despite his managerial title, Jonah experiences a persistent sense of diminishment from upper management when he tries to perform his role. Yet when you challenge this social minimization by asking about the skills his job requires and the importance of the work he does, Jonah's eyes light up. He says he and his crew have to be problem-solvers to get stalled machines going as quickly as possible. He takes pleasure not only in fixing the problem but in helping the machine operators. However, the "guys upstairs" have power over how Jonah experiences the value of his work. You notice and are curious about this social divide between the college-educated "upper management" and Jonah's crew:

Therapist: The guys upstairs, they don't know what you do—how does that happen? What do you think makes this divide?

Jonah: Charlie—he's my boss—he's a pretty good guy, I guess. But he gets his orders, you know. Doesn't matter if the orders make any sense! I tell him what we need to do the job, to work more efficiently. He says he tells them and it goes nowhere . . . no one understands, no one cares, [expletive] we could save 'em money!

Therapist: Like there's no way to communicate between you on the ground and the guys upstairs—more than that, what you say, what you know from your work day after day, doesn't count. You don't matter.

This sensitive reflection of the educational and social class power divide Jonah navigates touches him. He exhales deeply:

Jonah: Is it asking so much to want to matter? There're other things I could do, but I've got to make a living, you know—support my kids. Just play the game. . . .

Jonah's experience of "not mattering," that his input doesn't seem to be sought or taken seriously, is an example of what Fricker (2007) described as lack of credibility or epistemic injustice. You will need to explore further, but it is likely that those "upstairs" seldom seek Jonah's perspective or advice, or if they do, they do not understand or prioritize it. Though the kind of knowledge Jonah possesses is important to the functioning of the company, social power processes in this workplace render his voice almost invisible. This is detrimental to Jonah's well-being and also limits optimal functioning of the company.

Race and Power Processes

◊ *Use curiosity to name power processes*

You are also curious about the gender and racial/ethnic aspect of Jonah's work context.

Therapist: So, the "guys upstairs," are they all men? White men?

Jonah: (pauses a bit, which suggests he may not have thought about this much) Yeah. Everyone's White—I think. There's a new contract manager that's a woman. I don't know her name. She might be Hispanic or something.

Therapist: So upper management are nearly all White men. What about your crew? Are they White men too?

Jonah: No. Most of the guys are Latino. Frank is Black. No women.

You note that Jonah, the crew manager, is White. You wonder aloud how this racial and gender context affects relationships at work:

Therapist: So, you're managing a crew that's mostly Men of Color. How do you think the fact that you're White affects your relationships with them?

Jonah: We don't pay attention to race. We have a job to do, and we do it. We all get along pretty well.

As the conversation continues, Jonah describes little awareness of the perspectives of the Brown and Black men in his crew. He assumes they are all on the same page, because they show up on time and follow his orders. He believes the crew respects him. The ability to not think about race is an example of White privilege (Gallagher, 2003; Yancy, 2012). According to Yancy, whiteness is only invisible to those who have it. Social power dynamics around race and position limit the communication and personal connections between Jonah and his crew. It is possible that what looks like "getting along" is accommodation on the part of the crew, which may mask potential conflict or discontent. Like upper management, Jonah may also be missing information valuable to the engagement and performance of his team. It also leaves Jonah disconnected and alone.

◊ *Ask how roles and decisions are made*

To delve a little further into the intersections of race and position in Jonah's work environment, you ask how he came to be crew leader:

Therapist: How did it happen that you are the one that got promoted to crew leader?

Jonah: About two years ago Bud, the former crew leader, left—got a job at another company. He recommended me to Charlie. He and Charlie went way back, and I always got along really well with Bud. We'd get together on the weekends sometimes—with our wives and kids.

Therapist: You had the advantage of a connection to the people who make the decisions?

Jonah: Yeah. I never really thought about it that way. It seemed like a logical next step for me. Bud said I had the skills for it. He introduced me to Charlie and it seemed like a good fit.

Even though some of the other crew members had been on the team longer, Jonah—the White crew member—was identified as having the skills needed to take over as crew manager. This is an example of social capital (Garcia & McDowell, 2010). Jonah's similarity and connection to Bud, who was also a straight White man, smoothed the promotion wheels and increased the likelihood that he would be viewed as qualified for the role by upper management.

You now have an emerging idea of the power contexts in Jonah's work environment. While this is especially important since work was the site of Jonah's panic attack, you will be interested in expanding the lens with all your cases to include community and work/school contexts, including race/ethnicity, education and social class, and other factors such as sexuality, gender, nationality, legal status, etc. You want to get a picture of the social world in which your clients—and their clinical concerns—live.

Power Dynamics at Home

Jonah did not spontaneously introduce the perspectives of others into the conversation. Earlier, when asked how "low energy" and "tension" affected his life, some people might respond by saying they know he must be difficult to live with right now or that his kids try to avoid him because he's irritable and grumpy. That Jonah did not suggests a possible power imbalance in which attunement to his wife and children may not be a top priority. You are interested in learning more.

Jonah and Joy married when they were young. Soon, Joy was pregnant. Like many heterosexual couples, they automatically fell into a pattern that reinforced stereotypic gender structures (Knudson-Martin & Mahoney, 1998, 2009). Even though Joy worked as a hair stylist, she organized her time and focus around Jonah and the family. In contrast, though Jonah felt a responsibility to provide and enjoyed playing with the kids, he protected his personal space and time with his buddies and resisted "being told what to do." This created a gendered power imbalance in which Jonah's schedule and interests tended to shape the family as Joy and the children noticed and accommodated to his emotional states and activities.

◊ *Notice whose interests are centered*

When you ask how his low energy and tension affect Joy and the kids, Jonah responds that "none of them seem to give a [expletive]." In his response, you notice that Jonah seems to expect to be noticed and attended, and you are curious about a possible shift in the flow of power over time:

Therapist: No one seems to care . . . is this a change from earlier times? Did Joy and the kids seem more focused on you before?
Jonah: Yeah! It wasn't always perfect, but they seemed to look up to me—care about me at least.
Therapist: And what do you think they are experiencing from you now?
Jonah: I don't think they think about me at all!

You continue to probe for Jonah's ability to imagine Joy and the children's perspectives; however, Jonah remains focused on what he has lost or wants. His lack of awareness of his family members' experience while seeming to expect them to pay attention to him is a sign that Jonah is probably used to being in a power position in relation to his family. Through a so-cio-contextual lens, this is not just a family dynamic; it is a societal pattern structured into how gender and other societal roles are defined.

What Societal Discourses and Values Are at Play?

The term "discourse" refers to shared ways of thinking and talking that give meaning to experience (Krolokke & Sorensen, 2006). Societal discourses connect individual meaning and action to social systems and structures and are reflected in what we feel. These patterns in how we speak and in-teract arise from social and relational engagement over time (Bava, 2023) and are reflected in people's life narratives and identities (Combs & Free-man, 2016). As in Jonah's workplace, they are also reproduced in organ-izational structures and social policies that reinforce and re-create social inequities, with socioeconomic, interpersonal, and health consequences.

◊ *Move from personal story to societal one*

Without a third order socio-contextual lens, social discourses are likely to be seen as only individual-level expectations, values, and priorities. Look for the societal discourses embedded in your clients' stories. Listen for social messages regarding what people expect from themselves and others, what they feel entitled to, ideas about togetherness and separate-ness, what constitutes success, and ideas about what is good or bad, right or wrong. For example, when you ask Jonah about his statement that he is "worn out and on edge," you listen for and identify the societal standards and expectations within his story:

Therapist: You said you're worn out and on edge. Could you say more about that?

Jonah: I can't seem to do anything right. I should be on top of my game, and instead I'm [hesitates] confused. I don't know which way I'm going.

The idea that Jonah should know what he is doing, that he should not be confused or uncertain, is a common Western discourse especially im-posed on and upheld by men. As you reflect this "should," your awareness of this common societal discourse helps you put words to it:

Therapist: (thoughtfully) So . . . you should do things right? Know where you're going, not be confused?

Jonah: My dad always said, "If you don't know where you're going, how can you lead?"

You will eventually want to know more about Jonah's family of origin, but for the moment you stick with a socio-contextual lens to understand his (and his dad's) experience:

Therapist: Sounds like a strong message, that you are supposed to lead, to know what you're doing. What does this message say about you if you are uncertain, confused?

Jonah: That you're not a man . . . that you're not on the ball, not worth much to anyone.

Therapist: Where do you think this idea comes from—that men have to be on top of everything?

◊ *Voice the underlying societal message*

By naming and exploring Jonah's confusion as a gendered idea that comes from somewhere, you stay close to his experience but shift the conversation from something wrong with him individually to something beyond him alone. You and Jonah are beginning to develop an expanded framework from which to approach his concerns.

Dominant Western discourses emphasize individualism, competition, and self-reliance at the expense of relational values (Combs & Freedman, 2016; Mehl-Madrona, 2010). The values, qualities, and interests of people and communities oriented toward relationships tend to be minimized or discredited. Jonah's anxiety and lack of energy are occurring in this sociocultural context.

How Are Identity and Well-Being Connected to Social Power?

There are many social discourses. As individuals engage with others and their worlds, they draw on the available discourses to assemble identities—a sense of who they are in relation to others. As we move from one discourse community to another, some stories of self are more meaningful or relevant than others. Saliha Bava (2019) offered "hyperlinked" as a helpful metaphor for this way of thinking about identities as both fluid and connected. Jonah resonates with some sets of identity discourses when he is relating to "the guys upstairs" and with a different set when overseeing his crew. He engages other social discourses at home with Joy and the children. All of these identities are in some way positioned in relation to larger heteropatriarchal discourses that support and maintain the dominant socioeconomic system. Some may be in opposition to the dominant discourse, such as when Jonah says, "I have always been a sensitive and artistic guy."

◊ *Listen for alternative/marginalized identity discourses*

Thinking of identity as fluid, multistoried, and created through relationships encourages you to be curious about the aspects of Jonah's sense of self that have been discounted or marginalized:

Therapist: In what settings was the sensitive and artistic guy welcomed?
Jonah: My mom used to call me her "little artist." She gave me lots of art supplies when I was a kid.
Therapist: You mother encouraged the artist when you were young. How did others respond to you as an artist? In what other settings were you welcomed as an artist?

◊ *Ask about social meaning*

Notice the contextual nature of these questions. They are asking about ideas and responses of others, expanding the lens outside Jonah and his family.

Jonah: Nowhere really—not as I got older. It wasn't really a guy thing. I didn't talk about it with my friends. I kept doing it though—at night in my room; just for myself, just scribbles . . .
Therapist: What would it have said about you to be labeled as an artist—and sensitive?
Jonah: That I didn't fit—that I wasn't serious. Not capable of doing anything that mattered.

Therapist: So . . . what you took in, the message you got, was that to matter, to do something serious, you had to hide your sensitive artistic
part? [Jonah nods]. How do you think this happens in our society?

Identity building is not a passive process in which we simply absorb
what the outside world tells us about ourselves. It is an interactive activity
in which some experiences are more emotionally meaningful and become
neurologically structured in our bodies (Mehl-Madrona, 2010; Zimmerman, 2018). For Jonah, knowing himself as "sensitive and artistic" was a
vulnerable position. His socio-emotional experience said he could not
uphold his role as a man—a man doing something that mattered—when
connecting to his sensitive and artistic qualities. This lifelong social marginalization of some aspects of his identity limited how Jonah could know
himself—and how others could know him. As you connect the personal
and the contextual, you wonder how this social experience relates to his
panic attack at work:

Therapist: How does the idea of you as a sensitive and artistic man fit
into your job at work?
Jonah: (pause) It doesn't fit at all. At work I'm playing the game . . . you
can't be sensitive or artistic and do that.
Therapist: How so? What do you mean, "playing the game"?
Jonah: Fitting into the mainstream. Doing what you have to do to get
the paycheck. Living that life like everyone else. Ever since the kids
were born, I really don't have a choice. I've got to be a good father.
I mean, I love the kids, but if it weren't for them . . .
Therapist: So, the way you've learned to be a good father—to fit into
those mainstream expectations about doing something [air quotes]
serious—means you have to cut yourself off from the sensitive artistic
part of you? It's not even a choice . . .
Jonah: I'm a smart guy. I could do anything—I never wanted to get
caught up in that merry-go-round . . .

◊ *Use queries and reflections to help clients expand their stories*

Jonah dropped out of high school because he didn't want to put up
with what he saw as superficial, meaningless expectations he associated

with "the mainstream." When he met Joy, he saw a fellow "free spirit." When they became pregnant, he studied for the GED so he could get a better-paying job. He thought of himself as a good employee and had been pleased to be promoted to crew manager. And in response to your questions, he told you that Joy and the kids were "everything" to him. He is irritated at himself for feeling tense and low energy. Applying a socio-contextual lens, you see that Jonah tried to resist many dominant social discourses for White heterosexual masculinity, but living outside them carried economic implications for his family. Over time, these dominant culture expectations regarding providing and fatherhood guided his life. You name this context around which Jonah's panic attack occurred.

Therapist: From what you're telling me, it seems that even as a kid you knew there were a lot of different ideas out there about how to live your life; you—probably more than some people—saw what you would have to give up to fit in the mainstream. [Jonah nods] I'm picturing you at work, this sensitive artistic guy doing your job—doing it well—and all of a sudden panic sets in.

Jonah: (thoughtfully) I hadn't thought about it like that, at least not for a long, long time; thinking about it now . . . it makes sense—Wow! [takes a deep breath] that's a lot to think about.

Therapist: It's a lot to lose.

There are, of course, more components to Jonah's story. You will be interested in how personal and family developmental histories interconnect with larger socio-contextual factors. As Sally St. George and Dan Wulff (2014) framed it, braiding macro-level sociocultural discourses together with micro-level (personal and family) patterns and interactions helps us see the meaning and complexity of our clients' dilemmas.

◊ *Connect social power and vulnerability*

Our research (Knudson-Martin et al., 2021) found that attention to the interplay between vulnerability and social power is especially important. The power context creates different kinds of vulnerabilities for all involved. The cultural discourses regarding masculinity and fatherhood that Jonah internalized and struggled with support a male-dominant social structure. Regardless of who plays the leadership roles, qualities associated with heteropatriarchy (assertive, competitive, nonemotional, etc.) are prioritized in these discourses. To identify as a cisgender male and not demonstrate those qualities is a vulnerable position. Jonah experienced this vulnerability throughout his life, with clear expectations of leadership/dominance modeled by his father and reinforced by his peers, school, media, work, etc. Helping Jonah address his anxiety requires that you apprehend his felt experience of vulnerability, even as he enacts a power position in relation to his children and Joy and judges himself (and is judged by others) by these "masculine/professional" standards in his work life.

Attuning to the sociocultural and power contexts of vulnerability enables you to recognize multiple ways vulnerability is expressed depending on the intersections of social power, marginalization, trauma, and developmental processes. Our research identified five ways clients express vulnerability.

- *Socialized vulnerability*: societal discourses encourage them to take a vulnerable position (maintains a submissive power position)
- *Socialized invulnerability*—societal discourses suggest they should remain unaware of their vulnerabilities and/or hide them from others (maintains a dominant power position)
- *Reactive (in)vulnerability*—a response to societal marginalization and/or trauma that protects the self by resisting and/or maintaining domination
- *Reactive vulnerability*—a response to societal marginalization and/or trauma that protects the relationship by taking on blame or responsibility
- *Shared vulnerability*—each person is open, curious, and willing to admit mistakes and express needs—promotes shared power

Socialized expressions of vulnerability tend to reproduce societal power structures. For example, women are expected to protect men from expressing vulnerability by knowing what they need and taking on responsibility for maintaining relationships; persons with marginalized identities and cultures are expected to silence themselves and conform to dominant culture standards and norms, so as to avoid making more privileged persons uncomfortable. Reactive vulnerability/(in)vulnerability are more nuanced and often exacerbate socialized power patterns despite an internal sense of worthlessness on the part of the dominant person (see Chapter 4). Sometimes a person (often female) may use anger protectively and look powerful, while actually having limited influence in the relationship.

Apprehending the connection between your clients' felt identities and their clinical concerns contributes to forming a therapeutic alliance. A third order socio-contextual lens also helps identify and validate previously marginalized social discourses that may be meaningful to clients and expand the possibilities available to them.

How Do Societal Power Inequities Affect Relationships?

From a relational perspective, power is not an individual property or characteristic; it is a dynamic process of influence between people and groups. When I refer to someone's power position, I am thinking of it as the outcome of a relational process—one that often involves many components and that may shift from context to context. People with limited social power are more vulnerable physically and emotionally. They experience less safety and security, are more likely to suffer mental and physical illness, and die earlier (Watson et al., 2020). Mutually supportive relationship bonds can be an important resource in dealing with societal stressors, including discrimination and marginalization (Bergeron et al., 2020; McDowell et al., 2023).

Because power imbalances limit trust and communication, they not only hurt the less powerful, they also harm those holding more power. As we developed SERT, we learned that the ability to interrupt and transform these power inequities and/or their relational impact was foundational to other clinical change (Knudson-Martin & Huenergardt, 2010; Knudson-Martin et al., 2015).

◊ *Observe power processes in session*

From your initial conversation with Jonah, you have a sense that he is not very attuned to Joy and the children, yet seems to expect them to be attentive to him. To learn more, you invite Joy to the next session. As you introduce yourself to Joy and welcome her to the session, she is clear that she loves Jonah, but thinks this a problem he needs to address himself. This surprises you a little, because stereotypic gender discourses tell women that they are responsible for the well-being of their families and partners.

According to Karyn Loscocco and Susan Walzer (2013), the culture of American heterosexual marriage is such that individualism is prized but gendered—men are entitled to and expected to enact individualism, while women are encouraged to support relational bonds and are held responsible for relationship troubles. You are curious to know more about Joy's seemingly more individualistic stance and wonder how it affects the couple's power dynamic:

Therapist: (to Joy) You say that Jonah has to address this problem on his own. Can you say a little more about that?

Joy: I don't mean he's totally on his own—of course not. But when we first got together, I followed Jonah in everything. He was a free spirit, so I was a free spirit. I've been there for him through everything! And now I need some space. Don't get me wrong; I love Jonah. I feel bad for him. I worry about him. But I've just finally begun to find myself. I've started working on a degree in social work. I've done some of my own therapy. The kids are older now. [sighs]

Therapist: (naming the power process) You followed Jonah in everything. What do you think told you that you should do that? Be what he wanted you to be?

Joy: It's how we were raised. All my friends were focused on our boyfriends. [pause] I even had sex with him before I really wanted to.

Jonah: What do you mean? You always said you wanted to!

Joy: I know. But I was afraid I'd lose you; that you would think I wasn't into you.

◊ *Explore egalitarian and relational ideals*

You see that what could look like partners both focused on themselves is actually a move on Joy's part to correct a long-standing imbalance in which one partner is focused on the other. Given the substantial research that shows most couples today hold egalitarian values and want to be emotionally connected but have difficulty achieving these ideals (Jonathan & Knudson-Martin, 2012; Knudson-Martin & Mahoney, 2009; Sullivan, 2005), you probe to identify Jonah and Joy's relational goals:

Therapist: Jonah, it sounds like it's a surprise to know that Joy's been following your lead for so many years. Is that what you wanted—a relationship where she follows you? Where you determine the direction for both of you?

Jonah: Of course not! I want us to determine things together. But now she doesn't seem to care about me. She just wants to go her own way.

Therapist: (to the couple) What you want is a relationship where you can both be there for each other and support each other's health and goals. Is that right? [both partners agree]

You recognize multiple societal discourses at work in Jonah and Joy's relationship—stereotypic gender patterns that put relational responsibility on Joy (until she resists) and discourage Jonah from focusing on or being aware of his need for others, as well as less well-developed discourses that invite shared relational responsibility and emotional connection. Your sociocontextual lens enables you to identify and highlight relational possibilities that the larger society (possibly including Joy's personal therapy) tends to minimize.

Therapist: If I'm understanding correctly, for a long time Joy was the relational glue that held the two of you together and supported you, Jonah, and it put Joy's needs on the back burner. Am I getting that right?

Jonah: I never meant to put Joy on the back burner!

Therapist: It's a common pattern that happens to a lot of couples. How do you think Joy on the back burner limited how the two of you could communicate? Your connection with each other?

Joy and Jonah's relationship was limited from the outset because societal discourses shaped their interactions such that Jonah's interests guided their relationship without either partner intending this pattern. When

Anne Mahoney and I studied nonclinical heterosexual newlywed couples and couples with young children (Knudson-Martin & Mahoney, 1998, 2005), we found this happened for most participants, primarily because they fell into these social patterns without discussing them. Couples with more equal relationships made more intentional decisions, which frequently also included expressing and working through more conflict.

Power imbalances constrain communication. Those in powerful positions can't risk appearing uncertain or showing their weaknesses; it is not safe or acceptable for those with less power to say or do things that upset those with more power. Clear and direct communication is impossible or risky. As long as the less powerful accommodate and/or day-to-day patterns are well-established, life can go smoothly, albeit with emotional intimacy compromised. But when changes happen, a crisis emerges, or social stressors like discrimination or a pandemic add to life's challenges, the ability to creatively respond is restricted. Conflicts are impossible to positively address, so they are either swept under the table or dealt with at only a surface level. Depression, substance abuse, or focusing outside the relationship are common coping strategies that maintain power imbalances.

When relationships are distressed—regardless of gender and sexual orientations—there is usually a power imbalance in who is able to influence the relationship and receive support and care. Jonah and Joy are both still committed to their marriage and family, but their ability to support each other is compromised. Their relationship is structured, in part, by destructive societal patterns they did not consciously choose. Individual symptoms, such as Jonah's, often arise in the context of relational power imbalances.

Societal power discourses also affect parent-child relationships. When we studied parents of young children, we found that when parents followed gender discourses that told them mothers had a natural connection with children, men tended to step back from regular child care tasks and ended up emotionally disconnected from their children despite their desire to be engaged fathers (Cowdery & Knudson-Martin, 2005). When Aimee and Nathan were younger, Jonah played with them and "helped" Joy with their care, but he was considerably less attuned to them than Joy. Jonah loves his children and has always enjoyed activities with them, but his relational connection with them is limited. It is harder for him to engage with them now that Aimee is a young adult and Nathan is almost a teen. He is not used to apprehending what they are feeling and need. The ability of Aimee and Nathan to know their father is also restricted.

How Is My Clinical Role Related to Societal Context?

The inequitable social structures and discourses that influence clients' lives are also present in the therapeutic space. When clients express familiar societal messages, they may seem so familiar that we do not question them. Or when clients do not conform to dominant discourses, we may view them through a pathological lens. When our clinical approaches emphasize individualistic outcomes such as autonomy or goal-directedness, we may not ask what other kinds of potential outcomes are being overlooked. Like clients, therapists enact societal discourses they do not intend. If you imagine you are neutral, you will likely reinforce the status quo.

◊ *Position your practices in relation to the dominant discourse*

Through a third order socio-contextual lens, neutrality is not possible. Therapists need to be intentional regarding how our words and interventions are positioned in relation to dominant discourses. The dialogues illustrated in this chapter were situated to open possibilities obscured by the dominant social system. Even though they flowed from client experience, the discussions of class, race, gender, and relational power did not happen automatically. They depended on how you responded to the clients' accounts and the questions you asked. In other words, as the therapist you are co-creating what is said and talked about and how problems are defined.

You could have focused primarily on Jonah's anxiety and helped him develop strategies for how to manage it (first order change). Or you could have helped Jonah share his struggles with Joy (second order change). While these strategies could be helpful, if not integrated into a larger perspective, they would reinforce the idea that Jonah's problems lie within him (i.e., that he is the source of the problem). They would also replicate the idea that women should tend to men (but not vice versa). Alternatives outside these systems would seldom come up. In contrast, you invite Jonah to reflect on the impact of his behavior on Joy, his children, and his crew. This sort of intervention interrupts dominant gender and race patterns and addresses client symptoms in a sociocultural context (third order change).

Most of us learn early in our clinical training that clients need to make their own decisions based on their values and what matters to them. This is sometimes interpreted to mean that therapists and counselors should take a passive, less influential role. In SERT, we agree that clients need to make their own decisions. The question is: What do we add to the clinical conversation? Who and what do our actions support? How can we position our work to shed light on what has previously been unseen? How can we facilitate an experience that opens new possibilities and connects personal and relational outcomes to systems of systems?

◊ *Ask what values your work supports*

Ivan Boszormenyi-Nagy's work (Boszormenyi-Nagy & Krasner, 1986) reminds us that as humans we have an ethical relationship to one another and to our environment. In SERT, we ferret out and validate skills and characteristics associated with relational values. We trust that when we ask people about relational aspirations, we will find them. When asked, Jonah said he did not want a relationship where Joy followed him. If the therapist had not opened this line of inquiry, it may not have come up.

Jonah also volunteered in passing that he had always been sensitive and artistic—probably as a way to explain part of "his" problem. The therapist's response highlighted the social context around this marginalized discourse and worded questions in a way that made room for a variety of possible masculinity discourses. Had Jonah not spontaneously raised this alternative, you would have listened for what was not said and invited other options. For example:

Therapist: You said you take your role as a father seriously—that this is why you work so hard. What other ways do you show your love as a father?

OR . . .

Therapist: Your father emphasized that men should lead. I'm curious about the other side as well. What have you learned that helps you take in or notice what others are longing for or need? For example, where Joy wants to go? What matters to her?

◊ *Be transparent about your relational and equitable values*

I make my relational position clear to clients from the outset. I tell them I work from a model that assumes that whatever problems people are facing, they are usually related in some way to the world around them and their relationships with others. People get this. I also tell them I work from the premise that relationships should mutually benefit and support each person and ask if they agree. I have never had someone say no.

Applying third order thinking will help you develop a socio-contextual lens to connect the dots between clients' personal experiences, larger social contexts, and your clinical role. Like learning to think systemically, once you begin to recognize these connections in clients' stories, you will see them regularly. They will no longer be able to remain invisible to you. In SERT we are especially interested in the connections between societal discourse, emotion, relational patterns, and power. We work with these in three inter-connected phases (see Chapter 8 and Appendix C):

Phase 1: Position—Position therapy to counter inequalities and orient toward relationality

Phase 2: Interrupt—Create relational safety by shifting in-the-moment-power processes

Phase 3: Practice—Embody new options and practices that pro-mote mutual support and equity

In Jonah's case, your initial contextually based questions and reflections have charted an emergent larger framework through which to approach his presenting concerns. As a result, Jonah will likely have begun to think about his panic attack and low energy and the options available to him in light of the societal messages that inform his identity and what he has lost personally and relationally. You will build on Jonah's relational desires by positioning therapy to interrupt power patterns that keep Jonah disconnected from others. Rather than viewing Joy as self-involved or disinterested in Jonah, you will help Jonah take responsibility for relational engagement that he previously left to her, beginning with attunement to her experience and accountability for the burden she has carried.

While you don't know what decisions Jonah and Joy will make as they go forward, you will help them make these choices from a more equitable foundation and expanded awareness of their social world and how they want to interact within it. The overarching SERT goal will be to help Jonah experience mutually supportive relationships with Joy and in the larger community. These will enable more intentional, just, and health-promoting responses to societal, work, and family stressors. In the next chapter we explore how the connections between emotion, relational engagement, and societal discourse serve as the foundation for this goal.

Therapist Checklist: Expand the Lens

☐ Connect client concerns to social power contexts
☐ Observe power processes in session
☐ Use curiosity to name power processes
☐ Ask how roles and decisions are made
☐ Notice whose interests are centered
☐ Move from personal story to societal one
☐ Voice the underlying societal message
☐ Listen for alternative/marginalized identity discourses
☐ Connect social power and vulnerability
☐ Explore egalitarian and relational ideals
☐ Ask what values your work supports
☐ Be transparent about your relational and equitable values

3

LINK EMOTION, SOCIETAL DISCOURSE, AND RELATIONAL PROCESS

You have expanded your lens to see the societal context. Now what? How can you facilitate third order change when social structures are so pervasive and largely out of our control? Once our team understood that emotion is the bridge to the sociocultural, developing a model of change became a lot easier. Meaning is socioculturally structured and created in social interactions, but it lives in the body and in our visceral connections with others (Siegel, 2019; Zimmerman, 2018). In other words, socio-relational experience literally changes our bodies. Change involves new relational experience. In SERT, third order change is an experiential process that involves the interconnections between societal discourse, emotion, relational engagement, embodied interactions and identities, social power, and relational justice and well-being (see Figure 3.1).

In this chapter we consider why optimal human development requires ongoing mutually supportive relational bonds. You will learn how emotion, societal discourse, and power connect to create lived experience and involve the neurobiology of the social engagement system. You will see how these socio-emotional processes relate to core clinical issues such as safety, identity, belonging, and mutual support and why reciprocity based on mutual care is a relational justice issue foundational for other clinical change (Knudson-Martin & Huenergardt, 2010).

DOI: 10.4324/9781003270232-3

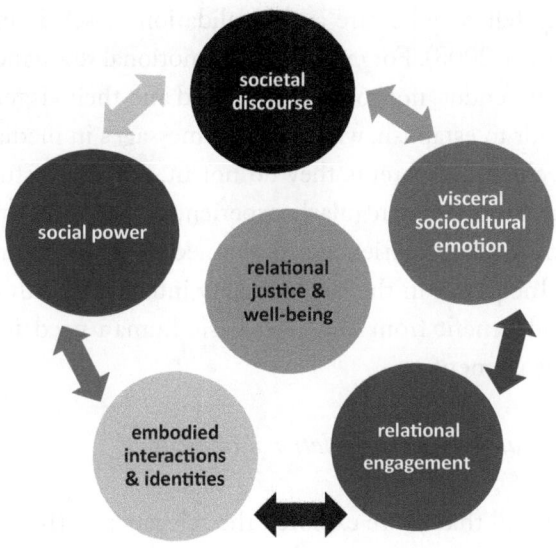

Figure 3.1 Socio-Emotional Experience

Why We Need Equitable Relationships

Socio-Emotional Relationship Therapy begins with the assumption that humans are fundamentally connected to each other and to their social worlds. People cannot thrive without reciprocally caring relational bonds. We need to love and be loved. How we respond to each other has substantial consequences, both positive and negative. Interpersonal neurobiologists and attachment theorists have documented why this is so (Gerhardt, 2004; Fishbane, 2007; Johnson, 2019). Their work helps explain the physiological aspect of what it means to be social creatures and the interpersonal nature of development and offers implications for optimizing the change process. Bottom line—in order to flourish, we need to "feel felt" (Siegel, 2012), to experience a sense of being known and belonging. This is both an interpersonal process and a sociocultural one. It is not a "would be nice if you can get it"; it is a core human need. Understanding this relational requisite involves rethinking emotional life and what we mean by justice.

Those whose personal experience does not fit dominant societal understandings and expectations live in an inherently unjust world in which feeling felt may be rare and invalidation of self is insidious and ongoing (Brown, 2008). For example, the emotional resonance between a transgender or gender "nonconforming" child and their cisgender parents may be difficult to establish, while societal messages in media and school also tell the child and parents they do not fit. A college student from a working-class family may regularly experience disconnection from peers at school, while also experiencing disconnection from their family and community. Inequities in the larger society intertwine with our capacity to receive and benefit from our most basic human need for connected reciprocal engagement.

◊ Identify and align with relational interests

You may recall that as we explored the relevance of the larger societal context to Jonah's clinical concerns in the last chapter, we saw that power processes left him alone and disconnected from others at home and at work, despite his relational desires and needs. He was even cut off from potentialities of his self. This disconnection from others and limitation in who one can become shows up in virtually every troubled client and relationship I see. This is why, along with attention to the larger context (see Chapter 2), SERT begins with identifying and aligning with relational needs and interests.

Imagine that you are working with another case, a distressed couple who seeks your help co-parenting their young child. The following five guidelines will help you connect emotional experience, social discourse, identity, and well-being as you get to know them and establish a therapeutic contract.

□ Reciprocal responsivity is essential to well-being
□ Emotional safety and connectedness are adaptive
□ Social discourse drives emotion
□ Identities and belonging are felt sociocultural experiences
□ Sociocultural value and emotional capital politicize well-being

Norma (age 32) and Simon (age 47) married when they learned they were pregnant with Tam (18 months). Following Tam's birth, the couple began experiencing escalating conflict and fights. Though their battles never included physical violence, the intensity scared them; it was not the environment they wanted for their daughter. About six months ago, as the pandemic abated, the couple separated, and each has been involved in individual counseling while they shared parenting approximately 50–50. They are seeking your help to work through what happened between them in the hope of being good co-parents. Determining whether they will reconcile or divorce is not their immediate concern. On the intake forms, each identifies as heterosexual and Latinx. Each indicates experiencing abuse in the past. Simon also reports a history of alcohol abuse, with 10 years sobriety. Both say religion is not important to them. Simon has a 19-year-old daughter, Sarah, with whom he indicates a limited relationship.

Reciprocal Responsivity Is Essential

A key point you keep in mind as you get to know Norma and Simon is that across the lifespan people need to be on the same wavelength as others, responsive to one another's inner states and what matters to them. This is not simply a matter of direct communication; it is more subtle and requires each person to attune to and take in the experience of the other (Siegel, 2007). Daniel Siegel emphasized that it is not enough for others to "get" our experience; we must also be able to empathically imagine what is going on for *them*. It is a two-way (or more) street in which the neural systems of each person reciprocally impact emotional regulation and the physiological response of the other, a process Stephen Porges (2009) called the social engagement system. Reciprocity and responsiveness are key.

Emotional connection based on attuned communication is an intentional act of openness to the internal state of the other (Siegel, 2007). Neurons in one's body viscerally mirror the other's experience. Each body is changed, activating metabolic processes that stimulate the neuroplasticity needed for flexibility and growth while reducing stress (Cozolino, 2016). When people are not able to—or will not—attune to the other, personal and relational development is thwarted.

Norma and Simon wanted to evolve as parents and lovers. But due to their histories and sociocultural contexts, including heightened tensions around togetherness due to the pandemic and life cycle changes, they resist this process by fighting. Neither is able to risk vulnerable engagement. Their internal physiology is also affected, including the likelihood of reduced serotonin and increased cortisol, which are associated with depression (Hanna, 2014), as well as decreased immune functioning and increased stress to nearly every part of the body.

◊ *Assess degree of reciprocity*

It is important to note that although both Simon and Norma are fighting and resisting engagement, this does not mean their positions in the relationship are equal. When you reflect that it seems hard for each of them to risk vulnerability, Norma immediately takes responsibility, while Simon focuses on Norma as the source of their problems. This means Norma is more vulnerable and burdened in the relationship:

Therapist: From what you are describing, I'm guessing it feels a bit risky for either of you to engage with each other.

Norma: That's on me. With my history, what I've been through, I just can't let myself get hurt again. [looks down] I wish I could; I know it would help, but not yet . . .

Simon: That's just it! She goes off the handle at everything! She won't listen. She's too sensitive.

Attuned engagement requires reciprocity. Norma shows signs of trying to attune to Simon, but when it is not reciprocated, she backs down or gets angry.

Norma: I know. It's hard for you when I get upset. I understand that. I get it. I try to stay calm, but . . . [closes her eyes]

Simon: I'm just frustrated. I raise my voice—so what? [louder] You make me out to be someone I'm not!!

Norma: I know. I can be hard to live with . . . I just need you to be patient with me.

◊ *Gently invite reciprocal relational engagement*

At this point, you know Norma demonstrates some empathy for Simon despite her distress. You need to know whether you can also access Simon's relational interests and empathy for Norma. You also want to send a message that you see their relational potentials even if they are not always able to enact them. You frame your response in terms of the reciprocal human need to know another and to be known:

Therapist: Simon, I can see how distressing it is when there is this gap between you and Norma. You want her to understand. You want this relationship to work and to be a good parenting team. [Simon agrees] It's hard when there is this distance [Simon nods]. It's hard for Norma, too.

Simon: Yeah. I know her history and all that. But I'm not her dad or [Norma's prior partner].

Therapist: You want her to see you as a caring, loving person—a caring, loving father. Can you say more about why Tam and Norma are so important to you?

Simon: (sighs) I messed up the first time.

Therapist: With your daughter?

Simon: Yeah. With Sarah, with everyone. [expletive] I was a real jerk, but that's not who I am today. Why can't Norma see that!

◊ *Name relational consequences*

We have learned that when therapists identify the relational desires of powerful partners, it is important to follow by also identifying the relational consequences of their actions (Samman & Knudson-Martin, 2015). Otherwise, the session tends to become focused on the needs of the dominant partner and inadvertently maintains the power imbalance. Therefore, you join with Simon's relational desires *and* also begin to address his accountability to be responsive:

Therapist: You're afraid Norma sees the jerk you used to be. [pause] What would it mean if she saw you that way?

Simon: That maybe I haven't changed. . . . That I'm not good enough. [quickly, emphatically] But I have changed!!

Therapist: (gently) It's hard to be the new man you're becoming, if Norma can't see it?

Simon: Yeah! She doesn't give me a chance!

You shift from his relational interests to his relational accountability:

Therapist: You get upset when you think Norma's not giving you a chance. [pause] How do you think it affects her when you get upset? When you raise your voice?

Simon: I don't know. [shakes his head]

Therapist: (calmly) Just think for a moment. You know Norma. You know your raised voice is hard for her. What do you think that is like for her?

Simon: (slowly) It can't be good.

Therapist: It can't be good and . . .

Simon: I suppose she feels like she's being attacked—that she could be hurt.

Therapist: I don't think you want to hurt her, do you?

Simon: No! I just want her to listen.

Therapist: What do you think you could do to make it easier for Norma to hear you? To show her that you care about her? To make it safe for her?

In this exchange, you are working with the couple to frame their experience with each other in terms of reciprocal responsiveness. You have aligned with their relational needs and desires, while also being mindful that this two-way flow of connection requires an equitable flow of power and taking care to avoid replicating imbalances.

Emotional Safety and Connectedness Are Adaptive

Humans are designed to constantly adapt to our changing environments through coordinated action. We need to pick up on each other's emotional states and respond accordingly. Emotions are both an early warning system and a source of security and safety. When this is working well, we adjust to each other, and this supports emotional regulation. It is a state of ongoing mutual influence (Gerhardt, 2004). While this intersubjectivity is key to developing a sense of security early in life, it evolves and remains important across the lifespan. According to the noted developmental psychologist Allan Schore (2021), the need for interpersonal connectedness extends beyond family to all levels of society:

> Throughout life interpersonal synchrony, operating beneath levels of awareness, acts as a fundamental interpersonal neurobiological mechanism not only within dyads, but also in all human group dynamics, and in the organization of all cultures.
>
> (p. 12)

The experience of being known, of neurological fittedness, creates emotional safety and catalyzes energy for change. It is not possible when power positions are not equal or when those who hold powerful positions (parents, teachers, public officials, etc.) do not intentionally open themselves to receive the experience of others and be influenced.

◊ *Attune to clients' felt sense of emotional safety*

Neither Norma nor Simon came to their relationship with consistent experiences of synchronicity in close relationships or in the larger social world. Such intersubjectivity does not necessarily require the agreement of others, but it does require that one's experience is felt and that the responses of others reflect this affective awareness. Norma has many female friends and is "close" to her mother, but has always presented a competent face that protects others from awareness of her interior worries.

This relational pattern likely started when as a child in a household with an unpredictable father who verbally (and occasionally physically) abused her mother, Norma's affective system responded by intuiting "trouble" and calming the situation by not adding to her worries. When her mother left her father when Norma was nine, she sensed her mother's overload as a single parent and tried not to increase her mother's burdens. Several years before meeting Simon, she ended a volatile relationship with a boyfriend when he threatened her with his upraised fist. To most observers, Norma is a confident, outgoing, and competent person who earned an MBA and excels at leadership.

Simon also grew up in an emotionally unsafe household. He describes his father as sullen, depressed, and emotionally distant. When he was young, his mother responded to this nonrelational environment by screaming at Simon and his siblings, slapping and hitting them when they "mouthed off." As a teen he avoided his family and his own feelings, using alcohol to mask his internal experience and as a social lubricant. He spent a few years in the military, but chaffed at the rigid authority structure. He had a number of primarily sexual relationships with women and fathered a child, Sarah. About ten years ago, after multiple DUIs and losing his job, Simon entered an alcohol treatment program. Though he has maintained sobriety since, risking his emotions with others remains challenging. He is self-employed as a contractor and regarded as highly responsible on the job, affable, and easy to get along with.

Backgrounds like these are familiar to therapists. It is probably clear to you that Simon and Norma need help building trust and letting each other in. They have developed protective "walls" that keep them "safe" but limit intimacy and the capacity to deal with the emotional substrate of daily family life, such as those inspired by parenting. It is easy to think of these as feelings *within* each partner that "come out" in stressful interactions. SERT approaches emotion differently. We view emotion intertwined with societal power contexts, as a braided link between the individual and the social world. As Margaret Wetherell (2012) put it, emotion is "where body possibilities and routines become recruited or entangled together with meaning-making and with other social and material figurations" (p. 19).

As Norma and Simon interact, socially meaningful patterns register and are felt. There are changes in their heart rates and blood flows and in the muscles that shift their facial expressions and posture. There is a push to do something. According to recent science integrating neurobiology and social processes (Burkitt, 2014; Wetherell, 2012), this is not a linear progression with one following the other. Neurology is involved, but the source is not internal. Social patterning is enlisted and informs meaning, but it is not determinative. It is not possible to separate mind/body/context. In any interaction, there are multiple possibilities. Body states are always situated in power milieus and infused with social meaning. The therapeutic alliance will be strengthened as you attune not just to the feeling but to the larger socio-emotional experience.

◊ *Attune to the mind/body/context of emotion*

Safety and belonging are both important relational needs. In optimal contexts they go together—we move toward our relationships for safety and support. Shelley Taylor (2006) called this affiliative response to stress "tend and befriend." For Simon and Norma there is a tension between safety and belonging. In order to maintain emotional safety, each of them limits relational possibilities and a felt sense of belonging. Their family environments play a part in this disconnection as a survival response; however, these family experiences and their personal reactions are supported by sociocultural discourses and include apprehending the power context.

Societal Discourse Drives Emotion

Emotion is a nonverbal form of communication that facilitates a quick response to one's environment. How bodies demonstrate emotion is similar across cultures—for example, sadness is expressed by downturned lips and squinted eyes, while anger comprises enlarged pupils and tightened lips; the *meaning* of these internal responses is derived from social discourses and power contexts (Burkitt, 2014; Siegel, 2012). Emotion signals, and is an indicator of, what is important. In SERT, you seek to know your clients by attuning to what resonates with them, apprehending their socio-emotional (mind/body/context) experience and the societal discourses that inform them.

◊ *Expand outward from emotion to social meaning*

For example, in a later session with Simon and Norma, they report that Norma seems to be angry "out of the blue." Norma says she doesn't understand her response, because things are going better between the two of them. Since you know that her bodily reaction is connected to social meaning, you are interested in the discourses that give rise to her anger. You attune to her felt experience and then expand outward to more fully apprehend it:

Norma: It doesn't make sense. Simon's being really good—better than he has ever been. He's good with Tam; he doesn't call me upset about things. He's respectful to me . . .

Therapist: Things are going better—and it seems like your body is a little scared.

Norma: That's it—I'm not scared of Simon. I know he's not going to hurt me. [pause] I should be more trusting . . .

Therapist: What would it say about you if you were more trusting? What would it mean?

Norma: (sighs) That I need a man too much. That I can't get along on my own. That I'm weak. Not strong enough . . .

You recognize social discourse about not needing men and refer to it as an "idea":

Therapist: The idea that you shouldn't need a man; that you should be strong; where do you think that idea comes from? It's a pretty common story I hear.

Norma: Well, I was raised in a feminist household.

Therapist: (reflectively) A feminist household. [pause] I'm trying to understand what that means. You are strong, it seems to me. What would it mean to be weak?

Norma: My sister was "girly-girl" and she was the soft one. I learned that only strong people get somewhere; that anger gets people's attention. [pause] I've told a lot of people about what went on between Simon and me.

Therapist: You don't want them to see you as weak—or even to see yourself as weak? [expands to discourse] To be one of those women who need men too much?

Norma: Yeah. I don't want to be one of those women.

◊ *Connect "gut reactions" to sociocultural values*

Emotions are mostly nonconscious. Norma's bodily expression of anger communicates social meaning. Exploring these "gut reactions" opens access to embodied sociocultural value systems and enables the client's experience to be more fully felt and recognized. As Norma's response illustrates, emotion is catalyzed within sociopolitical contexts at particular historical times, places, and cultures (Burkitt, 2014). The meaning of Norma's anger and its connection to feminism is located where personal, familial, and social meaning come together.

◊ *Explore emotionally salient words*

Emotionally salient words provide a window to larger societal discourses. Exploring them helps raise clients' awareness of their felt experience and the circumstances that invoke it. You know you are on track when clients are more responsive (Pandit et al., 2015). For example, you noticed that when Norma talked about needing a man, she became more engaged. She sat straighter and her voice raised. This was a clue to follow this emotional thread *outward*, listening for societal expectations and standards in her responses.

Therapist: It's like you can't be a strong woman if you let yourself need— or trust—a man? [Norma nods]. How does that work in the relationships you know? Among your friends? Relationships that you see out there?

Norma: Women are always put down. [shakes her head] I don't know anyone who has a good relationship and her own life.

Therapist: It's hard to imagine a mutually supportive relationship with a man where a woman could thrive?

◊ *Listen for multiple possibilities*

There are always multiple possible discourses in a given situation (Winslade, 2009). We remember those that are personally salient and emotionally evocative and solidify them when we relationally name and narrate them (Mehl-Madrona & Mainguy, 2015). As social connotation changes, new experience is possible and neuro-memory evolves (Zimmerman, 2018). Expanding outward from what was emotionally salient opened a conversation about relational expectations that validated Norma's experience and also allowed exploration of alternative possibilities. It is interesting to note that Norma's feminist identity still operates within dominant cultural discourses that privilege strength and rationality, discount relational needs, and encourage power-over relationship structures (i.e., not third order change).

Identities and Belonging as Felt Sociocultural Experience

When social discourses are recognized as personally meaningful, they are embodied as felt identities. As discussed in the previous chapter, these identities are not fixed or innate to the individual. They are specific to sociopolitical contexts and change across time and settings (Bava, 2023; Combs & Freedman, 2016). Listening for and exploring discourse enables you to attune to your clients' felt identities and patterns of belonging. You move from simply being aware of structural inequalities and your clients' social locations to apprehending their uniquely felt experience of their places in the world—their felt identities.

◊ *Seek to apprehend a felt sense of place in the world*

As narrative therapists Gene Combs and Jill Freedman (2012, 2016) admonished, identity-making processes are not neutral and usually echo the values and interests of the dominant culture. Though dominant discourses reflect only some of the possible values and meanings in the situation, they tend to be applied to everyone. This creates injustices in how people judge themselves and are judged by others and limits access to shared social meanings that promote neuro-fittedness, interpersonal attunement, and a sense of belonging. Clinical symptoms are often signs of these injustices.

◊ *Look for marginalized identity potentialities*

Both Simon and Norma know themselves in relation to the dominant discourses associated with heteropatriarchy and Western capitalism.

Aspects of these ways of knowing may be helpful, especially as they navigate their work environments. But they are also incomplete and frequently destructive. In SERT, we are on the lookout for potential aspects of self that have been marginalized or invalidated, especially those that promote relational engagement, reciprocal responsivity, and connection to community.

As we have seen, Norma's felt identity around being a "strong woman" cuts off many qualities often associated with femininity, such as needing others and sharing vulnerable emotions. Simon also identifies with discourses that reject "soft" emotions and weakness. You discover that being a "protector" is especially evocative to him:

Therapist: Simon, I'm curious what you took from our session last week. What did you find yourself thinking about?

Simon: When you said I needed to make it safe for her—Wow! That really got to me. That's what I'm all about; keeping people safe. That's a big part of my job—of who I am.

When you initially asked Simon what he might do to make it safer for Norma to listen to him, you didn't realize you were tapping into a core identity discourse. Finding this resonance is very helpful. It helps you connect with him and opens possibilities for expanding what it means to keep people safe:

Therapist: (empathically) It's important to you to keep people safe. Can you say a little more about that?

Simon: All my life, I solve people's problems. I'm a fixer. People appreciate it. Just today, Norma's car wouldn't start. I took her where she needed to go and got her car to the shop.

Therapist: You feel valued when you fix things for people—make them safe.

Simon: Yeah. [nods] Big time. It's just who I am. I like that about myself.

Therapist: I imagine your customers like that about you too. [Simon smiles and agrees]. What does being a fixer—making people safe—mean to you as Tam's father?

Simon: I'm her protector. It's up to me to keep her safe! To be there for her, to guide her. I want her to know she can count on me!

◊ *You can validate one identity while also exploring others*

While validating Simon's felt identity as a protector, you are also curious whether Simon's identity includes a sensitive, emotionally nurturing part:

Therapist: You want to protect Tam, to keep her safe. [Simon nods] Is it also important to sense her feelings? To have an emotional connection with her?

Simon: Yes. Of course! I want her to know I love her. I tell her "I love you." [looks down] Norma's better at knowing feelings . . .

◊ *Expanding to discourse reduces shame and blame*

Therapist: How do you think that happens? How does society make it hard for men to know feelings?

Simon: You mean, why is it hard for me to deal with feelings?

Therapist: You—but not just you. I see it with a lot of men. How does that happen?

Simon: Oh man—they just wash that stuff right out of you!! [proceeds to tell a number of examples from his life]

◊ *Look for and name egalitarian ideals*

Like most clients, though Norma and Simon enact dominant societal values that work against relationships, their identities also include egalitarian values and an image of partnership (and co-parenting) based on mutual respect. A key part of SERT is helping clients identify and develop these egalitarian values and related, but previously marginalized, identities.

Therapist: I'm curious. What attracted you to each other? Simon, why Norma?

Simon: Well. She's beautiful, of course! [looks at Norma] I was really attracted to her—still am.

Therapist: You were physically attracted. [pause] There are a lot of beautiful women. What was special about Norma?

Simon: We worked really well together. We made a great team.

Norma: We worked together on a construction project for my company. When we put our heads together, ideas would flow. He was working for me, actually.

Therapist: So you worked well together as a team. Simon, what was it like to work with, for, a woman? A younger woman?

Simon: It was like there was no age difference. I was like—Wow! This woman is really smart. She has a lot on the ball. I loved talking with her, hearing her ideas, strategizing together on how to make the project work.

Therapist: Norma, what was your experience? Did you feel respected by him?

Norma: Totally. In fact, that's what attracted me to him. Here was a guy who wasn't afraid of a smart woman. I felt respected by him in a way that's unusual—and I work with a lot of men in my job.

Therapist: It sounds like you were attracted as equals. Norma, you felt heard and valued [Norma nods]. And Simon, you liked that she could work as a real partner with you in the project?

Simon: It was a kind of relationship I had never experienced with any woman before!

This is an example of identities synchronizing around a felt sense of commitment to a new gender discourse. Therapy will not be as much be about changing their identities, as experiencing and embodying their relational and egalitarian ideals.

◊ *Promote mutual identity validation*

Identity development is a relational process. Mutually supportive relationships validate and confirm positive personal identities. Simon and Norma experienced validation of who they want to be when they collaborated at work. Marriage and co-parenting have had the opposite effect. Leslie Greenberg and Rhonda Goldman (2008), who addressed the dynamics of emotion, love, and power in emotion-focused couple therapy, related struggles for identity validation to power and dominance processes. For Norma and Simon, the battle to retain their identities and the diminishment they felt when they were challenged were so painful that they separated. Therapy is an opportunity to reclaim positive identity validation in their co-parenting roles and interactions together.

◊ *Promote identity-affirming connections*

Identities are about who we connect with and find ourselves. Intimate and family relationships are important; so are larger communities of belonging, including ethnic and spiritual connections. Such communities can be a positive source of belonging, safety, and health. As Elisabeth Esmiol Wilson (2018) identified in her justice-informed framework for religious and spiritual resilience, spiritual/religious engagement can be empowering and healing; it may also be hurtful. Similarly, as Monica McGoldrick (2016) so aptly described, connection to one's cultural "home" or "people" provides safety to develop self-esteem and resist oppressive forces. On the other hand, affiliative communities can also constrain development.

As part of getting to know Simon and Norma and their connections in the world, you inquire about some of their ethnic and spiritual experiences. You learn that when Norma's mother left her father, she also left her extended family, Dominican heritage, and Roman Catholic faith. When Norma's mother reached out to members of these communities, they minimized her abuse and distress, encouraged her to work harder at keeping her husband happy, and did not accept divorce. As a result, Norma grew up disconnected from her ethnic background and holding negative connotations regarding religion. She knew her extended family only peripherally.

Simon describes his family of origin as isolated from the community in general. He knows that his Mexican American roots extend generations but little else about his Latinx legacy. He did not find the "higher power" part of his alcohol treatment helpful, but occasionally participates in a 12-step group. Your curiosity about these aspects of their lives raises communities of belonging as possible therapeutic resources.

Therapist: You both said you are pretty disconnected from your Latinx roots. How do you think that part of your background influences your identity—how you know yourself?

Norma: I'm White-passing. But when I look in the mirror, I still see a
Dominican gal. I guess it's like I have more to overcome to get where
I want to go.

Therapist: More to overcome. How so?

Norma: Like I don't have a solid foundation to stand on. [pause] Like
my background is shameful somehow.

You follow these experiences of diminishment to take them in and
acknowledge them. Then you also turn to positive connotations that
Norma may carry:

Therapist: From what you're saying, you've been pretty alone with making sense of your Dominican heritage—it's been an extra load to carry. [Norma nods and sighs] I'm wondering, are there any aspects of
your Dominican background that you appreciate or value?

Norma: Hmm. Yes! I think my mother's perseverance is what so many
Dominican woman do. They stick with things and are not deterred.
For my mom, that meant leaving and going it alone no matter what.
But you know, the women who stayed, they had to be strong too.
[looks up] I have that too. I don't give up.

Therapist: When you look in that mirror and see a Dominican woman,
there's also pride in who you are.

Norma: Yes. I don't think about it much, but it really is extraordinary
what Dominican women do.

Therapist: Have you and your mother ever spoken about this characteristic of Dominican women? To not give up? [later] What other
women in your family or Dominican community do you admire?

◊ *Ask relational questions*

Relational questions get relational answers. Norma is used to describing strength as a personal quality. Now she is also seeing her Dominican heritage as a potential source of positive identity, empowerment,
and community. You ask similar questions regarding Simon's Latinx
ethnicity. You also inquire about the connections that support his
recovery.

Therapist: Simon, you said that you didn't find the "higher power" part of treatment helpful. [Simon nods] When you think about the connections you experienced in treatment, what was helpful or valuable about them?

Simon: Just knowing I wasn't alone. All my life, everything was on me—I was the bad guy, the mess-up. In treatment we were all messed up!

Therapist: It was helpful to not be the only one.

Simon: Yeah. Like if other people could go through this [expletive] and stay with the program, so could I.

Therapist: You said you go to meetings sometimes, but it seems like you also carry some kind of community inside with you? [Simon nods] How is that? What is this community you carry with you?

Simon: You know, I'm never really alone. I don't have to be, unless I want to.

Therapist: Even when you're on your own, you're not really alone. You've got this connection inside . . .

In the process of leaving wounded identities behind and striving for acceptance and success, Simon and Norma each adhered to dominant culture stereotypes that emphasized strength, autonomy, and independence and minimized many of their attachments to others. Their fights with each other were dominance struggles over identity—over who has the right to determine reality as the nature of their intimate and parenting relationships took shape. In these moments, their needs to protect their identities tended to override their needs for connection. A positive part of their identity battles is that there are still two voices. Neither is willing to give up or silence themselves to maintain stability, a condition associated with depression (Greenberg & Golden, 2008; Jack, 1991).

Sociocultural Value and Emotional Capital Politicize Well-Being

Politics refers to the processes by which power relationships are determined and maintained. Whose identities have value and are socially validated is political. Which emotions can be expressed, who can express them, and how are also political—all of which have consequences for health and well-being. Norma's competitiveness and personal achievements were recognized and validated in her work environment and friendship groups. When she expressed these qualities, she felt a sense of belonging. Simon was validated when he hid his fears and sensitive emotions and presented himself as one with answers, a problem-solver. Both felt shame when they presented aspects of themselves that were met with social disapproval and disconnection (Cozolino, 2016).

How emotions are expressed is often gender-related and intersects with other social identities and developmental experiences. In most cultures, men are permitted—expected—to exhibit anger while women are not. Recall that Simon expects to be able to "raise his voice." He is confused and irritated when Norma responds negatively. Anger is more ambivalent for Norma. On the one hand, she sees that people who "get somewhere" use anger and is determined not to show signs of weakness. Yet she is repeatedly apologetic about her expressions of anger and believes she should be able to control them—and Simon agrees. Taking the political (power) context of emotion into account will help you develop clinical responses that counter the dominant narratives that sustain them.

◊ *Identify the power context of emotions*

Here is an example that makes the sociocultural power context of emotion more explicit:

Therapist: How did it go between the two of you last week?

Simon: Norma went off on me again the other day. [He describes a situation in which he was frustrated by Tam's tantrum. When she continued to cry and wouldn't let up, he "tapped her on the butt," put her in her crib, and left her alone until she finally fell asleep.] When I told Norma about it, she got all upset . . .

Norma: I probably overreacted, but you wouldn't listen to me. You won't even read the parenting book [friend] recommended.

There are many ways you could respond to this story, depending on your focus. You begin by moving from emotion to the power context:

Therapist: It's distressing to you that Norma was upset. What was that like—for Norma to be upset at you? She said you wouldn't listen.

Simon: I was frustrated enough without her adding to it! Without her telling me what to do!

Therapist: (naming the stereotypic masculine discourse) You felt like you should know what to do? That you shouldn't need help?

Simon: This isn't my first time through this! I did raise a kid before. I do know something about being a parent.

Therapist: It's hard for you to need—to welcome—some advice from Norma?

Simon: Well . . . [he calms] I guess it just seemed like she was picking on me when I was already down.

We can now see that Simon's response to Norma's input came from a patriarchal power context in which he is supposed to be "on top," to have the answers; he's not supposed to need help. His reactive response to Norma's input is to feel challenged and diminished. As Tim Baima and Elizabeth Feldhousen (2007) detailed, emotional expressions often serve to maintain male dominance; they can also "hijack" therapy sessions (ChenFeng & Galick, 2015). It would be easy to focus on how to contain Norma's anger and not diminish Simon. Instead, you make Norma's side of the power context visible and connect to their egalitarian ideals:

Therapist: Norma, you said you probably overreacted. Simon says you were trying to tell him what to do. What was it like for you?

Norma: We agreed we were never going to hit Tam. I know he didn't hurt her . . .

Therapist: You believe it was "just a tap"?

Norma: Yes, I do. It was just a tap on the diaper. But he could have called me. We could have talked about it. We could figure out another way. I could have come over.

Therapist: You felt like Simon wasn't interested in your input? That he was ignoring what you might offer?

Norma: He does this a lot when it comes to Tam. It's upsetting. I've done a lot of reading and I took a class on parenting.

Therapist: You want to feel that Simon values your input, especially when it comes to Tam.

Norma: Yeah! I know he's older and he's been a parent before, but I feel like he treats me like a child!

Therapist: (to the couple) These emotional reactions seem connected to those old messages that say "father should know best"—a hierarchical way of relating you're both trying to overcome.

Simon: (laughs self-consciously) That can be hard to get away from . . .

Therapist: I know—you want to parent as a team and support one another in that. It's helpful to become aware of what's getting in the way.

Norma's "overreaction" is not just about the moment between the couple. It is also related to the persistence of patriarchy in society in which "not being listened to" is a regular occurrence. Simon's discomfort at not feeling competent and "being put down" are also part of larger gender patterns. You can now explore the social scripts that inspire these emotional responses to each other and/or invite them to engage from a mutual power position.

◊ *Attune to the political nature of emotion*

The couple's reactions, even in a private incident like this, may be magnified by living in a society in which, as Latinx, they must constantly work harder to prove their worth due to ongoing, and often subtle, racial discrimination. These effects of marginalization often operate at an unconscious level, yet are woven into bodily responses and "rational" thought. Recognizing the political nature of emotional reactions helps you attune to and validate client experience. For example, as you get to socio-emotionally know Simon, you are able to understand the pressure he feels to get things right:

Therapist: You feel a lot of pressure to get it right—to not make mistakes.

Simon: You can't make mistakes in my line of work. People want it done right—no excuses!

Therapist: That sense that there's no excuse for a mistake, do you think that would be different if you were Anglo?

Simon: [expletive] Yes! Some of those [Anglo] guys mess up a lot—but they can have a do-over. [sits up straighter and looks you in the eye] My dad wasn't great, but one thing he taught me, with a name like ours, you have to get it right the first time. There are no do-overs.

Therapist: And yet, here you are—a testimony to do-overs. Your recovery, your business, and your new daughter. [pause] There's a lot you're working hard to get right.

Simon: [sighs] You got that right!

By attuning to the socio-emotional salience and inquiring about race, you are now able to access and validate parts of Simon's experience that he may otherwise not raise or be able to put into words.

What emotional expression is considered proper varies across sociocultural contexts. As illustrated by Jessica ChenFeng and colleagues (2017), in Asian cultures outward expression of emotion may be experienced as an inappropriate burden on others, a need for them to attend to your emotions. In a collectivist context, expressing vulnerable emotions may feel or be judged selfish. It is important to validate this felt experience, identifying the relational goal of protecting others from worrisome emotion. When you attune to the sociopolitical nature of their emotion, you will work gently and respectfully to tap into emotional experience without forcing emotional demonstrations.

Implications for Facilitating Change

Living with ongoing powerlessness and social invalidation impairs access to health-affirming social engagement systems and affects the body physiologically. It increases stress hormones, compromises the immune system, and affects genetic expression (Mehl-Madrona, 2010). In contrast, mutually supportive, identity-affirming relationships increase oxytocin and the ability to respond to stressful circumstances. Socio-Emotional Relationship Therapy zeros in on reciprocally responsive relationships as a foundation for physical, emotional, and relational health and focuses on the need for relational and societal power contexts that equitably validate and support positive identities and a sense of belonging. This is facilitated from the outset of therapy by an engaged, validating, and responsive therapist (Seedall et al., 2016).

◊ *Attune to felt identities*

SERT practice goes *toward* the felt sense of our clients' intersecting identities. You may need to overcome internalized ideas that it is not appropriate or respectful to explore differences such as race, class, religion, and other sociocultural contexts. When we therapists are willing to socioculturally engage from a position of openness and curiosity, clients feel felt and less blamed. They are more able to engage in the therapeutic process. As the clinician, you are more able to fully apprehend the social meaning of the presenting issues and develop appropriate clinical responses.

◊ *Direct interventions toward mutual support*

Power disparities undermine relational engagement. As a foundation for other change, SERT interventions (a) shift power imbalances that limit reciprocal responsive engagement and (b) facilitate relational experience from positions of mutual support. To do this, you must be intentional about the effect of your clinical actions on underlying, often subtle and taken-for-granted societal power processes that affect who is open and receptive to the experience of others and who is able to benefit from neuro-fittedness and social validation from partners, family members, friends, and the larger community.

◊ *Engage emotion, relationality, and reflection*

As Sue Gerhardt (2004) described, emotion was cut off from rationality as part of the enlightenment, industrialization, and expansion of capitalism; to focus on productivity, people were treated as "extensions of their machines, not people with feelings" (p. 6). Emotions were viewed as a hinderance. Cognition and emotion were separated. In SERT, we reconnect them. Clients become aware of the discourses they have internalized (though they probably will never use that word), and they embody alternative relational patterns through affective, relational, and reflective engagement.

Embodied change is a relational process that arises from new, emotionally resonate experiences of self and other. As Simon and Norma are able to share the positive consequences of mutually responsive engagement, even around difficult topics, they feel closer and more connected. Neuroplastic processes that stimulate creativity are activated, and they are more able to reflectively make decisions about their parenting and how to negotiate their personal and interconnected lives. This change goes beyond words to relational action that "our whole body learns and absorbs" (Mehl-Madrona & Mainguy, 2015, p. 206). Gradually, neurobiological physiologies that correspond to these new experiences and understandings are established (Ewing et al., 2017). Change is facilitated by an active and engaged therapist mindful of the flow of social and relational power in clinical decision-making. The next chapter will help you address these complexities.

Therapist Checklist: SERT Change Principles

- ☐ Well-being requires affirming, neurological fittedness with responsive others
- ☐ Access to emotionally responsive others is a power issue
- ☐ Direct interventions toward mutual support
- ☐ Changing societal scripts or patterns involves accessing and embodying felt experience
- ☐ As social meaning changes, the body develops corresponding neurobiological physiologies

4
IDENTIFY THE FLOW OF POWER

Power is reflected in access to being known, feeling felt, and being viewed as credible and in the ability to have an impact on others and one's own social world. Power imbalances are likely among distressed clients and relationships, yet identifying and tracking power processes can be confusing. In part, this is because people think about power in a variety of ways and in any given situation there are likely to be multiple sources of power. It is also because those in more powerful positions often are not aware of their power. As therapists, we may not see power imbalances, or if we do, we may be unsure how to appropriately respond. This chapter provides a guide.

From a structural perspective, power is embedded in social roles and identities; simply by virtue of social location and collective socialization processes, norms, and patterns, people in "higher" roles are imbued with power that is often taken for granted or beyond conscious awareness. From a social constructionist view, personal identities are created within and reflect these structural power processes, but are enacted and experienced in unique ways. The relational perspective of SERT takes both these views into account and emphasizes power as a process *between* people, rather than a personal position or characteristic. We focus on the flow of power; how the experience of being attended to and the ability to influence the relationship moves from one to another or accumulates toward one person or group.

DOI: 10.4324/9781003270232-4

We introduced the concept of power in Chapter 2 and in Chapter 3 considered how emotion and power are connected. In this chapter we focus on how to recognize and track the flow of power in relational systems, with attention to the implications for trust and vulnerability across varying cultural contexts and how this intersects with trauma, oppression, and marginalization.

Gender, Power, and Relational Attunement

Determining the relational impact of an action requires knowing the power contexts. For example, when our research team was coding video of couple therapy sessions, a husband reached out and touched his wife while she was speaking. Without more information, we could not tell whether this action was meant to silence and limit her voice or if it was a demonstration of support. Exploring history is also important. In the case of Jonah and Joy described in Chapter 2, we could not understand Joy's apparent disinterest in Jonah's experience without understanding that until recently of the flow of power between them had focused almost exclusively on Jonah.

◊ *Look for reciprocal relational focus*

In mutually supportive relationships, the flow of power is reciprocal. As the therapist, you start getting a sense of power dynamics as you listen for and observe who is focused on and responsive to the other and who is attending to the relationship. Sometimes these actions are overt—you observe a person tell another what they can or cannot do, or a client recounts an experience in which a partner directly controls where they can go or who they can see. But in most cases, power processes are much more subtle and covert. Imbalances in the flow of power may be reflected in whose interests determine which topic gets discussed, who accommodates, who notices or takes the other into account, who listens, or who minimizes the other's point of view.

For example, Theo and Andrew seek therapy to address "communication and intimacy issues." When you ask how they hope therapy will be helpful to them, Theo appears impatient and dismissive of Andrew's concerns:

Theo: I work really hard. We've been together for three years. I don't know why Andrew can't just let up on me. It's irritating. I've told him I am giving what I can.

Therapist: You're giving what you can—can you say more about that?
Theo: My job is very important to me. When I get home, I need to relax!
   I don't want to talk about my day. I just need to be left alone!

After following up with Theo a little more, you turn to Andrew:

Therapist: Andrew, how do you hope therapy will be helpful?
Andrew: Theo works in a very high-pressure environment. It's not a
   welcoming place—I understand why he does not want to come out
   about our relationship there, and it's OK. Believe me, I get it. But
   I wish he would share more about his life with me. I'd love for us to
   have more of a relationship.
Theo: I've told you—this is me. Take it or leave it.

Though you barely know this couple, you observe what is likely a significant
power difference between the two men. Andrew demonstrates a fair bit of
attunement to Theo, while Theo appears closed to taking in Andrew's perspective. You will need to explore the flow of power more fully and attune to
the intricacies of their unique socio-emotional contexts, but already you are
aware that the dominant heteronormative culture is having an impact on how
this gay couple relates to each other and that the flow of power within their
relationship makes it difficult for Andrew to have an influence on Theo or to
experience support from him. The back and forth needed for clear and open
communication and intimacy is thwarted. Though power imbalances are not
always this obvious, focusing on the degree of reciprocity in who is attuned to
the other and open to influence helps make the flow of power visible.

◊ *Notice whose interests take priority*

The flow of power in heterosexual relationships tends to be masked.
When observing heterosexual couple therapy sessions, we see how readily
they became organized around the interests of male partners (ChenFeng &
Galick, 2015). Therapists are frequently instrumental in perpetuating this
imbalance. This includes sessions conducted by therapists in our own
research group!
   For example, Doug Huenergardt and I were co-therapists working
with Daryl and June, a couple with obvious power differences. June had

perspectives and opinions, but shared them hesitantly, in a soft voice, and often questioned her own perceptions. Daryl spoke with certainty—not only about his own experience, but about what "really" was happening for June and what she should do. To counteract this imbalance, Doug and I worked to create space for June's perspectives and validate her credibility. Even so, when Daryl minimized her account during discussion of an emotionally salient event, we began to explore June's experience, but just as she started to speak with more certainty, Daryl jumped up and went to the window, saying, "It's hot in here." Doug and I immediately dropped our focus on June and began to address Daryl's concerns. It can happen to anyone. When it happens regularly, therapy supports power imbalances rather than disrupting them.

◊ *Look for "hidden" power*

When we were studying how nonclinical couples manage power, Anne Mahoney and I developed a guide to assess the balance of power (Mahoney & Knudson-Martin, 2009). It is illustrated in Figure 4.1. We were especially interested in the ways power stays hidden from view, enabling partners to interact with the implicit assumption that they are equal, despite demonstrating inequitable relational patterns that limited the intimacy and connection they said they wanted but were not able to achieve (Jonathan & Knudson-Martin, 2012; Knudson-Martin & Mahoney, 1998, 2009).

A landmark study by Jessica Ball et al. (1995) helped show how hidden power works. In this study, heterosexual couples were asked to discuss a problem of concern to them. Their conversations were recorded, and the researchers then interviewed each partner separately regarding what they were thinking at the time. They found:

> [W]omen tended to raise the issues and draw men out in the early phase of the discussion, while men controlled the content and emotional depth of the later discussion phases, and largely determined the outcome. The women's accounts emphasized that their influence in the early phase was often illusory: their behavior was shaped primarily by the effort to choose strategies that would avoid upsetting their husbands.
>
> (p. 303)

WHAT IS THE BALANCE OF POWER?

RELATIVE STATUS
- Whose interests shape what happens in the family?
- To what extent do partners feel equally entitled to express and attain personal goals, needs, and wishes?
- How are low-status tasks like housework handled?

ATTENTION TO OTHER
- To what extent do both partners notice and attend to the other's needs and emotions?
- Does attention go back and forth between partners? Does each give and receive?
- When attention is imbalanced do partners express awareness of this and the need to rebalance?

ACCOMMODATION PATTERNS
- Is one partner more likely to organize his or her daily activities around the other?
- Does accommodation often occur automatically without anything being said?
- Do partners attempt to justify accommodations they make as being "natural" or the result of personality differences?

WELL-BEING
- Does one partner seem to be better off psychologically, emotionally, or physically than the other?
- Does one person's sense of competence, optimism, or well-being seem to come at the expense of the other's physical or emotional health?
- Does the relationship support the economic viability of each partner?

Figure 4.1 Assessment of the Balance of Power

Source: Knudson-Martin, C. (2015). When therapy challenges patriarchy: Undoing gendered power in heterosexual relationships. In C. Knudson-Martin, M. E. Wells, & S. K. Samman (Eds.). *Socio-Emotional Relationship Therapy: Bridging Emotion, Societal Context, and Couple Interaction* (p. 17). AFTA Springer Briefs in Family Therapy (used with permission)

These power differentials in communication processes affected participants' marital satisfaction, with concordance in accounts especially important— unacknowledged male dominance was particularly problematic.

◊ *Consider how power is tied to emotional responsiveness*

In happy relationships, each partner is responsive not only to positive expressions but to expressions of negativity such as hurt, anger, disappointment, or distress. They are open to being influenced by the felt experience and concerns of the other. According to John Gottman (2011), this creates a foundation of safety and trust. Gottman's research showed that women tend to be better at this than men; that is, they are more likely to emotionally attune to their partners and seek repair. His conclusion emphasized the detrimental nature of gendered power in heterosexual relationships:

> Mistrust and betrayal are more likely to occur in marriages in which the husband has more power than his wife, specifically with negative affect, and in which she does not have very much power to influence him with her negativity.
>
> (p. 432)

When women in Gottman's research were able to influence their partners through negative expressions, their husbands were more likely to look out for her concerns as well as his own. Women's ability to influence by expressing their concerns—and anger—in early years of marriage predicted relational success down the road. While a "soft start-up" on the part of women may be somewhat helpful, this is only to the extent that it helps her partner attune to her—and it replicates the gendered nature of power, with women responsible for protecting men and the relationship.

◊ *Distinguish power and gender*

Though the findings noted earlier are gendered, they are really about the flow of power. In Gottman's research, heterosexual couples who stayed happily married demonstrated less gender stereotypy and more equal power to influence the other. Gottman's research, like others, showed that same-sex partners tend to be more equal, to reciprocally attune to and influence the other. Studying same-sex couples helped our team distinguish between gender and power.

My colleague Naveen Jonathan (2009) studied how 40 same-sex couples (20 male couples and 20 female couples) in committed long-term relationships organized and handled issues of power and equality. Qualitative analysis showed that 30 of these couples organized around reciprocally understanding each other and concern for each other's needs, which Naveen labeled "attuned equality." These couples described attending to fairness in communication, with a primary concern that each partner was "heard."

Six other same-sex couples practiced "attuned inequality," in which they were dealing with power differences relating to situations such as unequal childcare or workplace responsibilities and/or economic disparities. These couples were highly aware of their inequalities and described ongoing efforts to mitigate them. In contrast, among the four same-sex couples categorized as "unattuned inequality," like Theo and Andrew, one partner's needs and interests appeared to be consistently overlooked or remained unaddressed. Naveen looked carefully to see if committed male couples demonstrated different relational processes than committed female couples and did not find differences between genders. Each organized around mutual attunement.

Naveen and I collaborated on a follow-up study (Jonathan & Knudson-Martin, 2012) with heterosexual couples that other team members had previously categorized post-gender, gender legacy, or gender traditional. Without knowing how they had been categorized, Naveen coded for mutual attunement. When asked about what they considered a good relationship, all couples in the study said they valued and sought relational connection; however, only those heterosexual couples previously categorized "post-gender," those that described discussing gender norms and making intentional efforts to relate beyond those patterns, were able to maintain a sense of attuned communication. Most, those we labeled "gender legacy," described their efforts to maintain relational connection as thwarted in ways that frustrated them and which qualitative analysis linked to stereotypic gender patterns that privileged male interests and autonomy.

Studies like these helped our team learn how to recognize power imbalances in the flow of communication and interaction. These imbalances are often tied to well-being. In a study in which one partner had diabetes (Knudson-Martin, 2009), I found that when men had diabetes, their partners took a "we" approach and shared responsibility for diabetes care. In addition to helping their partners monitor their blood sugar levels and diets, they also supported them by changing their own diets and participated in their partners' new exercise regimens. In contrast, when women had diabetes, their male partners described concern for them but saw her diabetes care as her responsibility. This gender disparity in the emotional and physical benefits of heterosexual marriages has long been known (Baber & Allen, 1992; Bernard, 1973; Kiecolt-Glaser et al., 1994). The unequal flow of power is reflected in inequities in the burden and benefits of care—a pattern accentuated in the disparate effects of the recent COVID-19 pandemic on women and minorities (Bucciarelli et al., 2022; Carli, 2020; Roesch et al., 2020; Watson et al., 2020).

◊ *Make hidden inequalities visible*

Most people today express egalitarian ideals but do not have a model of what a mutually supportive relationship would look like (Gerson, 2009; Mahoney & Knudson-Martin, 2009). Behavior frequently does not match ideals (Sullivan, 2005). For example, Dorine, a mother of two young children and director of a local nonprofit, called to schedule an appointment with me. She said she was worn out and thought she was depressed. She hoped therapy would help her manage her stress. When I learned she was married, I said it would be helpful if her husband, Michael, came to our first session. At this meeting, Michael expressed considerable concern for Dorine and suggested she might need medication or hospitalization. Both agreed they had a good marriage. I noticed that he seemed full of energy and vigor and commented on this disparity:

Therapist: Dorine, you are so worn out that you're wondering if you can go on, and Michael, you seem so healthy, so full of energy. [both nod] I'm wondering how that happens? How you are doing so well and she is at the end of her rope?

Michael: Her job is really stressful. She needs to relax and have better boundaries!

Dorine: When you have a day off, you go skiing or golfing! When I have a day off, I spend it with the kids and getting the house in order.

Despite their egalitarian ideals, Dorine and Michael had fallen into stereotypical gender patterns without discussing them. They did not intentionally place more burden on Dorine than Michael. Yet though Michael was an involved parent and the couple said they shared household tasks, enjoyed time together, and communicated well, he felt entitled to time for himself and expected that if Dorine needed "help," she would say so. Dorine always had the children and Michael on her mind and orchestrated and attended to their schedules. She felt guilty about not being "there" for them as much as she "should." This is an example of how inequality is still structured into gender roles and socialization.

Once Dorine and Michael discussed these patterns, they were able change their power dynamic so that "shared" responsibilities did not leave most of the burden on Dorine. Though Dorine also made changes, correcting the imbalance required Michael to be more attuned to the family and relationship and not expect Dorine to be the invisible glue that holds the family together and make most of the changes.

You might think therapists would readily recognize these relational power imbalances. They do not. In their review of how therapists and other relationship guides address the imbalance created by cultural norms that leave relational responsibilities to women, Karyn Loscocco and Susan Walzer (2013) found that nearly all change advice is directed toward women. And of course, like Dorine, women tend to blame themselves and step forward to make changes. The changes they make may be helpful in the short term, but if they happen without addressing the larger social and relational contexts, the power imbalance—and its effects—widens and continues.

You might also think that the gendered flow of power is an old issue that doesn't apply to younger people. Unfortunately, this is not so. As expectations that relationships *should* be equal increase and gender roles evolve, the gendered nature of power imbalances is often more subtle and so beneath the surface that their profound negative impact on communication, intimacy, and relationship dreams tends to be overlooked or concealed.

A recent study highlighted the persistence of gendered power. Olga Smoliak (2022a) and her colleagues conducted a critical thematic analysis of 30 couple therapy sessions conducted by well-known therapists. They found that expressions of a "softer" masculinity tended to obscure the ways they remained embedded in larger patterns of male dominance:

> Male-identifying participants typically took up features associated with femininity (e.g., dependence, relational orientation, vulnerability, emotionality, domesticity) while continuing to enact hegemonic ideals of stoicism, self-reliance, aggression, control, and non-domesticity. These masculinity norms seemed reconfigured in less obvious, that is, egalitarian, universalizing, and softer terms. For example, whereas physical aggression was rejected, verbal aggression was retained as acceptable. Domesticity was embraced but packaged as a choice in a way that concealed the maintenance of male privilege and material gender inequality. The focus on male partners' emotional pain and displays of progressive, caring, and sensitive masculinities seemed to obscure the dynamics of dominance and to absolve men of accountability for injustices.
>
> (p. 441)

In Michael's case, his ability to express his feelings and concern for Dorine and his contributions to [some] domestic labor and "shared" decision-making masked an inequitable flow of power in which his independence-directed focus and Dorine's gratitude for Michael's "help" and softer relational style left the burden Dorine was carrying unacknowledged and unaddressed.

A grounded theory analysis Kirstee Williams and I conducted of articles and books on treatment of infidelity (Williams & Knudson-Martin, 2013) illustrates how therapists can miss and perpetuate underlying power dynamics, especially when powerful partners are in emotional pain. Language such as "you both" or "each of you" masked disparities in who did what and seemed to presume partners were equal; authors suggested the same interventions without any attention to the power context around the infidelity. Though some discussed gender differences in the etiology of affairs, none integrated this information into an assessment of the flow of power—whether the affair stemmed from a relatively powerless position or from a position of entitlement—or directed interventions with the flow of power in mind.

Intersections of Power and Sociocultural Context

People of Color and other minoritized populations often develop the capacity to read the interests of those in power and strategically suspend their own reality when necessary. According to Aída Hurtado (1996), sometimes this means silence; other times it may mean being outspoken. Sometimes it means withdrawal, and other times intentionally transgressing dominant culture expectations—or, alternatively, accommodating them. Client behavior needs to be understood as responses within multiple intersecting power contexts. What can look like symptoms may be better understood as resistance; for example, emotionally shutting down rather than expressing anger or argumentatively standing up for oneself in ways that seem at first glance "out of proportion."

In a society based on heteropatriarchy, the gendered nature of power interacts with other power positions in varied and complex ways. Many men do not experience much power in the larger society due to their social locations. Others have themselves been the victim of abuse or other traumas. Yet their responses (and the reactions of others) may still result in power flowing to them in family and intimate relationships. Dominant societal norms tell men they *should* be in charge and in control. When this is not possible outside the family, they may seek it inside the family.

Women who understand what their partners or sons experience as Men of Color may protect them or try to sensitively navigate around enactments of male dominance (Hill, 2005). When a Black man in Randi Cowdery and colleagues' (2009) study of middle-class African American couples described "dummying up" at work "because nobody wants a Black man who knows more than they do," his wife reported "dummying up" to him to help him feel like he has power, "if not in society, at least in their relationship" (p. 32).

◊ *Beware of role reversals*

In minority or immigrant populations, women may have more access to better-paying jobs than men, especially in times of an economic downturn. This was the case for Marco and Juanita, who sought couple therapy because of ongoing anger and arguments. Each identified as second-generation Mexican American and grew up in the same neighborhood. Juanita, who had a college degree, had a job with an insurance company that included health care benefits for the family. Marco, who graduated from high school, was unable to find a job that paid better than minimum wage. As a result, he was a stay-at-home dad for their three children. As such, he took on childcare and household responsibilities while Juanita was at work. Juanita handled most of these tasks when at home.

When our team met the couple, we noted that Juanita was highly verbal and expressed strong opinions and emotions. Marco seemed disengaged. At first, it appeared that the flow of power accumulated toward Juanita. A closer examination showed this was not the case. Despite her anger, Juanita expressed considerable understanding of Marco's position and appreciation of his contributions to the family. Marco seemed unable to attune to Juanita and was uninterested in her experience or perspectives. Juanita had very little ability to have an impact on Marco, and neither partner experienced a sense of emotional connection or intimacy. They were able to manage on an economic front and appeared to be caring and engaged parents, but their marriage was at risk.

◊ *Consider how work and resources are valued*

Though access to financial resources may increase opportunities for influence over one's life and the credibility and respect one receives, money alone usually does not trump gender or race—in society or in intimate relationships. When Veronica Tichenor (2005) studied nonclinical heterosexual couples in which the female made considerably more money, she found that rather than giving women the ability to exercise more power, partners communicated and organized their relationships in ways that maintained male dominance and put additional stress on women. "Men continue to exercise a great deal of control over money and decision making . . . and continue to benefit *as men* from the privileges they enjoyed under the conventional marriage contract" (p. 179). Their earnings actually created an extra burden for women:

> Women seem to bear the brunt of the work to maintain peace and harmony in the home. They often work to bolster their husbands' masculinity by deferring to them . . . and avoiding displays of power. This can entail tremendous psychic costs for women as they monitor their behavior and sensor themselves to avoid looking too powerful.
>
> (p. 185)

◊ *Don't back away from culture or religion*

Collectivist values can support equity in mutual attunement, since socialization emphasizes a focus on others and the well-being of the group as a whole; however, this requires overcoming hierarchical gender structures (Quek & Knudson-Martin, 2006, 2008). Karen Quek's research of dual-career newlywed couples in Singapore found that when men valued their wives' work, they described learning to better attune to her needs. Couples also described active negotiation. Some women voiced their wishes forcefully; others described being softly persistent. In the end, the extent to which the power structure shifted was controlled by men:

> Over and over again we heard husbands say "I give up" in response to wives' outright resistance to a male-only decision-making process. Li Ben recalls: "We spend a lot of time arguing . . . I'd say, no, no, no, don't do that. And she'd say . . . no I want to. I just give in. She wants to do, I just let her". . . . Paradoxically, the processes that shift power in couple relationships are embedded within systems of implicit male dominance. Thus changes in their power relationships occur when husbands decide to "give up" or share power.
>
> (Quek & Knudson-Martin, 2008, p. 524)

People often claim religious or cultural justifications for a power imbalance. Yet, if you ask, nearly every religion includes principles of love, justice, and responsibility to others.

Sometimes when clients' ethnicities, cultures, or religions are different than the therapist's, therapists pull back from full engagement (Vargas & Wilson, 2011). They want to be "respectful," so they do not invite clients to reflect on these areas. However, sociocultural attunement to power contexts and the potential for change require that we move *toward* cultural and religious experience.

For example, when Seddigheh (Sandy) Moghadam studied how Islamic couples in Iran manage gender and power (Moghadam & Knudson-Martin, 2009), she found that while male dominance structured into Sharia law was reflected in most relationships, Iran's history of values that emphasize justice and women's rights was also present. She discovered considerable variation among the couples. One was especially noteworthy. They organized family roles traditionally, with a marked division of labor. Yet both partners clearly described how attuned he was to her and how much he valued and relied on her perspective—not only relative to family affairs but in business as well. Insofar as our analysis could find, the flow of power in this "traditional" marriage was mutual. This study helped convince me that there are nearly always multiple discourses and potential relationship patterns within any culture or religion, and some of these are likely to invite a more equal flow of power than others.

◊ *Transform power within religious and cultural contexts*

In most cases, you will be able to help people interrupt and transform power imbalances by working *within* their cultural and religious ideals, making space for equity based on love, compassion, and justice. Justine D'Arrigo, Beth Patrick, and Chris Hoff offered an example of working with an evangelical Christian family whose religion interpreted biblical text in opposition to LGBTQ identities (D'Arrigo-Patrick et al., 2018). The family sought help following their son's recent coming out and suicide attempt. The therapist (Chris Hoff) used the power of his role to interrupt the power of dominant discourses by affirming the young man's gay identity, while also engaging the moral complexity of the family's situation and helping them draw on their values of love and family unity to attune to and support their son. Identifying and expanding the flow of power to include the discriminatory power of larger oppressive discourses was essential to this family's capacity to acknowledge and love their son without necessarily giving up their religion.

In a different kind of example, Guy and Charnell, a White heterosexual couple in their early 20s, were referred to me. Charnell had been sexually abused in early adolescence, and her parents, in line with their understanding of church teachings, had prohibited her from finishing high school. As Guy and Charnell spoke, it was clear that their church actively supported male dominance, and both partners had been taught that faith meant obedience and not questioning. Many of their issues related to sex. Given Charnell's experience of abuse, I suggested they refrain from sexual activity in the early phase of our work.

After a few sessions, Charnell reported that Guy forced her to have sex; he framed it as her wifely role to accommodate him. I immediately saw each partner separately to track and name the power and accountability issues. They also saw a church elder who reportedly told Charnell she had to submit to her husband. Since I was no longer willing to see the couple together and Guy felt vindicated by the church, he stopped participating in therapy with me and refused a referral. I continued to see Charnell.

As I respectfully explored Charnell's religious ideas and the sociocultural world in which she lived, she grew to trust me. I was able to attune to how important her religious community was to her and also validate her own knowledge and wisdom. The excerpt that follows grew out of a discussion of our progress. It illustrates how to focus on the flow of power in an individual session while going toward religious and cultural values:

Charnell: I know you think I should leave Guy.
Therapist: No! What matters to me is that you make your own decision.
    I think you are the best judge of what is right for you.
Charnell: (pause) Really! [softly] You trust my judgement?

Therapist: Of course. I experience you as honest to yourself and thoughtful about your life and your options. . . . You grew up being told not
to question or think for yourself. Now you're questioning; thinking
things through. You church is very important to you. Your marriage
is part of that. I understand and respect that.

Charnell concluded that if she left Guy, she would also have to leave her
church. We discussed the loss this would mean and what religious/spiritual
values would be important to retain if she left the church in which she
was raised. Eventually Charnell did leave Guy. She completed her GED
and enrolled in college. Years later, Charnell—who now held a graduate
degree in religious studies—tracked me down to tell me how important
it had been to have a therapist who helped her name the power processes
she was experiencing and validated her ability to think for herself.

Power, Marginalization, and Trauma

People who have experienced trauma and/or social marginalization may
be especially sensitive to power. Some may seek more control; others may
relinquish control. However they respond, the trauma experienced typically includes an assault to the self, powerlessness, and fracturing of one's
sense that the world is just and predictable (Brown, 2008). Trauma may
result from an identifiable event such as rape, an incident in war, a natural
disaster, or a fire or accident. But as Laura Brown has described, trauma is
often insidious. Like "drops of acid falling on stone," many live with daily
threats to emotional safety and assaults to self as a result of "everyday
racism, sexism, homophobia, classism, ableism and so on . . . ever present
pulls of energy toward a survival level of consciousness . . . that someone
somewhere is trying to make you and people like you less welcome on
the planet" (p. 103). Trauma may also be historical, with the effects of
family, cultural, and sociopolitical traumas passed from one generation to
another (Glebova & Knudson-Martin, 2023).

◊ *Connect vulnerability and power*

Experiences of trauma, abuse, and societal marginalization and discrimination combine with cultural discourses, socialization, and family

developmental processes to affect the relational flow of power. Melissa Wells and colleagues studied how gendered power intersected with part-ners' ability to trust and mutually support each other in sessions of SERT therapy with heterosexual couples in which one or both partners had experienced childhood abuse (Wells et al., 2017). In contrast to "entitled power" built into stereotypic male socialization such that men assume they are entitled being attended to and their needs met, the abused men in this study demonstrated "disentitled power." While expressing feelings of worthlessness and self-deprecating remarks, they also aligned with "male discourses that privilege a focus on their own needs and autonomy rather than the relationship" (p. 129). They were unreceptive to influence from their female partners and appeared disinterested and dismissive of her experience.

Thus, while not coming from an experience of power, the flow of power in the relationship still moved toward the men, while they showed little responsibility toward the relationship or relational repair. Women often responded with "reactive power," that is, self-protective responses that defended her own safety through arguing, emotional distancing, hyper-criticism, or sarcasm. When the therapists shifted the flow of power by helping male partners align with their relational needs and take the lead in engaging through vulnerability, female partners engaged.

In the one unsuccessful case, the therapist's efforts could not engage the male partner in taking the risk to let his guard down sufficiently to accept or reflect on his relational intent or to appear in any way to be at fault, i.e., he maintained his power position:

> The men in our sample with a positive relational outcome became able to listen to their female partners about relationship issues, but Burt seemed so sensitive to appearing at fault with Cassie that any comments from her typically led to his use of disentitled power to deflect her concerns.
>
> (Wells et al., 2017, p. 137)

In the case example that follows, consider how to make hidden power vis-ible, connect clinical concerns to power, link power and vulnerability, and begin situating your clinical actions in relation to these power processes.

Identifying the Flow of Power: A Case Illustration

Imagine you are working with a female-identified couple, Sokha (26) and Marie (32). Marie called for an appointment regarding "trust and communication issues." She said each of them have mental health diagnoses and have had considerable personal therapy. As you review their intake forms, you note they have been partnered for seven years. Sokha lists her ethnicity as Cambodian, and Marie identifies as biracial, Haitian/Puerto Rican. Sokha is employed as a lab technician. Marie works part-time in a group home, has a degenerative eye disease, and is not able to drive. Each indicate they are pansexual.

To identify and track how power flows between Sokha and Marie, you apply the following guidelines:

1. Raise mutual support as a guiding principle

You approach Sokha and Marie with the assumption that people do better in mutually supportive relationships (see Chapter 3). You share this with them as you introduce yourself and get to know the couple:

Therapist: I'm so glad to meet you. I know for most people the decision to see a therapist is big and not easy. In the first session, I usually jump right in and get to know you and why you are here. And you get a sense of me and how I work. Then toward the end, we can talk more about what to expect; you can ask any questions you have about me or how this process works. Will that be OK with you? [both agree]. I don't know anything about you yet, except that you are here to work on your relationship [both nod]. I always begin with the assumption that people do better in mutually supportive relationships—that your relationship should be good for each of you; not benefit one more than the other. Does that fit for you?

Marie: Of course. That's what we've always been about—being there for each other.

Sokha: I agree. I wouldn't want our relationship to be bad for either of us.

Therapist: OK. So, that's something I'll be paying attention to—how the back and forth works between the two of you and what we might be able to do to make it better. [pause] Marie, you called to make the appointment. How did that come to be? What were you hoping would happen by coming here?

People instinctually understand the notion of reciprocity. Sociologists consider it a deeply internalized, universal social norm (Burger et al., 2009; Gouldner, 1960). Naming it early in the therapy provides a general, agreed-upon framework for identifying and focusing on the flow of power during sessions. As the couple's story and process unfold, you explore the degree to which focus on other and the relationship is reciprocal.

2. Explore reciprocity in relational focus

Marie begins with a focus on what she can do to correct hurt she has caused Sokha:

Marie: Sokha can't trust me anymore. [looks at Sokha] I hurt her. I can see that. I didn't mean to. I gave money to a friend . . .
Sokha: A friend she knows I don't like!! I don't know how she could go behind my back like that!! [to Marie] I told you Corine is bad news—to stay away from her!
Therapist: Marie, you said you hurt Sokha. Can you say a little more about that?
Marie: Corine and I go way back, since we were kids. She's kinda messed up—she's been through a lot. Sokha has never liked her. She thinks I protect Corine—and she's right, I probably do. But what she's really upset about is that I went behind her back. I shouldn't have done that. Sokha is the love of my life! [looks at Sokha] I'll do anything, whatever you want, to get back your trust.

Marie describes a strong relational focus, including awareness of her partner's perspective, accountability for her behavior, and interest in what is needed to repair the relationship. To get a sense of the degree to which this is reciprocal, you explore Sokha's relational stance:

Therapist: (to Sokha) Marie expresses a lot of concern—and regret—that she hurt you by going behind your back and giving money to Corine. She says she'll do anything to get your trust back. What about you? Why are you here? What are you hoping for in your relationship with Marie?

Sokha: We were planning to get married, to have a baby. I don't know how I can do that with someone who goes behind my back. She knows I don't like Corine. I don't see how I can trust her again!

Therapist: Your trust was really violated by this incident with Corine. It's hard to picture going forward with your plans for your life together. [Sokha agrees] Marie says she'll do whatever it takes to earn back your trust. What about you? What are you willing to do to get through this together?

Sokha: She needs to stop seeing Corine!! I've moved out for a while. I don't know if I can ever trust her again.

Therapist: So at this point it's pretty hard to imagine trusting Marie again. [softly] and yet you're here. What are you hoping will happen?

Sokha: I've invested a lot of years in this relationship! I feel really stuck. I love her, but I can't trust her.

It appears Marie is more focused on the relationship than Sokha. She is willing to take responsibility for her part in the impasse and anxious to work toward repair. Sokha resists accountability on her part and shows limited openness to Marie's perspective. You don't know if this difference is primarily a reflection of this particular incident or if it is a larger pattern in their relationship. After exploring each of their perspectives a little more, you address the power imbalance present in the room.

3. Explore in-the-moment power processes

One of the best ways to identity the flow of power is to explore and make visible the patterns of relating demonstrated in session. By naming what you see and inquiring about what is happening, you avoid prematurely drawing conclusions about the behaviors you are witnessing, and clients are part of the interpretation and naming process. Instead of an abstract pronouncement from on high, it is a collaborative activity. Though those in more powerful positions will still likely have difficulty taking in the power they hold, it is hard to disagree with or refute the immediacy of the process. You simply name what you have observed and your curiosity about it:

Therapist: I notice that now, as we talk about this incident regarding Corine, Marie, you describe a lot of responsibility, not only for what happened but also for making things better. Sokha, at this moment you do not express much interest in what Marie needs or what you could do to help rebuild trust. I'm curious, is this a common pattern—that Marie takes the lead in efforts to fix or strengthen the relationship?

Sokha: Marie is a giver. She's always giving to people and trying to make their lives better.

Marie: I suppose I might be too co-dependent, but I care about people. I want to see them happy. I want to see Sokha happy!

Therapist: (to Sokha) So if Marie is a giver, how does that work in your relationship? What is your role as a giver?

Sokha: Well, I want to give too, of course. But it seems to come more naturally to Marie. I think she gives too much. She needs to think about herself more.

Therapist: So in the balance between the two of you, do you think it's fallen into the expectation that Marie is the giver, the one to focus more on the relationship—that's she's been the one to hold things together [pause] and you've been sort of used to having her do that?

By naming the immediate process of giving and receiving, you begin to highlight the flow of power while opening conversation about how the couple functions together. In so doing, you notice that both Sokha and Marie seem to discount the value of giving and consider it a less healthy attribute. You recognize this as a possible societal discourse that perpetuates relational power differences by making caring work—and those who do it—invisible and less regarded.

4. Connect relational power processes with larger contexts

Therapist: Both of you describe Marie as a "giver." Sokha, you said she gives too much. Marie, you said you might be [finger quotes] co-dependent—as though caring about others is a problem in some way. [pause] We all need to be cared about. Where do you think the idea comes from that people who care a lot are somehow [finger quotes] sick or not self-sufficient enough?

Marie: My therapist said I was co-dependent; that I need to think more about myself. I've been trying to do that. But it's hard. My family and friends mean a lot to me.

Sokha: I think people take advantage of her.

Therapist: There are a lot of messages from society that sort of put down caring about others as a bad thing. The idea of co-dependency can be helpful sometimes, but I worry that we don't give credit to the value of caring work. I think the problem comes when caring isn't a two-way street, when it's out of balance.

Marie: (smiles) I think so too! I feel good when I care about others. I have a lot of friends and family, and I get a lot from that . . . Sokha doesn't have that. I think it's hard for her to understand what it means to me.

By expanding the conversation to include a "societal idea," you introduce societal context as part of the couple's power processes. You are transparent about your thinking in a way that reduces blame and opens dominant discourse for reflection and alternative possibilities. This immediately validates and supports Marie, whose caring and giving have previously been constructed as a problem.

5. Explore the history of power in the relationship

You now have a sense that the violation of trust experienced by Sokha occurred in context of a relational flow of power in which Marie typically focuses more on Sokha's needs and the relationship than Sokha focuses on her. Marie's act of giving her friend Corine money without consulting Sokha appears to challenge their power [im]balance. But you need to know more. As you get additional background on their relationship and each of their histories, you watch for power processes embedded in their life stories and in the formation of their relationship.

Therapist: To understand what's happening in your relationship today, it's helpful to back up a little and get a bigger picture—discuss some of your history. Is that OK? [both agree]. So tell me, what attracted you to each other?

Marie describes being interested in Sokha (i.e., beginning with a focus on other):

MARIE: Sokha was so cute, and so interesting to talk to—I was just enthralled with everything she said. She was different from everyone I grew up with. I wanted to know more.

Therapist: You were really interested in Sokha.

Marie: Yeah! [smiles] She had a good sense of humor, too. What really impressed me was her certainty about what she wanted and how hard she worked to get where she is. We met at the JC [junior college].

Sokha: I was just 19. She was like an angel. Really—an angel! She was so interested in me. I'd never been able to talk to anyone like that before. She made me feel special. And she laughed at my jokes [chuckles]. I fell in love right away.

Therapist: She listened to you; made you feel special. This was new?

Sokha: Very new. I'd always been a loner. Just kept my head down and my eyes on my goal.

Therapist: And your goal was . . . ?

Sokha: To make it on my own. To leave my past behind; to be where no one knew me.

Marie: We both have things in our past; we both have mental health diagnoses. We can understand that about each other.

Though recognition of shared traumatic histories was—and continues to be—a common bond, Sokha and Marie began their relationship with an imbalance in relationship focus. Sokha was attracted to being listened to, to being the center of someone's attention. This was new for her. In contrast, Marie was focused on Sokha as an interesting partner. Over time, this difference solidified as an organizational pattern between the partners. It creates a power imbalance in whose needs and interests are attended to and has the opportunity to feel felt. Marie's declining sight adds to the power difference, as she must either take the bus or depend on Sokha or others for transportation. Marie is also only able to work part-time, which limits her ability to contribute economically.

6. Link power and sociocultural vulnerability

Without attending to the flow of power, it would be easy to organize therapy around the intense hurt Sokha experiences and Marie as the cause of her pain. After all, going behind Sokha's back to give Corine money is a betrayal of their relationship. However, understanding Marie's behavior in context of her one-down power position and limited ability to influence Sokha changes the meaning of this action, with implications for how to address it so that "repair" does not simply put the power discrepancy back in place. Our research has shown that to successfully understand and transform power disparities, it is necessary to attune to each partner's vulnerability within societal contexts (Knudson-Martin et al., 2021).

Sokha's mother (Chanthou) was born shortly after her parents escaped the Cambodian genocide by the Khmer Rouge and came to the United States as refugees. Chanthou is developmentally disabled—perhaps due to the harsh and unspeakable conditions her family experienced during the pregnancy. Sokha was born when her mother (Chanthou) was only 15 years old, probably as the result of rape. Sokha lived with her grandparents and mother until she graduated high school and left. She describes growing up in poverty with grandparents who provided physically but were emotionally disengaged and with a mother who loved her but was not able to care for her. She never knew her father. You seek to understand Sohka's felt experience in light of this traumatic sociocultural family history:

Therapist: I'm trying to picture what it was like for you growing up, with the trauma your family experienced. What was it like for you in the community? In school?

Sokha: We were in a pretty small town. My grandparents kept to themselves. They just worked. I was on my own. I was different—you know how kids are.

Therapist: It was hard to be so different from the other kids.

Sokha: I was like a pariah. Everyone looked down on me [angrily] like I was nothing!

Therapist: Everyone looked down on you. That must have been hard. How did you deal with that?

Sokha: I stayed away from everyone. Didn't care about them. [looks up] I learned to be independent and take care of myself.

Therapist: It sounds like you were very alone. Who did you turn to for support?

Sokha: Teachers sometimes. But then they leave you at the end of the year.

Therapist: You learned to depend on yourself? To not need others?

Sokha: Yeah. The only person I could depend on was myself!

Sokha's power position in relation to Marie stems from a history of experiencing herself as less than, worthless in the eyes of others. She did not have a community she could trust, and everyone in her family of origin suffered from sociopolitical trauma that left them immeasurably wounded and unable to provide an emotionally supportive haven for her. As a result, Sokha demonstrated *reactive (in)vulnerability*—a response to societal marginalization and/or trauma that protects the self by resisting and/or maintaining domination (Knudson-Martin et al., 2021). Falling in love with Marie was a new experience, one that required letting her guard down enough to risk needing someone but did not necessarily include opening herself to take in the perspective of others and be influenced by this awareness.

Marie also approached relationships from a history of marginalization and trauma; however, her experience and response were quite different. Marie's Puerto Rican mother worked two jobs to support Marie and her sister. Although her father died when Marie was only two years old, she remains in close contact with his Haitian family. Living in a close-knit community where "people looked out for each other," Marie looked after her sister and tried to make her mother's life as smooth as possible. When she was raped at the age of 13, she did not tell her mother:

Therapist: You didn't tell your mother—what stopped you?

Marie: I knew how upset she would be by what happened to me. I couldn't do that to her. She already had so much on her plate.

Marie also learned to keep things smooth for others at school, where she was one of the few Students of Color:

Therapist: What was it like for you at school? You said most of the other students were White.

Marie: I just always smiled. I could get along with almost anyone.

Therapist: You had a way of getting along with others. Did you feel welcomed and accepted? That the other kids understood you?

Marie: I could keep the peace and get along—keep people happy. My life was pretty different than the rest of the kids. I didn't expect them to understand.

Therapist: Did some people understand?

Marie: A few—sort of. My eyes were bad even then, and most people had a lot more money. Corine had struggles too. We sort of understood each other.

Marie's felt experience of trauma and marginalization was *reactive vulnerability*, to protect relationships by taking on blame or responsibility (Knudson-Martin et al., 2021). Apprehending this helps you "get" Marie's willingness to do whatever Sokha needs to regain trust and why she felt compelled to both help Corine and avoid upsetting Marie by telling her about it.

7. Connect power responses to clinical concerns

Now that you have developed a picture of the flow of power between Sokha and Marie, you will use this awareness to guide clinical decisions. You will address the current breach of trust in context of the power imbalance in which it occurred. This means that while attuning to the hurt Sokha experienced, you will help her resist the temptation to protect herself by dominating and controlling Marie. While attuning to her pain, you will also help Sokha apprehend Marie's relational fears and needs and to understand what Marie's relationship with Corine means to her. You will validate what Marie does to maintain relationships and the relational bind Corine's need represented. You support Marie's accountability for the breach of trust and efforts to repair, but not without also helping Sokha be accountable for her part in the repair. It will also be important to first create a context in which Marie's experiences and interests can be heard by Sokha and then help Marie share more about issues in which they may disagree, such as her lifelong relationship with Corine.

Your awareness of the connection between the flow of power in the relationship and the presenting issues—and how this is influenced by larger power processes at the societal level—guides how you frame your suggested approach to the therapy:

Therapist: I am struck by how much each of you has had to overcome. You each grew up in settings where you were marginalized for many reasons—being different than most of the people around you, the color of your skin, your race and ethnicity, having fewer economic resources, your sexuality, your own or your family's disabilities that others don't understand. [both nod] You said one of the strengths of your relationship is that you are able to understand each other's mental health issues. It makes sense to me why you fell in love. [both smile] But you responded to your social circumstances in very different ways. Sokha, you turned inward and focused on yourself. You didn't let the denigration of others hold you back. You survived by not letting anyone in and not letting anyone put you down. [Sokha nods] Marie, you learned to get along by being attentive to others, by knowing what they needed and being able to smile and keep the peace. [Marie nods] When you got together, you continued these patterns. Sokha, you described how wonderful it was when Marie focused on you—an angel, you said. And Marie, you were used to focusing on others. You didn't necessarily expect much back from Sokha. But it created an imbalance that is affecting how to deal with this trust issue. I think as we work though what happened and go forward in a way that makes it safer for each of you to be vulnerable with each other, trust will grow.

Marie: That's what I'd like—what I was hoping for. That we can work through this and that it could make us closer.

You are not surprised that Marie took the lead in responding. In terms of the power imbalance, it is important that Sokha is also engaged and does not just passively agree:

Therapist: Sokha, what do you think? You've been hurt, but I've been touched by how important Marie is to you. [you touch your heart] What I'm suggesting can be emotionally risky. Is continuing to work on this together something you're willing to do?
Sokha: (slowly) I think you understand us. I'm willing to come back.
Therapist: You want to be able to trust Marie. You're willing to open your heart a little and take some steps toward that?
Sokha: I'm willing to give it a try. [pause] Marie is the love of my life. I don't want to lose her. [jokingly] Who would I be without my "angel"?

Depending on the responsiveness of clients and length of the session, you may not be able to detail all this information in one session. However, you will begin to see the flow of power relatively quickly once you look for it. You will continue to track and detail it, and the connections to sociocultural vulnerability, throughout the therapy. You will develop and direct your clinical actions with their impact on the power balance in mind. Using the Circle of Care described in the next chapter will help organize the clinical process.

Therapist Checklist: Identify the Flow of Power

- ☐ Raise mutual support as a guiding principle
- ☐ Explore reciprocity in relational focus
- ☐ Explore in-the-moment power processes
- ☐ Connect relational power processes with larger contexts
- ☐ Explore the history of power in the relationship
- ☐ Link power and sociocultural vulnerability
- ☐ Connect power responses to clinical concerns

5

CENTER THE CIRCLE OF CARE

Most of us want equitable, mutually supportive relationships, but few have a vision of what it looks like day-to-day. We fall into taken-for-granted patterns that limit relational options and personal well-being, usually without intending to do so. The Circle of Care is an interrelated set of four principles—mutual vulnerability, mutual attunement, mutual influence, and shared relational responsibility—that serve as a guide to equitable relationships and a framework for clinical assessment and treatment planning (see Figure 5.1). Rather than skills to be taught, they are orienting values and aspirations that clients enact and make their own, depending on their contexts and interests. Enacting the Circle of Care fosters mutual support that makes it easier to positively respond to developmental and societal stresses, challenges, and inequities.

In this chapter, you will see how the conceptual foundation for Socio-Emotional Relationship Therapy laid out in previous chapters—attention to societal context; the social construction of emotion; the effects of power disparities on self-worth, communication, and intimacy; the ethical balance of give and take—all come together in the Circle of Care. This is how the societal becomes personal and how therapy (intended or not) becomes political. The Circle of Care counters individualism-centered discourse and makes abstract concepts regarding equity

DOI: 10.4324/9781003270232-5

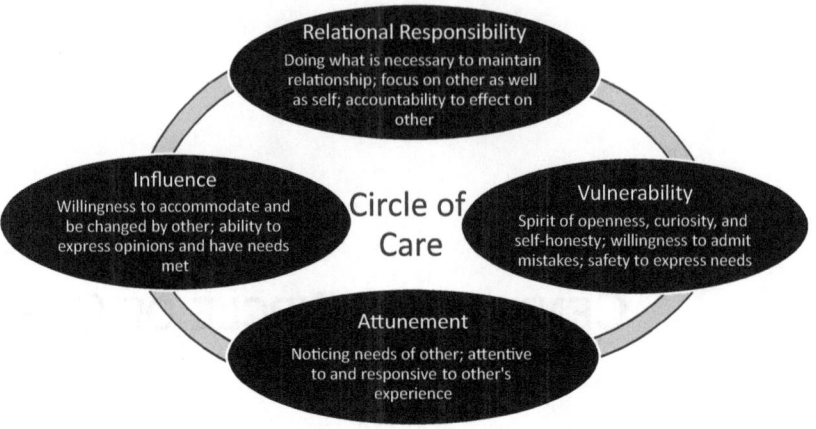

Figure 5.1 Circle of Care

Source: Knudson-Martin, C. & Huenergardt, D. (2015). Bridging emotion, societal discourse, and couple interaction. In C. Knudson-Martin, M. E. Wells, & S. Samman (Eds.). *Socio-Emotional Relationship Therapy: Bridging emotion, societal context, and couple interaction* (p. 6). Springer. Used with permission.

real and what each of us experiences in our daily lives, not only in our most intimate couple and family relationships but also at work, in the community, and in the larger social sphere.

Mutuality in the Circle of Care

To explore the Circle of Care and how to use it as a guide to clinical decision-making, imagine you are working with Bobbi (42) and Armand (49). Bobbi called for an appointment, saying their family is facing a lot of stress and she is afraid their marriage won't make it if they don't get some help. She says they are arguing a lot and that she is "exhausted by it all." Bobbi reports that Armand is skeptical of counseling but willing to come. On the intake forms Bobbi indicates she identifies as White and has a Native American grandmother. Armand identifies as White/French Canadian. The couple has been married for 14 years. It is a second marriage for Armand. They have three children—Zoe (age 18, Bobbi's daughter from a prior relationship), Heather (age 10), and Jaden (age 12). Armand owns a real estate business; Bobbi is a stay-at-home mom who used to be a model. They list no religious affiliation, but the children go to a private K–12 Episcopalian school.

You bring your socio-contextual lens and attention to power dynamics to your efforts to understand the issues with which Bobbi and Armand are grappling. Your goal is to promote mutual vulnerability, mutual attunement, mutual influence, and shared relational responsibility. This organizational template helps you and your clients keep a relational focus while connecting the dots between larger social influences and each partner's felt experience. The four Circle of Care principles are interrelated and enhance each other; one does not necessarily come first, and more than one may be involved at a given time. We will take them one by one here, beginning with vulnerability.

Mutual Vulnerability

Relational engagement involves vulnerability. Vulnerability, as used in SERT, refers to a spirit of openness, curiosity, and self-honesty that people bring to their relationships. It includes willingness to make and admit mistakes and seek repair, as well as space to express one's relational needs and innermost feelings and thoughts. While everyone experiences vulnerabilities, i.e., sensitivities that may cause emotional pain, risk, or threat (Scheinkman & Fishbane, 2004), the nature of them and how they are expressed vary depending on one's social context and personal history (Knudson-Martin et al., 2021).

In cisgender heterosexual relationships such as Bobbi and Armand, societal discourse and socialization processes tend to make *expression* of vulnerability a "female" characteristic. Masculinity discourses require the appearance of invulnerability. In terms of power dynamics, those in less powerful positions carry more vulnerability. Those in more powerful positions experience less vulnerability and may fear that expressing vulnerability is a sign of weakness or loss of power; rather than expressing vulnerability, they tend to present their needs and interests as demands or expectations. Cultures also vary in how vulnerability is typically expressed and the circumstances that give rise to it. For example, trust needed for openness to others—even among family members—may be compromised for those who live with totalitarian histories or regimes or who have experienced sociopolitical oppression (Glebova & Knudson-Martin, 2023). In collectivist cultures, expressing emotion may be seen as placing an undue burden on others (ChenFeng et al., 2017).

Vulnerability

☐ How able is each to let down their guard to take in the other's experience?

☐ How willing is each to admit weakness, uncertainty, or mistakes in the other's presence?

☐ How safe does each feel to share innermost thoughts and feelings with partner(s)?

☐ How able are partners to seek relationship repair by expressing a feeling or concern? Who is more likely to do this?

☐ How are each of these expressions of vulnerability related to social identity/norms and/or trauma and marginalized experience?

When you meet Armand and Bobbi, they describe conflicts about raising their children, money, household management, and time. Discussion of these struggles quickly escalates to anger and personal attacks on both sides. From a vulnerability point of view, neither is able to let their guard down to take in the other's experience. The need to protect their identities from fear, shame, and powerlessness overtakes their needs for connection and affiliation (Greenberg & Goldman, 2008). However, when you intervene to reflect your emerging attunement to each of them, Bobbi and Armand respond with very different expressions of vulnerability:

Therapist: Whew! You're both expressing a lot of emotional intensity here. Armand, you're carrying pain and hurt from an affair that happened over four years ago—well before the pandemic. Can you help me understand what's important to you now about that? Why you raised it today?

Armand: I don't want to talk about it! I don't even know why we're here! [looks at Bobbi with anger] After what you've done to me, [raises voice] why should I even care about you!!

Bobbi: (visibly deflates and looks down) I don't know what to do. I was wrong—so wrong. I've said I was sorry so many times. We went to therapy. I try to make it up to him [heavy sigh] but no matter what the issue, he just puts that over me. I tell him I love him, that the affair was a crazy, acting-out thing . . . [appears to have trouble breathing]

◊ *Look for openness to take in other's concerns*

As you explore and track what is happening between these partners, you observe that when his point of view is being aired, Armand appears engaged, but when Bobbi raises current concerns, he cannot—or will not—approach the conflict with openness to hearing them. Instead, he expresses anger about the past affair in a way that avoids the vulnerability of taking in his partner's negative experience (Gottman, 2011) while drawing on his hurt to maintain a power position. For example, when discussing household management issues, Armand is clear about his expectations, but not open to Bobbi's:

Armand: I like the house picked up—Bobbi knows that. I like to cook. When I'm home I do that. I don't think it's asking too much to have some order in the house!

Therapist: What does it mean to you to have order in the house? Can you say more about how that's important to you?

Armand: My mother was an alcoholic. I never knew what to expect when I came home. Most of the time the house was in complete disarray—and she was drunk.

Therapist: When the house was in order, it was calmer? Your mother wasn't drunk?

Armand: Right.

Therapist: The house in order was a sign of safety? At least for the moment? [Armand nods]

Bobbi: I know that, and I get it. I do my best to keep the house clean and orderly—for it to be a good place to come home to. But I have other things to do too. I can't be picking up after everyone all the time. The kids could help! [raises her voice slightly] When I get on them, you support the kids over me.

Armand: (angrily) You have an easy life. I give you this beautiful house and you don't even take care of it! You go slutting around instead!!!

Armand demonstrates what our research termed *reactive (in)vulnerability* (Knudson-Martin et al., 2021). His childhood wounds interact with middle-class White male discourses that tell him his needs and interests should take priority and that it is shameful to feel his attachment to and need for Bobbi. Bobbi sometimes reacts in kind, also demonstrating reactive (in)vulnerability that protects her from a history of denigration by men in her life. But in the end, she shifts into *reactive vulnerability* (Knudson-Martin et al., 2021). She capitulates and appears defeated, feeling shame and helplessness at not being able to fulfill societal gender expectations that tell her she is responsible for Armand's emotions and the quality of their relationship—an experience intensified by an emotionally abusive father and prior exploitive relationships during her work as a model.

◊ *Attune to the sociocultural nature of vulnerabilities*

My research with Lana Kim, Emily Gibbs, and Raquel Harmon found that to successfully interrupt power dynamics, therapists had to attune to the sociocultural nature of each partner's vulnerabilities and use this awareness to guide clinical actions (Knudson-Martin et al., 2021). To understand the sociocultural nature of Armand's vulnerability around Bobbi's affair, you go toward his emotional reactivity and then expand outward:

Therapist: Armand, you said that you believe that Bobbi regrets the affair and will not do it again. You also said that you know she loves you and is committed to you and your family. And yet when another concern comes up, like Bobbi saying she can't keep the house as orderly as you would like, you lash out at her and use the affair like a club. What is your sense of what is going on for you—inside [you touch your chest]—at that moment?

Armand: It's like how could she do this to me? I don't know—like she's dissing me; like what I want doesn't matter to her!

You could stay with the internal. Instead, you want him to get in touch with the sociocultural context of feeling diminished:

Therapist: You feel diminished, like she's dissing you. [Armand agrees]

That idea that if your wife doesn't meet your needs, it says something negative about you—where do you think that idea comes from?
I hear a lot of men say similar things.

Armand: My mother never respected my father. He was a laughingstock! That he would put up with her behavior, her drinking, her
laziness—what kind of man does that!

As you continue this line of exploration, staying with his experience while
encouraging him to reflect on its sociocultural meaning, you and Armand
come to see his response to Bobbi—which has the effect of dominating
and invalidating her—in the context of messages about masculinity and
social value that he internalized while growing up with few socioeconomic
resources in a generally upwardly mobile White community. He learned
to idealize the provider/leader/savior father portrayed in media and felt
embarrassed by his parents rather than loved and protected. Armand studied hard and worked his way through college in an effort to attain social
respectability. He adopted social discourses that to be respected, one must
be in control and not questioned or appear weak. When he met Bobbi,
who was physically attractive and grateful for his attention and support,
Armand felt validated with her at his side.

Bobbi was delighted to meet a "respectable" man who admired her,
treated her "like a queen," and could talk about his feelings. He was a
contrast to the "coarse and crude" men who "only cared about her body"
that she had known. Having also grown up with very limited economic
resources and on her own as a single parent, Armand offered Bobbi the
chance to be the kind of stay-at-home mother she had thought was out
of her reach. Like Armand, her image of worth and respectability is tied
to living up to social discourses that support heteropatriarchy and the
dominant—and inequitable—socioeconomic structure and judge her
identity and worth by her ability to please her partner and protect him
from shame (ChenFeng & Galick, 2015).

While both partners bring multiple sociocultural vulnerabilities to
their relationship, Bobbi is in a particularly vulnerable position that
places all relational responsibility on her and tells her she is "lucky" to
have a man like Armand. Her vulnerability is apparent in her worn-out
demeanor—the color literally drains from her face and she visibly shrinks
when Armand is upset—and in the depressive symptoms (low energy,

hopelessness, and despair) she describes. When Armand expresses his (in)vulnerability through anger and blame, her vulnerability increases.

◊ *Link vulnerability to power and accountability*

It is important to not let the emotional pain and vulnerability expressed by the more powerful partner dominate the session, which will exacerbate the imbalance in vulnerability. This is challenging because despite his willingness to direct harshly disparaging anger toward Bobbi when confronted, Armand frequently demonstrates what Olga Smoliak and colleagues called "soft masculinity" that can mask dominance still inherent in masculinity discourse (Smoliak et al., 2022a). He cooks most of the meals, he shares his inner feelings (so long as they are not in regard to Bobbi's criticism/concerns), he enjoys spending time with the children, and he can be a sensitive lover. So long as Bobbi maintains peace and plays her role as loving wife, Armand can seem comfortable expressing vulnerability. In session, he is willing to address his childhood pain, his worries about his performance at work, and the hurt he carries from Bobbi's affair.

Without accountability, validating the more powerful partner's hurt may reinforce the less powerful partner's relational burden. Thus, after validating Armand's sense of being dismissed, you also move toward the effect of his reactions on Bobbi (see Samman & Knudson-Martin, 2015):

Therapist: It's hard when you feel dismissed by Bobbi. Her respect is important to you [Armand nods]. What worries you when she raises a concern about something you do? [tentatively] That you'll be a "laughingstock" like your father? That you're not a good enough man? [pause] What do you think that feeling is about for you?

Armand: I try to be a good husband—and to be a different kind of father than my dad was to me.

Therapist: And your fear is . . .

Armand: (looks down, sighs) That I'm not a stand-up kind of guy—that she's not happy with me, with what I can give her.

Therapist: Bobbi is really important to you. You care what she thinks—and, I'm assuming, you care about her. How do you think it affects her when you when you lash out at her, when you call her names?

Attuning to the sociocultural nature of each partner's vulnerabilities reduces blame. It enables you to better identify the salient vulnerabilities and help each partner recognize them in themselves and their partner and take accountability for how they respond. This line of questioning moves Armand toward expressing his underlying vulnerabilities, thus taking a more vulnerable position in the relationship. Directing his attention to his impact on Bobbi also engages Armand in attuning to her and being accountable for his impact on her.

Mutual Attunement

As described in Chapter 3, mutual attunement—being known and feeling felt—is central to healthy relationships and mutual well-being. Daniel Siegel described this as an *intentional* process of engaging with the experience of another (Siegel, 2007). Rather than being a passive observer or waiting for someone to clearly state their wishes, it involves seeking to take in—to apprehend—another's felt experience and responding from that awareness. I think of it as noticing and listening with one's whole body. Mutual attunement results when each person focuses on the other and the well-being of the relationship overall, as well as themselves. It includes being interested in negative experiences and feedback, not only positive ones. Attunement is thus connected to openness to taking a vulnerable position.

Attunement

- How interested is each in knowing and understanding the other's experience and perspective?
- Who listens to the other? About what? In what circumstances?
- To what extent does each notice and respond to the other's feelings and needs?
- How able is each partner to accept and respond to the other's negative emotions?
- To what extent is the focus on what is good for the relationship overall, compared to what is good for the self?
- How are these attunement processes related to social identity/norms and/or trauma and marginalized experience?

◊ *Look for intention and desire to attune*

Mutual attunement is at the bedrock of intimacy, but is important to all kinds of relationships. When one is in a position of power—parent, employer, teacher, civic leader, etc.—the intention to attune is especially important. As noted in previous chapters, those holding less power tend to attune to the more powerful for survival. Women and those from less individualistic cultures are also socialized to orient to others (Silverstein et al., 2006). It's not surprising that John Gottman's research found women better at attuning than their male partners (Gottman, 2011).

Sociocultural contexts interact with attunement processes in nuanced ways. There are times when neither Bobbi nor Armand are attuned to the other. Reactive (in)vulnerability takes over, and each is so focused on protecting themselves they don't risk apprehending the other. However, most of the time Bobbi is quite attuned to Armand. It is a relational orientation she learned well as a young woman. In her environment, attunement to others was literally necessary for her safety. It also helped her navigate the competitive world of modeling. From the beginning of their relationship, Bobbi automatically attuned to Armand and did not notice that he was not reciprocally attuned to her (or expect him to be). As you track their attunement to each other in session, this discrepancy is still present:

Therapist: Bobbi, you said you understand that an orderly house is important to Armand. You also said you wished he would support you in expecting the kids to learn to pick up after themselves. Could you say a little more about what his support regarding the kids means to you?

Bobbi: I did a lot as a kid. I had to be responsible—so did Armand. I'm glad our kids have it better, I appreciate that. But I worry that we are spoiling them; that they're not learning to look after themselves. When we argue and don't have a united front . . .

Armand: (interrupts) They're just kids, Bobbi. Give them a break— you're too hard on them!

◊ *Track and facilitate attunement in session*

With the Circle of Care in mind, your clinical response focuses on identifying and facilitating their attunement process, rather than the content of the disagreement.

Therapist: Armand, Bobbi was explaining why your support in making the kids more responsible is important to her. You jumped in with your perspective before she'd finished. What do you think it was like for her when you didn't seem interested in what she was saying?

Armand: I've heard it before. I see it differently.

Therapist: And from her perspective, what is important to her about your listening to her concerns?

Armand internalized social expectations that as the husband/father he should have the answers. He knows how to listen to people and does it well with clients looking for a house, but he has not learned to orient to Bobbi or take her input seriously. Over time, this lack of attunement has left Bobbi invalidated in ways that are hard for her to put to words but leave her feeling lonely and empty. Processing Bobbi's experience of attunement helps Armand recognize the potential for him to have a positive impact on her—something he actually does care about.

Armand: I suppose she wants me to understand what matters to her.

Therapist: What do you think it will be like for her when you show her you understand?

Armand: Good, I suppose. [pause] Maybe that I care about her.

◊ *Identify the relational impact of attunement*

It was important to persist in encouraging Armand to imagine his impact on Bobbi. You follow by helping him attune to Bobbi's parenting concern. When Armand does this successfully, you ask Bobbi what it was like for her to be heard:

Therapist: Bobbi, do you feel like Armand got what mattered to you just now?

Bobbi: Yes. [softly] I felt heard by him.

Therapist: (softly, to match the emotional tone) What is it like to feel heard by Armand?

Bobbi: (tearing up) I feel closer to him. I know I matter to him—I always know that. But this makes me feel more connected [touches her heart].

Attuning to another not only has a positive impact on that person, it changes the nature of our own connection as well. Armand also feels less distant from her.

Therapist: Armand, Bobbi says she feels closer to you, more connected. What is it like to know you have that impact on her, on your relationship?

Armand: (thinks) I feel closer too. I didn't know I could affect her so much—so easily. I understand more where she's coming from. I still think she can be too hard on the kids, but I didn't realize how important it is to her to be together as parents, to present a united front.

Bobbi: (to Armand) One of the things I've always loved about you is how much you love the kids. You were so kind to Zoe when we first met. You've had a big part in making her a confident young woman who respects herself.

Armand and Bobbi still approach parenting from different perspectives. Mutual attunement makes it possible to address the conflict in a way that brings the couple together rather than divides them. Effective conflict resolution and intimacy will require that each is open to influence from the other. Since Bobbi may be socialized to automatically accommodate Armand once she feels understood, it will be important to not let Bobbi's prior concerns get lost.

Mutual Influence

Mutual influence means each can engage the other in issues that matter to them and that each person's interests are expressed and reflected in how the relationship is organized. Openness to influence is related to the other elements of the Circle of Care. Doing what another wants without willingness to be vulnerable, have attunement to the other, or have a shared sense of responsibility for the relationship can leave one feeling resentful or controlled. It can seem begrudging, formulaic, or transactional to the other person, as though "checking off a list" or saying "I did what you wanted, but am not happy about it." Mutual influence is thus a mindset and orientation to the relationship, not simply a behavioral act.

Influence

- ☐ How able is each person to engage the other in addressing issues of concern?
- ☐ How free does each feel to directly express their opinions or make requests?
- ☐ How open is each to being impacted by the other(s)?
- ☐ Whose interests determine daily routines?
- ☐ How are these influence processes related to social identity/ norms and/or trauma and marginalized experience?

◊ *Notice and explore openness to influence*

Armand does many things for Bobbi and the children. But he does them based on his image of what they should want or like. He is "giving," but his giving is not influenced by attuned awareness of them. If Bobbi does not seem to like his offerings or suggests something different, he gets upset. When Bobbi shares a concern or differs in her opinion, it feels like criticism to Armand. When Armand does what Bobbi asks, such as agreeing to put stricter limits on the kids, he does not experience it as a shared decision and feels like he has lost stature; that she is controlling him.

Influence is not just about who makes decisions. Hidden power affects decision-making processes. Bobbi tends to take Armand into account when making her decisions. She will often "choose" to do what she thinks Armand wants or what will make him happier. This is important to her relationally oriented sense of self. My colleagues and I (Silverstein et al., 2006) created a typology that considers how relational orientations relate to power and influence (see Appendix B). Regardless of gender identity, when people are individually directed, they expect others to speak for themselves and stand up for their rights—relationships are a negotiation of interests. Relationally directed persons do not see themselves and their own needs separate from others; they take others into account in determining what they want. This was one of the important findings of early studies of female development—women tend to define themselves through their connections to others (e.g., Belenky et al., 1986; Gilligan, 1982). Being influenced is a natural part of the connection.

Western psychology and clinical practice have been built on the primacy of the "separate" or individuated self, with a bias against depending on or focusing on others and an emphasis on boundaries between self and other (Jordan, 2010). In the separate-self model, being "overly" influenced by others is a problem, a developmental flaw. From this point of view, therapists would encourage Bobbi to care less about what Armand wants—to be less influenced by him.

From a relational perspective, influence processes are more complex and depend on mutual attunement and responsiveness. For example, the illusion of self-sufficiency tends to mask the supports necessary for individual competence and resilience. Rather than confidence from within, Judith Jordan suggested *confidence in the relationship* as the foundation of empowerment (Jordan, 2004). Strength, and one's sense of efficacy, is rooted in awareness of relationship. From this relational viewpoint, the question is not: Does Bobbi depend too much on Armand? It is: How mutual are sensitivity to the relationship and openness to influence? When Bobbi approaches decisions with awareness of Armand in mind but Armand expects Bobbi to represent herself, an imbalance occurs. This imbalance is reinforced when he discounts what she says or expresses anger at her "demands."

◊ *Explore the emotional experience of influence*

Differences in the emotional experience of influence affect every aspect of Bobbi and Armand's lives and are tied to power. When Armand lets himself take in Bobbi's experience (as he did in the previous example) and considers accommodating to her position, he feels an emotional tug of war.

Therapist: (to Armand) You said you feel closer to Bobbi, that you get how important a united front with the kids is to her. How does this affect what you're feeling right now about joining her in insisting the kids be more accountable about picking up their things?

Armand: Well, I feel for Bobbi. She wants the kids to see that I respect her and stand with her. I'd like to do that . . . but, I can't just give in.

Therapist: So on one hand, taking in Bobbi's perspective makes you want to support her in that way. And the part that says "I can't give in," what's that about? What's that part say?

Armand: (pauses to think) That I'm weak, that I'm not sticking to my guns. [looks down]

Therapist: So, being responsive to what Bobbi needs or asks feels like weakness? [Armand agrees] Where do you suppose the idea that you shouldn't [air quotes] give in comes from?

It is now possible to engage Armand in reflecting on the societal discourses he has learned regarding what it means to accept influence and to be able to consider other, more relational ways of responding. This struggle between wanting to be relational and socialization to maintain power is a dilemma for many men (Baima & Feldhousen, 2007; Smoliak et al., 2022a).

◊ *Look for subtle power and influence processes*

Emotion related to influence also affects how Armand and Bobbi respond to and heal from the affair. Bobbi's affair occurred in context of an imbalance in the Circle of Care. She did not feel felt or emotionally supported by Armand. At the same time, it was hard for her to find fault with Armand, who did so much for her and the children. It was very difficult for her discuss these concerns or to have an impact on Armand, who seemed impervious to her experience. In the moments of the affair, she felt resonate with her lover and connected with him. She also felt deep shame at violating her marriage and letting down the family. After a few months, she ended the affair and confessed to Armand. Four years later, every time she thinks of the affair, she feels shame—unworthy of connection.

Had Armand been more open to taking in Bobbi's experience and being influenced by it, it is possible the affair may never have happened. Or if it did, it would have been easier to repair. But Armand fit the pattern described by Reed Larson and Maryse Richards, who asked family members to record what they were feeling at various times of the day and studied how the emotion of one family member affected the flow of emotion across family members over time (Larson & Richards, 1994). They found that what fathers described feeling during the day affected what wives and children felt later. Children and wives did not have similar influence on the fathers—the men seemed largely unaffected by their experience, uninfluenced. Bobbi's internal experience of loneliness and disconnection prior to the affair was not apprehended by Armand and did not affect him or how he responded to Bobbi. Once he learned of the affair, he was humiliated by her action. He saw himself as a good man who did not deserve to have his wife cheat on him.

Whenever Armand reminds her of the affair, Bobbi feels shame and remorse again. Though neither partner feels good, Armand's power position is reinstated, and humiliation that she had the power to hurt (influence) him is temporarily overridden by anger. Bobbi needs to be accountable for her impact on Armand and their marriage—as she tries to be—but healing also requires Armand to take in and be influenced by Bobbi's experience, both in the past and present. The partners have to share responsibility for their impact on each other and the well-being of their relationship.

Shared Relational Responsibility

When responsibility for maintaining or improving the relationship is shared, each person monitors the state of the relationship and does the emotional work necessary to repair and enhance it. Each is sensitive to the well-being of the other and what needs to be done in the household and in childrearing or other responsibilities for the group as a whole. Responsibilities equitably shift from one to the other, so that the burden does not fall primarily on one person and the positive effect of supportive relationships is reciprocated. When power and responsibility are shared, each person is able to bring an open and authentic presence to the relationship, which facilitates mutual engagement and stimulates positive growth and change (Porges, 2009).

Relational Responsibility

- ☐ To what extent does each focus on what is needed to maintain or improve the relationship(s)?
- ☐ Who keeps track of what needs to be done in the home? For the children? For the relationship?
- ☐ Who does the emotional work in the relationship(s)? What does that look like?
- ☐ How responsible does each feel for the relationship(s)? How is this experienced?
- ☐ How does responsibility shift from person to person? When?
- ☐ How is the balance of relational responsibility related to social identity/norms and/or trauma and marginalized experience?

◊ *Notice who takes responsibility for care*

Despite social change, responsibility for maintaining relationships and caregiving tends to remain socioculturally gendered (Loscocco & Walzer, 2013; Smoliak et al., 2023). According to Olga Smoliak and her colleagues, not only is caring work devalued, who is considered deserving of care is inequitable. Bobbi feels shame for betraying her commitment to Armand and failing to be fully there for him. Armand's anger and humiliation regarding the affair—and most other concerns Bobbi raises—are linked to discourses that minimize his accountability for the quality of the relationship and promote expectation that his needs should be met, while obscuring hers.

In their analysis of a video exemplar of an emotionally focused couple therapy session published by the American Psychological Association, Smoliak et al. (2023) found that subtle sexist meanings and enactments reinforced female responsibility for giving care and maintaining relational processes throughout the session, which were largely overlooked by the therapist. For example, the male partner's lack of showing care for and about the female partner was framed as "her not expressing her distress and needs effectively" (p. 7).

◊ *Make responsibility for harm visible*

Another study by Smoliak and her research team (2022b) focused on denials of responsibility in videos of 40 couple therapy sessions published for training purposes. The researchers coded line by line what was happening regarding attributions of responsibility by each partner. Virtually all of the 500 codes involving denying, deflecting, and diffusing responsibility for their actions were made by men, both heterosexual and gay. Rather than outright denials, these responses tended to draw on gender discourses and male privilege to justify, shift, or minimize their own responsibility for the hurt or harm they caused, which therapists usually ignored. In contrast, when Armand does something similar in your session, you use it as an opportunity to name and reflect upon the imbalance in relational focus:

Bobbi: I wanted to talk with Armand about what is happening with Jaden and his friend Ethan. When I brought it up after dinner, he just ignored me and turned on the football game.

Armand: Come on, Bobbi. I was tired—I had a long day. Jaden and Ethan can sort things out.

Therapist: (to Armand) How did you decide to not discuss Bobbi's concern about Jaden and his friend?

Armand: (pause, seems a little taken of guard). I don't know. It just didn't seem important.

Therapist: So you took it upon yourself to determine whether or not Bobbi's concern was important?

Armand: When you put it that way. Yah, I guess. I never thought about it. The boys don't need a referee.

Therapist: How would you like it to work—in terms of deciding whose issues to focus on?

◊ *Consider who has choice regarding responsibility*

As gender roles shift, the sense of who has choice tends to maintain male dominance and reinforces the feminized nature of overall responsibility and care for the relationship (Smoliak et al., 2023). For example, Armand cooks because he chooses to. He does few less glamorous household tasks. Like men in the earlier study by Larson and Richards (1994), Armand usually feels relaxed at home, enjoys presiding over the kitchen when he decides to, and experiences little sense of responsibility for other family members when he is watching television or engaged in other activities he likes, such as golf or soccer.

On the other hand, Bobbi is always attuned to where other family members are and what they need, as well as holds in her head the schedule of what needs to be done in the household. She seldom "relaxes" from this responsibility, even when she is watching television or otherwise engaged. It falls on her to check with Armand regarding what food supplies he would like or to notice whether the children are doing well. This pattern is not unique; it is a common imbalance in relational responsibility and was exacerbated during the COVID-19 pandemic (Dean et al., 2022; Zimmerman et al., 2002).

◊ *Address relational responsiveness and parenting*

According to Smoliak and colleagues (2023), responsiveness to others is at the core of an ethics of care. Dana Matta and I found that the degree of responsivity of fathers determined whether they were engaged parents or "helpers" to mothers (Matta & Knudson-Martin, 2006). Most fathers in the study were not directly responsive to their children's needs and emotions and tended to rely on mothers to monitor these for them, citing work schedules and gender socialization and roles as the reason. In contrast, high-responsivity fathers tuned directly into their children's needs and did not endorse stereotypic gender discourses that place responsibility to care for children on mothers. Engaging in childcare tasks also enhances relational connection with the child (Cowdery & Knudson-Martin, 2005).

Like many men who demonstrate softer masculinity and contest certain aspects of traditional masculinity, Armand wants to be a "fun or cool" dad (Smoliak et al., 2023, p. 5). But he actually engages in few of the other responsibilities that go along with parenting. Despite spending time with children's activities, he is not well-attuned to Heather, Jaden, or Zoe. As a result, he is also not teaching the children to attune to and be accountable for their impact on others, and his relationship with them is more superficial than he probably would prefer.

Developing reciprocity in relational responsibility begins early and evolves over time. In an article examining parenting styles through a relational lens, Amy Tuttle and colleagues posited that relational parents authentically engage as a person and listen and attune to their children while maintaining developmentally appropriate responsibility for the child's welfare; children learn that they have an influence on their parents—and on others—and to be sensitive to them (Tuttle et al., 2012). This framework for understanding parenting styles is consistent with attachment theory (e.g., Siegel & Bryson, 2016) and also takes the societal context for which parents are preparing children into account. For example, working-class parents are likely to emphasize the need to obey and follow direction, while professional parents tend to teach their children to speak for themselves and question authorities such as teachers or physicians (Lareau, 2011).

Applying the Circle of Care

The Circle of Care principles apply broadly across sociocultural contexts. When mutually enacted, they enable each person to express the range of their feelings, interests, and concerns—those that inspire joy and optimism as well as disappointments, what is not working, and fears—and to also take in another's perspective and empathically respond. This involves openness to vulnerability and influence, as well as a sense of responsibility for the well-being of others and the relationship/family/group as a whole.

The Circle of Care is rarely equitably applied, especially in distressed relationships. Moreover, mental health professionals and clinical models tend to presume mutuality and proceed without assessing power dynamics. SERT prioritizes attending to and establishing mutual care as a foundation for addressing other clinical issues. Appendix J provides a checklist that may help raise awareness of how partners practice the four elements of the Circle of Care. This activity may also help identify differences in perceptions regarding how they apply these relational practices. Though more evident when significant others are involved, exploration of the Circle of Care is equally important when working with individuals.

◊ *Make expectations about care visible*

Working with the Circle of Care is a sociocultural intervention that makes visible and addresses taken-for-granted social discourses and assumptions about what kinds of care are expected, when, and by whom, as well as who is entitled to care and who is not (see Smoliak et al., 2023). Applying the Circle of Care principles without actively connecting them to clients' unique cultural niches (e.g., Falicov, 2014) may be inappropriate and fails to address the formidable influence of gender, race, socioeconomic status, sexuality, culture/religion, and other intersections of power and identity in relational life.

Like most of us, Bobbi and Armand approach the Circle of Care through multiple social contexts and discourses that frequently contradict each other or interact in nuanced ways. Both grew up with limited economic resources and social capital. Each experienced discrimination and internalized dominant culture discourses that equate personal value with economic standing and how one looks and presents. Armand's French Canadian family did not discuss his mother's alcoholism and felt judged by the larger community. Seeing his family through dominant Anglo standards, Armand was ashamed. Though he rejected Catholicism and many of his culture's more conservative values, the primacy of family and aspects of traditional gender roles remain salient to him.

Bobbi also learned to evaluate herself through dominant cultural discourses and "capitalize" her looks; however, her Ojibwe grandmother provided an island of calm and support in her otherwise chaotic life. Her indigenous cultural heritage emphasized the value of relationships, not only among family and the community but also to the natural world. When Armand and Bobbi met, they were drawn by their shared family values and desire to rise out of the socioeconomic situations and wounds of their childhoods.

◊ *Encourage intentionality regarding the Circle of Care*

The couple's success in figuring out how to play by dominant culture rules has been good for them in ways not to be discounted. They have been able to secure a stable economic foundation for themselves and their children. This enables options previously unavailable, including the time and resources for good health, access to green space, educational opportunities, and choice regarding work and family roles, among others. At the same time, the value of care has been compromised and its benefits not equally shared. Therapy is an opportunity for Armand and Bobbi to correct this imbalance and be more intentional regarding their values and how they enact them.

Your role as a SERT therapist is to center the Circle of Care, focusing on relational process and facilitating mutuality. This involves positioning your work in ways that challenge supremacy of the dominant culture's individualistic mindset. In the next section we will discuss assessment and treatment planning from this perspective, beginning with the ethical and practical implications of your clinical role.

Therapist Checklist: Center the Circle of Care

□ Look for willingness to express vulnerability and admit mistakes
□ Attune to the sociocultural nature of vulnerability
□ Track and facilitate attunement in session
□ Identify the relational impact of attunement
□ Notice and explore openness to influence
□ Notice who takes responsibility for care
□ Make responsibility for harm and positive impact on others visible
□ Consider who has choice regarding responsibility
□ Address expectations regarding who merits and provides care
□ Encourage intentionality regarding the Circle of Care

PART II

CLINICAL ROLE, ASSESSMENT, AND TREATMENT PLANNING

6

THIRD ORDER ETHICS AND THE CLINICAL ROLE

How therapists use power is an ethical question implicit in our clinical choices. Socio-Emotional Relationship Therapy is grounded in reflexivity regarding how we position our therapeutic roles and the ethical consequences of these decisions. In this chapter we examine how to responsibly use our influence as therapists. With third order ethics (McDowell et al., 2023) as our guide, we consider how to manage the tension between collaboration and leadership and the distinction between imposing one's agenda and opening space for alternatives to the dominant discourse. We begin with the myth of neutrality.

Myth of Neutrality

Challenges to the notion that therapists can and/or should be neutral are not new. For more than four decades feminists, critical theorists, and social constructionists have critiqued the assumption that therapists are impartial actors and called upon practitioners to examine how the values inherent in clinical models impact what happens in therapy—which statements are addressed, what questions are asked, how problems are defined, what interventions are made, what outcomes

DOI: 10.4324/9781003270232-6

are reinforced, and who benefits (e.g., Hare-Mustin, 1978; Goldner, 1985; McGoldrick et al., 1989; Leslie & Southard, 2009). Yet the assumption of therapist neutrality remains popular. I hear it all the time. New therapists often come into the field having absorbed this message.

That we have an influence on our clients can be worrisome. The reasons for this fear are important—we do not want to impose our values on another; we want to respect differences and empower clients to make their own decisions. Yet the world is not neutral; language is not neutral (Larner, 2015). What we name things and who has naming privileges make a difference. Context makes a difference. For this reason, SERT uses language carefully and intentionally, with an emphasis on transformative experience, in how the therapist's and clients' voices are positioned in relation to each other and how to bring forth new knowledge or understanding. This is not a neutral project. It is an influential one—one that is inevitably value-laden and political.

Imagine Alina is seeking your help. When she tells you what has brought her to therapy, you could respond in multiple ways. Notice how the two therapist responses in the following scenarios move what happens next in different directions:

Scenario 1

Alina: I'm just so down these days, feeling bad about myself. I thought coming here would help me feel less depressed—feel better about myself. Maybe you can give me some ideas about what to do.

Therapist: How depressed are you? Are you depressed every day?

Alina: Yeah. Most days. I mean, I'm not suicidal or anything. I just feel blah. Like it doesn't matter what I do.

Therapist: So most days you tell yourself, "It doesn't matter what I do." When you think that way, what do you do?

Scenario 2

Alina: I'm just so down these days, feeling bad about myself. I thought coming here would help me feel less depressed—feel better about myself. Maybe you can give me some ideas about what to do.

Therapist: What would it mean to feel better about yourself? How could others tell?

Alina: It would mean that what I'm doing is worthwhile. People would see me as worth something.

Therapist: What would the people in your life see that tells them—and you—that you're worthwhile? Could you think of an example?

Neither therapist has done anything "wrong," but the focus of the therapy and how the problem is defined are headed in quite different directions. The first therapist's response focuses on the symptom and encourages the client to look inward. The second therapist focuses on the relational meaning of the symptom and invites the client to see her problem in a larger context. Either may be helpful, and both sets of questions stimulate important information. But what the client says and how she presents her troubles are influenced by what you ask. Your role as therapist is not neutral—that is not possible.

◊ *Develop reflexivity regarding clinical decisions*

Stephen Scher and Kasia Kozowska highlighted the therapist as a link between knowledge and action (Scher & Kozowska, 2015). This involves "seamlessly" (p. 100) recognizing patterns, organizing information, and making inferences that translate into clinical decisions moment by moment. We have to "read" clients, consider the stakeholders, and respond. Due to the values inherently involved, these are not neutral or objective decisions; they are ethical and moral choices. It is an ethics applied all the time—"on the fly" (p. 102)—and involves the embodiment of ethical principles honed through reflexive practice.

Henry Grunebaum's description of "practical wisdom" is helpful in considering the value-laden, non-neutral nature of a therapist's clinical role (Grunebaum, 2006). According to Grunebaum, wise clinical decisions are fundamentally ethical because they "involve questions about how human beings should live their lives" (p. 117). "One must not only apprehend the current viewpoint of the various parties but also the narrative, historical, and cultural matrix from which these viewpoints arise"

(p. 121). Grunebaum argued that professional knowledge and clinical skills are necessary, but not sufficient; that wise decision-making requires contextual thinking and clarity about the values we espouse:

> It is clear that our theories emphasize goals that embody values.
> . . . We face the challenge of helping our clients to know and find what can be a good life for them, the life that will most enable them to thrive. And this means being clear about what we value and what they value.
>
> (p. 128–131)

◊ *Position your work through third order relational ethics*

As Megan Murphy and Lorna Hecker emphasized, ethical decision-making must also always include an analysis of the power relationships between therapist and client(s), as well as among those affected by the therapy and in the larger social context (Murphy & Hecker, 2020). I share Murphy and Hecker's view that ethical positioning is an ongoing and collaborative relational process in which therapists bear responsibility for the possibilities engendered within the clinical conversation:

> From a relational ethics frame, therapists continually work to listen to the narratives generated in the therapy room and listen for what is made possible by such narratives and what is made less possible. . . . Ethics, then, become a part of the conversations therapists have with clients, instead of a separate entity to consider when a clear ethical violation has occurred.
>
> (p. 544)

Ethical positioning is not about having the answers for clients; it is about comfort with uncertainty and complexity and being able to responsively use our roles to open understanding of our clients' worlds and generate transformative clinical dialogue that envisions and promotes relational justice. Through reflection on one's practice, this kind of clinical action can move from being deliberate (and thus slow) to being more intuitively responsive (Rober, 2021). See Chapter 12 and Morrison et al. (2022) for more on this learning process.

Third Order Ethics

As discussed in Chapter 2, third order thinking takes a meta-perspective that sees clinical processes embedded within systems of values-based systems. From this lens, the systems that we are involved in—the collective ways of thinking and organizing ourselves—are not set in stone; there are alternatives. By developing an in-depth understanding of how clinical frameworks, societal systems, and power structures operate, we are able to identify how our therapeutic stance may serve to benefit some at the expense of others.

SERT applies third order thinking to professional ethics to guide moment-by-moment practice and help us be accountable for the impact of our clinical decisions. Teresa McDowell, Maria Bermudez, and I developed a set of six reflexive practices that enable clinicians to ethically position our work to support relational justice (McDowell et al., 2023). We refer to them as ANVIET—attune, name, value, interrupt, envision, and transform. In what follows, I apply each of these to your work with Alina, drawing on reflexive questions from our discussion of third order ethics (pp. 69–70). These questions stimulate awareness of your context and assumptions as a therapist, the client's sociocultural experience, and the ethical impact of the therapeutic context and your clinical actions.

Attune to Sociocultural Context

Attuning to clients' experience within their sociocultural context is foundational to third order ethics. This involves trying to take in what it is like for this client to live in this world, seeking to apprehend what they have learned about what is good, right, and important and their sense of how others view them. While we can never fully know another's experience, openness to learning and curiosity go a long way. The goal is to go beyond cognitive understanding to a felt sense of your client's lived experience. SERT therapists often describe it as visceral awareness in which your neurons mirror theirs.

Sociocultural attunement also simultaneously involves awareness of your own experience and taken-for-granted "realities" based on your social locations, how these may have been influenced by the dominant culture, and assumptions you may have developed about persons with sociocultural backgrounds like your client's. Ethical positioning necessitates attunement to the potential impact of these and related societal power processes on your relationships with clients and the clinical goals you develop with them.

Reflexive Practice 1: ATTUNE

Understand, resonate with, and respond to experience within societal contexts

- ☐ What is it like for this client to live as [insert social locations] in this world?
- ☐ How do others in their community view him/her/them? How do they respond?
- ☐ What messages about what it means to be successful or good may this client have received?
- ☐ What is it like for me as [specific social locations] to interact with this client?
- ☐ What assumptions or ideas about [people in client's social location] do I bring to the therapeutic encounter?
- ☐ How may power differences in our social locations affect the therapist-client relationship?
- ☐ Whose interests are supported by potential clinical goals? Whose are suppressed or overlooked?

With these questions in mind, you seek to apprehend the world in which Alina (married, age 26) knows herself and others. You wonder what it is like for her as a young White cisgender woman in her environment and about her relationships with her husband and others. You consider how your own context may influence your responses to each other. For example, I am also a White woman and have a daughter somewhat older than Alina. It would be easy for me to assume similarities that may or may not be there and to take a protective maternal stance toward her. Alina may presume she knows some of my attitudes, especially since

I may represent dominant culture expectations to her. Acknowledging your social positionalities helps orient you toward Alina.

You begin much like the second scenario earlier, asking what it would mean to her to feel better about herself and using a relational lens that invites Alina to portray her sense of those around her. She says that feeling better about herself would mean that she is "worthwhile," that others "care whether she is there or not." She describes graduating from college because her parents expected it and a job where she feels "unappreciated" and "like everyone's lackey." She's not sure what she wants in life or how her husband fits in. As you expand your lens outward (i.e., third order thinking), you wonder how her sense of worth and purpose relates to her context as a young, White, middle-class woman. Ethically, you don't want to collude with external forces that tell her she is not worthwhile or that the problems lie solely within her. You also want to be transparent about your own social position.

Let's imagine you are a White woman just a little older than Alina. Speaking about your own social location invites openness to difference and the opportunity to reflect on the contextual nature of expectations:

Therapist: You're feeling unappreciated and taken advantage of at work—and in the world in general. Am I getting that right?

Alina: (vigorous nod) Yes! [sighs and shakes her head] I probably expect too much. I thought I'd be happier . . .

Therapist: I'm just a little older than you. A lot of people our age struggle with some of the same issues. I hear it from other clients and friends too. But I don't want to assume your experience is the same. You said you might expect too much . . . can you say more about those expectations? And where you think these ideas may come from?

You learn that at the age of three, Alina and her parents immigrated to the United States from Romania. Your professional training and interest in the influence of the larger context suggest that her immigration story is in some way connected to her expectations and current symptoms. As with all clinical actions, pursuing this line of conversation is an ethical choice, one in which you use your clinical judgment to determine how to position the therapy. Though you know immigration is often about opportunities for the next generation, you do not know if or to what extent this is true for Alina's family. You know many other contextual factors likely also intersect with her immigration experience (e.g., gender, societal division, impact of climate change, and so forth). You attune from both a knowing and not-knowing position (Falicov, 2014), using what you know to inform questions that guide the dialog and are also responsive to Alina (Sutherland et al., 2013).

Let's imagine that all you know about Romania is that it used to be a communist country. You have learned that dissent was not allowed and that many lived in fear and mistrust inspired by the totalitarian regime (György, 2023). But you don't know Alina's family experience, why they emigrated, or how these circumstances have affected her. Your questions about it inevitably shape the direction of the therapeutic dialogue:

Therapist: I don't know much about Romania, except that it used to be a communist country. What do you know about your family's experience living there?

Alina: My parents almost never speak of it. I know my grandfather "disappeared." He was a professor or something and one day he never returned home. My mother's family never learned what happened to him.

Therapist: How do you think your grandfather disappearing like that, without ever knowing what happened, affected your family?

Alina: He wasn't the only one [who disappeared]—I know that. My mother was about ten years old. She says she learned to say nothing to anyone about anything—to keep everything private. But that's all I know.

Therapist: (you make a relational values-based response) I imagine it was not safe to trust—or that one could not know for sure who to trust. [Alina agrees].

You probably have some assumptions or feelings about communism. Acknowledging these to yourself makes it easier to distinguish your stereotypes from Alina's family experience and what it means in her life. You learn that her mother and father immigrated to the United States "for a better life" and "financial opportunity." Though you still have a lot to learn about Alina's social world, you are beginning to have a sense of what it is like for her to internalize ideas about the "American Dream," prosperity, and achievement on the one hand, while also carrying forward collective mistrust in social relations and a sense that you must be cautious about what you say or present to others. You are aware that all this is happening while also being raised in the United States with societal assumptions of equal opportunity; that anyone can be "successful" if you work hard enough—and that this should be one's purpose and produce happiness.

Name What Is Unjust or Marginalized

Clients in marginalized positions feel the effects of oppression but may not give voice to them directly. They may express them indirectly or to select groups or just to themselves. Often, they internalize the injustice as self-blame and deprecation. Naming what is unjust or overlooked and amplifying silenced voices or perspectives is an important aspect of ethical positioning. It validates that which is central to the client but has been obscured or discounted rather than societally acknowledged.

Naming injustice requires third order thinking that recognizes power processes and inequities and credits skills or qualities overlooked or discounted in the dominant culture. Since we and our clients may not otherwise recognize or appreciate them in ourselves and others, practicing reflexivity identifies power realities, brings them to the surface, and makes it possible to see their impact. To be effective, naming arises out of dialogue, rather than a pronouncement from the therapist.

Reflexive Practice 2: NAME

Identify what is unjust or has been overlooked—
amplify silenced voices

☐ What societal inequities have the clients experienced? How may these influence their response to clinical concerns? How they feel about themselves?

☐ How may my experience with social privilege and/or inequities influence my approach to this case?

☐ How could power differences between therapist and client(s) silence voices and perspectives?

☐ What injustices or masked power differences need to be made visible?

☐ What skills or qualities of the client(s) are likely to be discredited or overlooked in the dominant discourse? By others? By the client?

☐ What skills or qualities in others may I tend to discredit or overlook due to the influence of dominant discourses?

☐ How could this therapy further discredit or pathologize skills and qualities not valued in the dominant discourse?

☐ What skills or qualities discredited in the larger societal context need to be validated within this therapy?

As you socioculturally attune to Alina, you begin to recognize many ways she is in a marginalized position and that she and her family continue to experience the traumatic effects of sociopolitical injustice (Glebova & Knudson-Martin, 2023), as well as gender disparities and inequities in the US socioeconomic structure. Naming these injustices helps position your clinical work to avoid replicating inequities and begins to create possibilities for addressing and transforming them. For example, you give voice to the collective trauma her family suffered and what it silenced and impeded:

Therapist: It makes sense to me that your family, and many others across Romania, had to keep to themselves, to trust no one. It was literally a matter of life and death.

Alina: It was. I can't imagine it really. [pause] I always wished my family could be more social—more a part of the community.

Therapist: (naming the loss and injustice). It was so wrong, so unfair to all of you. In order to survive, your family had to lose what so many take for granted—trust that the world is a safe and just place.

Though her family does not speak of it, Alina has always "known" that the world is not safe or just. Yet hearing it named helps establish a therapeutic alliance directed toward safety and justice. Alina has never before considered the ways she lives in fear or how the loss of family members and socioeconomic resources in Romania affect what could be valued and appreciated in her life as a young, 1.5 generation (born in another country but substantially raised in the US culture) woman in the United States.

Value What Has Been Minimized

Like most clients, Alina has spent little time examining the expectations that guide her life or considering their source and alternatives. SERT therapists highlight and expand upon values and characteristics that the dominant culture tends to overlook. This includes acknowledging and being responsible for the values we (therapists) choose to support and looking inward to recognize values and standards so taken for granted that we do not see them or reflect on them. If you grew up in the dominant US culture and/or absorbed values associated with achievement, financial success, and goal-directedness, you might unthinkingly join with Alina in supporting these values, without considering what other values Alina and her family may have masked to immigrate and survive in the United States. Third order ethics prompts you to reflect more broadly on both your own values and Alina's.

Reflexive Practice 3: VALUE

Acknowledge the worth of that which has been minimized or devalued

- ☐ What values do I choose to support in order to promote justice?
- ☐ What values and characteristics do I struggle to validate? How may these relate to internalized values of the dominant discourse?
- ☐ What societally overlooked values may my client(s) endorse when space is created for them?
- ☐ How can I validate the worth of what has been minimized or devalued in this client's life?
- ☐ Whose values do our clinical goals represent and support?
- ☐ What do we need to value so that our therapy promotes justice?

SERT's emphasis on relational values informs your exploration of the values influencing Alina. You have learned that financial success has been a driving value for Alina's immigrant parents and are curious how collective sociohistorical trauma in communist Romania may have impacted relational trust and connection among members of her family (e.g., György, 2023). Ethically, you are up-front about values that you bring into the conversation.

Therapist: As a therapist, I've learned that we need connections with others to thrive and that being open with each other—even with family members—can be risky in a social environment where it is not safe to trust others, as it must have been for your parents and grandparents. [Alina nods] I'm wondering how emotional closeness has been expressed in your family? I've heard you talk about hard work and the importance of financial stability, but I have not heard much about how love and emotional connection are communicated.

Alina: (pauses, appears to be thinking) We're not an emotionally communicative family. Love is . . . our commitment to each other. We don't talk about it . . . we just know it.

You use this opportunity to expand upon Alina's values around love and family, which she may not have overtly expressed if you had not raised the issue. Alina holds relational values—as does her family—but has not been in the habit of considering how these values guide her life (or not). Instead, she has been measuring herself by accomplishment and financial success, which seem not to inspire her and contribute to feeling "down," bad about herself, and worthless in the eyes of others. By continuing this conversation, you make a choice to help her explore the relevance of relational values in her life—in her family, in her marriage, and in her relationships more broadly:

Therapist: From what you said, your families lost their businesses, their professional standing, their homes in Romania. I can see why they focused on financial success here. What do you remember about what it was like in your family when you came to the United States?

Alina describes her parents working all the time, at multiple jobs. She recalls learning to speak English more quickly than her parents and figuring out what teachers, other children, and people in the community expected—what she needed to do to not only fit in but be successful. Through conversation focused on relational values, Alina begins to see how skilled she became in meeting the expectations of others and of the US society and how she never expected much back from others. She learned to not need or depend on people and to trust primarily in her own resourcefulness. At home, hard work equated with love. From an ethical positioning perspective, you validate values of hard work and resourcefulness as important strengths but also maintain a focus on the role of relational values in Alina's life.

When you ask about her marriage, you learn that she met her husband Dan at work while in college. He was somewhat older, had a good job, and seemed to like her. Now, Dan seems less interested in her, and she hesitatingly reveals that they "opened" their marriage about a year ago—each has another partner. This poses another values question. Let's imagine that you identify with monogamy but have been trying to learn about polyamory. You know that advocates of polyamory often view it as promoting agency for women and a shift from the patriarchal idea of men "owning" women and power over women but that societal privileging of monogamy discourse can also result in stigma, shame, and isolation (Jordan et al., 2017). You want to be supportive of Alina's relational orientation, and you also know that power imbalances and other problems may trouble any relationship, including polyamorous ones (Jordan et al). As you listen to Alina describe the relationships in her life—at work, in her family, and her intimate relationships—you notice that virtually all them seem organized around a power imbalance. You want to position therapy to intervene in power imbalances while validating and supporting Alina's values and relational choices.

Intervene in Inequitable Power Processes

You use third order thinking to recognize when oppressive power dynamics are present and having an impact on your clients. Then you consider the effect of your actions on these power process in your clinical decisions. You are careful that your choices do not inadvertently send the message that the sources of clients' problems are primarily internal—that something is wrong with them. One way to intervene in societal power processes that devalue aspects of clients' identities or mask the importance of reciprocal relationships is to ask questions about context and draw on this information to connect the dots between client concerns and the social world in which they live. Then, with your support and guidance, clients can make more informed choices about how to address them.

Reflexive Practice 4: INTERVENE

Support relational equity; disrupt oppressive power processes

- ☐ How can I create awareness of power dynamics present in the processes between clients or in their descriptions of interpersonal dynamics?
- ☐ How may the larger context of therapy inadvertently replicate oppressive power processes?
- ☐ What is required in my clinical role to ensure that therapy does not reproduce power inequities?
- ☐ How can my in-the-moment clinical interventions take into account and interrupt power inequities and support equity?
- ☐ How may my internal responses to the presence of societal power processes interfere with my ability to intervene in oppressive power dynamics?
- ☐ What will help me have the courage to intervene in oppressive societal power processes?

SERT therapists consider the impact of their interventions on the workings of power at all levels—which societal discourses are privileged, power dynamics in the client's relationships, and the power dynamics between the therapist and client(s). When making decisions about to whom to direct questions, who to ask to attune to another, what processes to name, etc., you do not assume that participants are equal. When working with an individual, such as in this case, you will need to bring interpersonal and societal processes into the conversation. One way to interrupt taken-for-granted power dynamics is to ask how a choice was made. For example, rather than simply assume that Alina and Dan made a shared decision to open their marriage, you ask how they came to that decision:

Therapist: How did you and Dan decide to open your marriage?

Alina: I thought it would make our marriage better. It was . . . low energy. Dan didn't want to go out or do things with me. I thought it would make him happier—that I couldn't be everything for him.

Therapist: So it was your idea?

Alina: Yes. I'd read a little bit about polyamory and I went to a meeting about it. So I suggested it, and Dan said it was a good idea.

Therapist: You suggested it. You had concerns about the marriage, thought it would make Dan happier. . . . And what were your hopes for yourself?

Alina: It was more about keeping Dan happy—and honestly, taking the pressure off me. It seemed like nothing I did was working. [pause] And I was a little curious about what it would be like; that it might be good to have someone else to do things with.

Therapist: It sounds like you felt some responsibility—pressure—to make Dan happy.

There are multiple options about where to move the conversation from here. You could explore societal messages that place responsibility for relationships on women. You could explore her ideas and experience around monogamy/polyamory. You could help her recognize and reflect on the theme of power imbalances that seem to cut across relationships in her life and the contextual factors that support it. You could help her explore and give voice to the values that she wants to prioritize going forward. And, of course, you could work with her to determine when and how it might be helpful to include sessions with Dan and/or other members of their polycule or help her open conversations with her parents. Any or all have the potential to interrupt power processes that are impeding Alina's ability to feel better about herself and help her envision a more satisfying future.

Envision Just Relational Alternatives

Countering dominant societal discourses and inequities doesn't happen automatically; we must create space for it. Clients need opportunities to envision and consider new options. Therapists find the "sweet spot" that provides leadership without imposing or dictating. And, of course, therapy itself must be envisioned. Therapists must believe change is possible and visualize it ourselves, so that we can illuminate reflective spaces previously obscured from possibility.

Reflexive Practice 5: ENVISION

Provide space to imagine just relational alternatives

☐ What will my practice look like when guided by my intentional values?

☐ How may my clients' preferred values support more just relationships?

☐ What is absent but implicit that suggests alternatives to societal inequities?

☐ What will clients' relationships look like when they are able to enact more equity?

☐ How do I make space to envision and support just relational alternatives?

☐ How do I envision my work with these clients will support justice in their lives and the larger mental health system?

It helps when envisioning is concrete. Ask clients to detail what changes or possibilities of change will look like. Help clients recognize and detail what they already know or value but have minimized or expressed as abstractions. As in solution-focused and narrative therapies, we can "thicken" preferred outcomes and stories of self and relationships by fleshing out and expanding upon what clients already know or are discovering. This is not accidental activity; therapists need to step up as creative, engaged partners. For example, you engage Alina in envisioning what a reciprocal relationship would look like for her:

Therapist: We've been talking about a lot of relationships in your life in which the weight of maintaining the relationship falls on you—is expected of you as a woman, as an immigrant, as an employee. What do you think it will look like when the responsibility is more shared?

Alina: Whew! That's hard to imagine.

Therapist: Which relationship would you like to imagine as more reciprocal?

Alina: Well, at work. I wouldn't be the one always taking the notes or getting everyone on board to get things in on time.

Therapist: When others are taking notes, what will you be doing?

Alina: Huh! [smiles] I'd be speaking more, thinking more about the project overall.

Therapist: You'd be speaking and thinking more . . . it sounds like you'd be more engaged in actually developing the project.

Alina: Yes! I'd have more say.

In this envisioning conversation, you do not tell Alina what a more reciprocal relationship should look like or mean to her, but you do take the lead in opening the conversation and actively respond in a manner that encourages her to reflect in generative ways. Your positioning role is to initiate new thinking and focus and fine-tune the image that emerges. It is Alina's image, but you are not a neutral player in its construction.

Transform the Imagined Into Reality

Awareness and questioning the status quo help make change possible. But changing internalized dominant narratives and habitual ways of thinking, behaving, and interacting does not usually happen simply by talking about it. More focused attention is required. Clients need to be affectively engaged so that the evolving new image or story of self and other is neurologically embedded (Zimmerman, 2018). People need to recognize and examine the positive effects of new experience and become aware of when they are off track. They need to share new felt experience with others so that it is not only internally held but relationally supported. SERT therapists position themselves to actively facilitate and share this focus.

Reflexive Practice 6: TRANSFORM

Collaborate to make what is imagined real—
third order change

☐ What enables me to maintain focus on just clinical processes, goals, and outcomes?

☐ In what ways are clients enacting their preferred, more just relational goals? What does this look like?

☐ What enables clients to maintain focus on their just relational goals? How do I use my therapeutic role to support this process?

☐ How do my ethical positioning and clinical interventions support just relational outcomes?

☐ How does our therapeutic process promote justice while taking into account complexities regarding cultural values, societal limits to autonomy, and potential costs of resistance?

In session, positioning toward transformation includes directing the conversation toward the envisioned goals and connecting the threads between the experiences or events clients describe in the moment and the sociocultural themes and third order goals previously identified. It is an active endeavor that can be surprisingly easy to derail. Let's imagine that you are meeting with Alina a few weeks after the conversation about power described earlier. If you begin by asking Alina something general such as how she's doing this week or what's been happening, you enable her to speak about whatever is important to her in the moment. Your role then is to listen for connections that link back to the goal of Alina being in a position to make more significant contributions to work projects or have more voice in her relationships (i.e., more power).

Alina: The big news at work is that my boss is leaving. We're all a little anxious because we don't know who will be taking her place. But I'm glad, because [boss] was always so hard to read—it was hard to know what she wanted.

From prior conversations, you know that focusing on what others wants has been helpful to Alina's success fitting in as a young immigrant, but also makes her susceptible to inequitable relationships where the flow of power is not reciprocal. While relationships with one's boss are always hierarchical, you decide to respond in a way that does not reinforce Alina's habit of taking a one-down position and instead helps her develop her image of what she has a right to expect:

Therapist: What do you think are the signs of good leadership? What will you expect from a boss?

Alina: I've not thought about that much. I think . . . someone who listens to everyone, who makes employees feel valued.

Since the overall goal you and Alina are working on is clarifying what she wants in life and making decisions based on a vision of relational justice, you link the conversation to this goal:

Therapist: So, as you make decisions about whether to stay in this job or what kind of position you are looking for, one of the things that will matter to you is whether it's an environment in which employees' input—your input—is valued.

Alina: Exactly!

You can now have a conversation about how she knows when she is valued and what she does when she assumes that what she has to contribute is worthwhile.

Alternatively, you could have begun the session with a more focused question based on prior conversations and goals:

Therapist: Last time we met, we focused on how you could be a more engaged, participatory member of your work group. You said you'd be doing less note-taking and contributing more ideas. What have you been noticing about the work group process in the last couple of weeks?

Alina: Well, not much different. Everyone just expects that I'll take the notes and organize all the pieces for the project.

You have a choice. You could respond by helping Alina recognize these supportive skills and why people appreciate them. While this could be helpful to Alina's self-image, it could also reinforce the current pattern rather than help her think more systemically about the role she finds herself in and where she would prefer to be. Instead, you ask a question that challenges the status quo:

Therapist: Last meeting you said that if you were not taking notes, you'd be speaking more; thinking more about the project. Did you find yourself thinking more about the project, your ideas about it?

Alina: I did. Yes! But it was after the meeting—while I was putting the notes together.

Therapist: Was this new? Thinking about your ideas when you're putting the notes together?

Alina: No. I always have lots of ideas. But I think what was new was that I was thinking [laughs a little], I was thinking that the project really would be better with my ideas.

Therapist: So you noticed more confidence that what you have to contribute would be worth sharing. How so? What specific ideas are you thinking about?

My point here is that there are multiple directions any session can go. And in each case, it falls on the therapist to provide leadership that is responsive to the client, while also acting in ways that avoid falling back into familiar narratives and patterns, and instead keep the focus on developing more just relational possibilities.

Ethical Positioning of Therapist Influence

Feeling comfortable with therapist influence can be challenging. In my supervision of new therapists, I find that this is often where they feel stuck. Many times, they see the inequitable patterns but hesitate to "push" clients. Or they make an initial intervention that names or interrupts the pattern, but when clients do not respond the way they hoped, they give up. Of course, not pushing or giving up also has consequences. Getting over this hurdle and actively engaging in a genuinely collaborative process—one that involves reciprocity *between* therapist and clients—is easier with clarity about the therapeutic role.

Justine D'Arrigo (D'Arrigo-Patrick et al., 2017) studied this conundrum—how do therapists use practices that promote social justice while taking their lead from clients and respecting their autonomy? Justine interviewed therapists known for integrating social responsibility into their work while drawing on critical and/or postmodern practices. They found that while all participants positioned their work as social action and emphasized socio-contextual issues, they represented a continuum in how they described their activist practice. On one end, some emphasized their role in countering injustice. At the other end, some emphasized activism through collaborating. Most moved back and forth between these two positions.

What I am suggesting integrates both perspectives. Therapists actively participate *with* their clients to form a collaborative effort that counters social inequities through socioculturally attuned engagement. They are transparent about their contributions and accountable for the consequences of their choices. Socially responsible therapists acknowledge the power implicit in their roles and practice reflexivity regarding how to use professional knowledge and influence to help clients achieve their goals. They maintain a curious, tentative stance open to editing and prioritize their connection to clients' experience and knowledge.

◊ *Provide leadership without imposing*

One of the challenges in ethical positioning of the therapist role is that most clients are not aware of how the societal context influences their expectations and goals, so seldom spontaneously raise this aspect of their lives. Therapists need to provide leadership that raises awareness of that which clients do not readily see or may take for granted. Much of this book is about how to use questions, observations about process, and naming to open socio-contextual dialogue that reduces individual blame and makes room for exploring possibilities. Such conversation will not happen if therapists do not invite it. Yet ethically and practically, such leadership is only appropriate and effective when it is attuned to and responsive to clients.

◊ *Responsively persist*

One of the best guides for how to do this is Olga Sutherland and colleagues' discussion of how therapists working from a collaborative perspective "can be persistently influential without becoming imposing or authoritarian," especially when clients do not immediately take up the therapist's line of thought (Sutherland et al., 2013, p. 470). They define persistence as "therapists staying the course they have chosen, despite facing conversational 'obstacles' that could thwart their intentions" (p. 471). Responsiveness is described as "the therapist's behavior being shaped by the emerging dialogical context, including clients' responses, and sensitively adjusted in light of that context" (p. 471). In the resulting dialogue, therapists and clients adopt and adjust to the other's input, while therapists are persistent about how they use their influence to achieve a particular purpose.

◊ *Identify the implicitly present*

Responsive therapist influence also involves being sensitive to what is "absent but implicit" in client narratives; "what is not being expressed but is lurking in the conversation" (Dickerson, 2013, p. 112). This kind of "radical" listening takes energy and action. Therapists hear what is in the background and identify values that are not said or expressed but are implicit in the client's depiction. Responsiveness also involves recognizing and naming felt experience, especially that which dominant discourses or inequitable power processes mask or minimize. We position ourselves to be influentially *with* clients, seeing them and engaging with them to experience new possibilities.

For example, when Alina said she was thinking the project would be better with her ideas, this implied that she was feeling more confident. You responded by tentatively naming her new-felt sense of confidence—to which Alina emphatically agreed, though she had not previously directly voiced it. And earlier, when Alina said she suggested "opening" their relationship because she thought it would make her husband happier, you named the implicit expectation in her statement that she is responsible for the quality of their relationship.

◊ *Recognize nuance and complexity*

And a caution—the impact of societal inequities and clients' responses to them are complex (see McDowell et al., 2023). Confronting injustice often involves costs and may affect various family members differently. Choice itself can be a privileged position, not equally accessible. Some things may be culturally common but not just. Our role is to help clients see what they are dealing with and determine how to respond. We cannot judge what the "best" choices are for our clients. To do so would itself be an imposition of power and not necessarily what is best. When clients leave us, they return to an unjust world. It is important to me that my work does not further replicate these inequities and that clients are able to take a more empowered stance in how they relate to each other and the larger society.

Therapist Role Across the SERT Clinical Sequence

The SERT clinical sequence (see Chapters 8–11) serves as a guide to clinical decision-making through the lens of third order ethics. In the first phase the therapist's role is to **position**. While positioning is ongoing, it is especially important as you form the therapeutic relationship and create a shared understanding about what the clinical issues are, how you are thinking about them, and what the goals of the therapy will be. Clients begin to see themselves in a larger contextual frame, and you form a socioculturally attuned therapeutic relationship.

In the second phase therapists **interrupt** and shift in-the-moment power processes to create relational safety. In this phase ingrained power processes are still very present. Interrupting them requires an active and persistent therapist role. Interrupting power processes makes it possible to experience new ways of seeing oneself and relating to others and is an important foundation for addressing other clinical issues.

Phase three is **practice**. As clients begin to see themselves contextually and start to envision just relationships, they gradually approach each other and their concerns through a new framework. Your role becomes primarily supportive, helping clients develop and embody new options and practices based on their evolving contextual understandings and vision of themselves. Your job is to keep them on track.

These phases are not discrete; they reinforce each other, and all are ongoing to some extent. However, thinking of therapy through this sequence will help you clarify your clinical roles along the way and guide ethical positioning. With this overall picture in mind, in the next chapter we explore assessment and forming a therapeutic alliance.

Therapist Checklist: Ethical Positioning

- ☐ Develop reflexivity regarding clinical choices
- ☐ Consider how your practice is embedded within systems of systems
- ☐ Apprehend the client's sociocultural context, values, and perspectives
- ☐ Attend to societal and relational power processes
- ☐ Be accountable for the consequences of your clinical actions
- ☐ Use your role to counter inequity and generate more just possibilities
- ☐ Practice ANVIET—attune, name, value, interrupt, envision, transform
- ☐ Demonstrate responsive persistence
- ☐ Recognize nuance and complexity in what is just and possible

---

7

SERT ASSESSMENT
AND THERAPEUTIC ALLIANCE

When you meet clients and get to know them, you are simultaneously developing a therapeutic alliance and joining in an assessment process that will set the stage for your work together. As a collaborative process, Socio-Emotional Relationship Therapy assessment is intertwined with forming an alliance that counters inequities and supports just relational possibilities. It is interactive and ongoing. Though assessment is never complete and will continue throughout the therapy, what you and the clients focus on in the early stages creates a shared understanding and socio-emotional framework that will guide the direction of therapy and the potential for third order change.

SERT therapists assume assessment and development of a working therapeutic alliance are "ethical sociopolitical issues that demand self-awareness, critical thought, and reflexivity" (Knudson-Martin & Kim, 2023, p. 275; see also Chapter 6). The meaning of clients' concerns and expectations for therapy must be explored in the context of their sociocultural niche (Falicov, 2014) and the nuanced power processes involved. As you engage in the synergistic assessment process, clients begin to see connections between their personal problems and larger systems and relationships and start to join with each other and the therapist to envision new possibilities.

DOI: 10.4324/9781003270232-7

◊ *Approach assessment with an expanded relational orientation*

In this chapter we consider how to begin therapy by engaging with clients to explore their concerns through a wider sociopolitical lens and relational framework (i.e., third order thinking, Chapter 2). The SERT Assessment Guide (SAG) detailed in Table 7.1 and Appendix F informs the curiosities you bring to the process; however, your most important assessment tool is your genuine interest in knowing clients in their

Table 7.1 SERT Assessment Guide (SAG)

Social Identities [Context and Discourses]
• In what kinds of societal contexts are clients embedded? How have these changed over time?
• What messages about gender, sexuality, and intimate relationships has each internalized?
• How do socioeconomic status and economic situation impact constructions of self, access to resources, and relationship patterns?
• How do social institutions (immigration, justice system, medical, health, social services, etc.) impact the client's sense of self and relationships with others?
• How do each person's religion, age, race, ethnicity, and disabilities impact constructions of self and experience in their relationships?
• How are the client's expressions of thoughts, feelings, and needs influenced by cultural, religious, or gender discourses?
• To what extent are the client's decisions determined by cultural, religious, or gender traditions?

Flow of Power
• How much personal, interpersonal, and institutional power does each client experience as a result of their societal positions?
• To what extent is each person equally able to express and attain personal interests/goals?
• To what extent do each expect to define what is "real"?
• To what extent does each person organize around what matters to the other(s)?
• Whose interests are most reflected in "shared" decisions?
• Whose interests and schedule organize the family's routines?
• How are differences in opinion handled?
• Who is more likely to accommodate the other person(s)?
• Does accommodation often occur automatically without anything being said?
• Does one person's sense of competence, optimism, or well-being seem to come at the expense of the other's physical or emotional health?
• Does the relationship support the economic viability of each person?

Mutuality in the Circle of Care

Vulnerability

- How able is each to let down their guard to take in the other's experience?
- How willing is each to admit weakness, uncertainty, or mistakes in the other's presence?
- How safe does each feel to share innermost thoughts and feelings with partner(s)?
- How able are partners to seek relationship repair by expressing a feeling or concern? Who is more likely to do this?
- How are expressions of vulnerability related to social identity/norms and/or trauma and marginalized experience?

Attunement

- How interested is each person in knowing and understanding the other's experience and perspective?
- Who listens to the other(s)? About what? In what circumstances?
- To what extent does each notice and respond to the other's feelings and needs?
- How able is each to witness and respond to the other's negative emotions?
- To what extent is each attuned to what is good for the relationship overall, compared to what is good for the self?
- How are attunement processes related to social identity/norms and/or trauma and marginalized experience?

Influence

- How able is each person to engage the other(s) in addressing issues of concern?
- How free does each feel to directly express their opinions or make requests?
- Whose expectations define standards in the relationship?
- How open is each to being impacted by the other(s)?
- Whose interests determine daily routines?
- How are influence processes related to social identity/norms and/or trauma and marginalized experience?

Relational Responsibility

- To what extent does each focus on what is needed to maintain or improve the relationship(s)? How do they do this?
- Who keeps track of what needs to be done in the home? For the children? For the relationship(s)?
- Who does the emotional work in the relationship(s)? What does that look like?
- How aware are each of the emotional work each one does?
- How responsible does each feel for the relationship(s)? How is this experienced?
- How does responsibility shift from person to person? When?
- How is the balance of relational responsibility related to social identity/norms and/or trauma and marginalized experience?

(Continued)

Table 7.1 (Continued)

Relational Ideals
• Do the clients seek relationships that mutually benefit and support each person?
• How valued is emotional work in the relationship?
• What relationship ideals and personal characteristics do clients endorse that support mutual engagement in the Circle of Care?

contexts. Each case is unique, and each person needs to feel felt. The SAG questions are effective to the extent they help you responsively attune to clients and stimulate them to reflect on their situations.

◊ *Responsive sociocultural attunement is your key assessment tool*

SERT assessment and alliance formation begin before you meet the clients and are central to the first sessions, in which your tasks are to:

- Expand the lens
- Be transparent regarding your approach
- Bring the felt sociocultural experience of each person to light
- Track the flow of power and relational safety
- Invite mutuality as a relational value
- Connect personal experience and larger social/relational systems
- Identify relational ideals and resources
- Encourage hope and a "we are confronting this together" attitude
- Summarize the agreed-upon clinical focus

Rather than a formulaic protocol, it is important to think of assessment as a process of relationship building. In what follows, I illustrate a guiding template for SERT's relational approach to assessment that creates the possibility of third order change.

Intake Sets the Stage

Imagine that Madeline (age 60) was referred to you because you are developing a reputation for working with couples and families dealing with medical issues. The intake report conducted by staff at the nonprofit agency where you work shows she identifies as a White cisgender woman of Northern European heritage. Madeline is married to Byron (age 62, also White). It is a second marriage for each of them, and both are Unitarian Universalist ministers. Madeline has two daughters (Genevieve, age 33, and Margot, age 36) and a 4-year-old grandson. Byron has one son (Denny, age 28). Madeline is seeking therapy following a heart attack about eight months ago. She says the heart attack brought up a lot of "unfinished business," that while she is physically recovered, she is having a hard time "being present" with others, and this is causing stress in her marriage and at work.

Pre-Session Reflection

As you read the intake report, you are aware of your internal responses to the information and pause to reflect on the larger context in which this new therapeutic alliance will evolve. What ideas do you have about people in their 60s? How may these ideas be gendered and/or connected to other social identities (race, sexual identity, socioeconomic status [SES], etc.)? How do these ideas reflect larger societal discourses? Laurel Salmon asks four orienting questions of all cases (Salmon, 2017, p. 14):

1. What are the common stereotypes about each of the groups that the client falls into?
2. What are the dynamics between us because of oppression?
3. How can I expect to oppress the client inadvertently if I am not careful?
4. How are the current presenting problems related to oppression?

Your responses to these questions depend on the intersection of your social identities and experiences and the clients'. They may also relate to your internalized personal and societal narratives about health and health care (Lawson et al., 2017). You are also aware that female heart patients are often misunderstood or minimized by providers (Galick et al., 2015). Depending on your age and social identities, your own family relationships, and professional experience, you may find yourself holding back from engaging with Madeline and/or Byron out of "respect for differences" (Vargas & Wilson, 2011). Or you may assume you have similar experiences and already "know" much about them and their family.

Initial Information

As is not unusual for women, Madeline took the first step in seeking therapy and owned the problem as hers. You begin to expand the lens in the intake process. How much control you have over this depends on where you work and the procedures involved. It is helpful to be as proactive as you can about what intake staff ask and say and what kinds of questions are on intake questionnaires and disclosure statements, as well as how therapy is depicted on the agency/practitioner's website. Figure 7.1 is an example of how I describe my clinical approach on my professional disclosure form. Note that it tells prospective clients that my work is premised on the idea that relationships are fundamental to health, that we will begin by looking at how what clients are experiencing is connected to the "bigger picture," and that it is often helpful to involve others in the work.

On my client questionnaire, identity questions (relationship/marital status, race, gender, SES, sexuality, ethnicity, religion, abilities, legal status) are open-ended so clients can use their own words. When data gathering requires discrete choices, look for ways to be as inclusive as possible and to also include open-ended questions to invite client preferences. In addition to questions about the presenting issues and hopes for therapy and screening for past and current experience with abuse and substance

---

Sample Professional Philosophy Statement

My work is based on the idea that relationships are fundamental to health and well-being. Whether your goal is to feel better emotionally, develop as a person, or address family and relationship problems, we begin by looking at the bigger picture—how what you are experiencing is connected to your stage in life, cultural and family background, gender expectations, and current roles and relationships. It is often helpful to involve significant others in our work.

We will develop the goals of therapy together, based on what you are seeking. However, one goal that is always important to me is that people are able to develop mutually supportive relationships. We are likely to work on communication and what you experience when you relate to others. I may ask you to speak directly to each other and help you experiment with new ways of approaching situations. We focus on what works and seek ways to help you expand what is possible.

Figure 7.1 Sample Professional Disclosure Statement

use, I also ask questions that expand the lens—for example, to list those persons who are important to them (not limited to family members or those alive), how important spirituality or religion is to them, concerns or satisfactions regarding work, and how safe they feel in their intimate relationships and neighborhoods. I also ask them to list strengths and relationships that have helped them get through crises or hard times.

Pre-Session Contact

Let's assume that the person who did the intake informed Madeline that you like to have a brief chat with clients to determine how best to proceed and who to invite to the session, and they have set up this call for you. In general, you prefer to include significant others in the first meeting, but you want to be sure clients are comfortable with this and you are not overpowering what they are seeking or setting up an unsafe situation. Recall that in Chapter 6, you met individually with Alina for a number of sessions before engaging significant others because it was clear that Alina sought space to reflect on herself, her relationships, and what she wanted in her life. In contrast, Madeline appears to appreciate the larger lens.

Therapist: A lot has been stirred up for you along with the heart attack. Who else is involved? Affected by it?

Madeline: Well, my husband Byron especially. He has to deal with me every day [pause] and he was there when I had the attack. My daughters too, of course—but they live quite far away and are busy with their own lives. And my congregation, I know they worry about me.

Therapist: (You introduce a framework of care) A lot of people care about you—and you care about them.

Madeline: Yes. Being close to people and caring about them has always been important to me.

Therapist: I find that when we're getting started in therapy, it's helpful to get the perspectives of all those who are most directly affected. It helps us get the big picture and then we can decide together how best to proceed. How would you feel about inviting Byron to the first meeting?

Madeline: That would be a good idea. What I'm going through affects him—and he might have a different take on things.

◊ *Notice indicators of power processes*

Not all clients respond as positively as Madeline to the suggestion to include significant others in a first session. But most see the logic of it. Their responses to the suggestion also provide a glimpse into the nature of their relationships. If Madeline had hesitated or appeared less certain, you could ask about the hesitancy and what she thinks it might be like to include Byron, which would give a sense of how free she feels to talk in his presence and an initial window into their power dynamics. Madeline wants Byron involved. She is concerned about what is happening between them, but had automatically assumed responsibility for her welfare and the marriage.

As you discuss a time for the first appointment, Madeline appears to know Bryon's usual schedule and sets an early morning time on a day they are each usually flexible. She says she will check with Byron and confirm, which gives you an impression that she expects him to be willing and that both partners have some autonomy regarding their schedules, something not available to many.

◊ *Preview a relational lens*

You conclude the short introductory conversation with a statement that reflects an initial, very broad interest in the relational context of her presenting concerns:

Therapist: I'm looking forward to meeting you and Byron. You've got a lot to deal with—this big shock to your health and its effect on you and your marriage, on your relationships with your daughters, and—I imagine—your congregation too.

Madeline: Yes, I've always been able to handle everything and be there for everyone; this [pause] has really rocked me—us.

First Session Creates a Shared Frame

If possible, you schedule a longer session for the first meeting. You introduce yourself to Madeline and Bryon; welcome them; and begin by asking about their presenting concerns, why they decided to seek your help now, and hopes for therapy. Madeline says the heart attack was unexpected, completely "out of the blue." While on medical leave, she had time to think about herself, to take stock of things. Now that she is back at work, she's having trouble "being there." She wants to feel "joy again" and to feel closer to Byron. Byron says he came because he is relieved Madeline has recovered and wants her to be happy; that their lives are both very busy—they are both drawn to a calling to be of service and make a difference in the world.

Attune to Contextual Meaning of Presenting Issues

As you delve into these presenting concerns with Madeline and Byron, you draw on the questions in the SERT Assessment Guide (Table 7.1) to bring a relational sociocultural perspective to the conversation, including each of the four areas (social identities, flow of power, circle of care, relational ideals). With sociocultural attunement as a priority, you go back and forth between these four dimensions and client responses.

◊ *Go toward the emotional energy*

The couple shared a lot in just a few minutes. You sense emotional energy for Madeline around "being there" and ask what that means to her.

Madeline: All my life I've been good at being there for others; people could count on me to be the steady one—to be emotionally present and supportive.

◊ *Notice and explore the contextual meaning*

You recognize "being there" as part of societal discourse regarding expectations for women and are curious how Madeline applies this discourse to herself:

Therapist: You've known yourself as a caring person who's there for others and emotionally present. The changes that you've noticed now— being less present—what does that say about you?
Madeline: I don't know. It's like I'm not me—and I'm letting others down.

◊ *Look beyond taken-for-granted discourse*

As you explore the meaning of "being there," you begin to take in what it feels like to be Madeline—a wife, mother, minister whose identity has in large part been oriented around her ability to connect with and support others. To avoid assuming that Madeline knows herself only through this stereotypic female discourse, you probe for additional meanings that may be less readily expressed. Looking beyond taken-for-granted discourse provides an expectation that the subsequent therapy will make space for the not-yet-said and conversations that expand possibilities:

Therapist: You don't want to let others down. That makes sense; being a caring person is a big part of how you—and a lot of women—have known yourself. Giving to those you love and to the larger community is important to you. [pause] And is what you give recognized by others?

Madeline: (pause) I don't know—sometimes. Since the heart attack, a lot of people have told me how much they appreciate what I give. Even my daughters.

Therapist: So when you couldn't [finger quotes] be there, people noticed what you do, what you give? [Madeline agrees] And what about the other side? What you would like from others?

With this prompt, Madeline has a lot to say about what she would like from others—to carry more of the load, to not take her for granted. She fears that if she goes back to her previous roles "as usual," nothing will have changed; she will still be the "responsible" one—though she quickly adds that it is not that she doesn't want to be responsible. You notice that speaking counter to the female responsibility discourse is a bit uncomfortable for Madeline:

◊ *Attend to in-the-moment [contextual] process*

Therapist: What is that like for you to say, "I don't want to carry all the load"?

Madeline: It's like I'm not supposed to say that. Or that it's selfish, that I'm not recognizing what others are doing or just want attention to be on me.

Therapist: It's as though you're breaking a rule. And yet it seems important to you. You have a lot of energy there. Perhaps that's something we'll want to look at some more. Are there other old "rules" you'd like us to discuss?

Observing and reflecting on the in-the-moment process is one of the best ways to bring relevant contextual meanings to the conversation. Note that when you observed what appeared to be Madeline's hesitancy to resist the female responsibility discourse, you created focus by stating what was happening, but did not jump right in to interpret the meaning; you asked her what she was experiencing. You could also have framed your observation as a question: "It looked like saying that you would like others to shoulder more responsibility was a little difficult for you, what was going on for you just then?" The key is to engage the client in noticing what they are experiencing and to help them begin to link it to the broader issues you are discussing.

◊ *Evolve an image of clients' multifaceted worlds*

Time management is a challenge in an initial assessment session. Expanding the lens around salient sociocultural discourse in clients' stories helps make sense of the presenting issues and can bring both complexity and focus surprisingly quickly, but it also raises more to explore. In the first session, you are trying to get an image and feeling for the pieces around the presenting issues and an outline of how they connect. Once you seem to have a shared initial understanding of one aspect, you need to move on to another. Clients understand this and experience it as part of a reciprocal process of discovery and possibility. The sense of reciprocity and engaging together is more important than getting every piece of the information.

◊ *Connect with clients' felt sociocultural identities*

You now turn to Byron. As with Madeline, you listen for his felt identities and seek to apprehend his socio-emotional experience in relation to the presenting issues:

Therapist: Byron, you said you are relieved that Madeline is recovered from the heart attack and that you want her to be happy. What is that like for you?

Byron: Oh my God, I was so worried when they took her in. I felt so helpless. It's like she said, Madeline was always there for me and for everyone. Those weeks right after the attack I didn't focus on much else but her. I'm glad we're back to normal now. There's a lot to catch up on, things that had to be put on the back burner.

Therapist: Her heart attack shook your world. [Byron agrees] She wasn't there in her usual way and you felt helpless. That feeling of being helpless, was that new for you?

Byron: I've always been a take charge kind of guy. Before seminary, I was the CFO [chief financial officer] of a company. Going into the ministry and meeting Madeline, they've made my life so much richer and meaningful. But helpless? Never. I've always had a plan for what to do.

Therapist: Being helpless—what does that say about you?

Byron: Whew! Not good. Not good at all. It's like I'm useless, not competent. [pause] I've read a lot of feminist literature. I know this is a guy thing, but I'm not good when I don't know what to do.

Assess the Flow of Power and Relational Safety

As in all relationship therapy, assessing for risk of harm to self or others is always a priority; however, in Socio-Emotional Relationship Therapy, establishing relational safety is a broader issue and is integral to development of the therapeutic alliance. As you are getting to know the clients you are also monitoring the flow of power. Relational safety in the session and in the clients' relationships depends on mutuality and the interconnections between power, vulnerability, and social context (Knudson-Martin et al., 2021; Wells et al., 2017). As Lana Kim and I stated earlier (Knudson-Martin & Kim, 2023):

> Conversation that brings the lived sociocultural experience of each partner to light minimizes individual blame and encourages a "we are confronting this together" attitude. Less powerful

partners are more able to trust because their experience is named and validated, while more powerful partners are able to engage without their feeling misconstrued or judged.

(p. 274–275)

◊ *Look for invisible or taken-for-granted power processes*

It would be easy to assume that the flow of power between Madeline and Byron is equal—they have similar jobs, appear to share household tasks, and both appear willing to be vulnerable in session. Yet though Byron and Madeline are "fluent" in social justice issues and appear committed to gender equality, you are beginning to see a familiar gender pattern in which she is oriented toward the relationship and Byron acts more autonomously and is used to being in charge. As you focus on the couple dynamic and Madeline's statement that she would like to feel closer to Byron, you are interested in how less visible power processes may be interfering with this goal.

Madeline: We talk about a lot of things—our work especially, what is going on in the world, our kids. We probably talk a lot more than most couples, but it doesn't really seem to be about us.

Therapist: (You are informed by relational theory) You don't feel the emotional connection that you'd like between the two of you?

Madeline: No. When we first met at seminary ten years ago, we were both starting fresh in our lives. We talked for hours. My first husband and I hardly ever talked, and certainly not about what I was doing. Byron and I set aside time to talk every morning. But we don't really share what is going on inside—and I want that. I need that.

◊ *Ask how conflict is handled*

Asking clients how conflict is handled or to identify and discuss an issue about which they disagree or is emotionally charged helps expose power processes. When the flow of power is equal, there will be room for multiple voices and disagreement. Notice *how* they respond, not just what they say. For example, Byron says that they usually agree on things and that there is not much conflict. Madeline starts to speak and then appears to hold back. When you prompt her to continue, she agrees that they have similar values and are on the same page about most things, then adds that Byron has strong opinions and that sometimes "it is not worth it" to disagree; that it's "easier to go along." When you ask what would happen if she didn't "just go along," she says they raise voices for a while and then usually she gives in—unless it's really important to her and then they work out something. But it takes a lot of energy. In their communication, Byron more readily influences Madeline than she does him. Responsibility for resisting this pattern appears to rest with Madeline.

Even with a couple as committed to equality as Madeline and Byron, establishing relational safety will require you to use your role to facilitate a more reciprocal flow of power. If you see signs that the flow of power is significantly inequitable or managed through violence, you separate the partners and meet with them individually to assess safety before determining how to proceed. Many therapists find it helpful to regularly schedule individual time with each partner as part of assessment in couple therapy.

◊ *Share what you are thinking and solicit feedback*

At this early stage of therapy, clients need to feel that you are genuinely interested in understanding them. It is also comforting to know what you think and why; that you see their humanity and are willing to be open and honest with them. You offer a tentative reflection about the gender pattern you are seeing:

Therapist: I had this thought; I'm wondering what you think about it. So long as Madeline was healthy and "there," neither of you focused on what she might need. The heart attack changed things. [to Madeline] You're longing for something new in your relationship with Byron. [to Byron] You're aware that masculine socialization limits how men relate, but you're not sure what that means in your life with Madeline.

Both agree with your reflection, so you share a little more about what you are thinking, which increases your transparency and commitment to relational safety:

Therapist: I'm just getting to know you, but I'm thinking that the gender patterns you describe might be affecting the way you communicate and how safe it is to be vulnerable with each other.

Byron: How do you mean?

Therapist: Well, I work with a lot of couples. Even when heterosexual couples set out to have an equal relationship, those old gender patterns often unintentionally give men more influence over what gets talked about and make their needs and interests more central—even when that's not what they want. And this makes it hard for either to express what is going on inside them. Do you think this might be happening in some way for you?

Byron: Maybe. But I always thought we have such a good relationship.

◊ *Begin to make power differences visible*

You must attune to each partner; however, if you attune to the more powerful person without also beginning to expose the power processes, you are setting the stage for the therapy to reinforce the existing power imbalance. Respectfully raising the power issue encourages Madeline to expand upon her experience. Your response develops the power issue beyond the individual couple in a way that supports each of them while inviting change:

Therapist: Madeline, what do you think? You said you'd like to feel closer to Byron.

Madeline: Yeah. I never, never think Bryon wants to dominate me. But something is keeping us from emotionally connecting. [hesitates] I feel like he can't handle hearing about my pain or worries. And if I do share them, he jumps in right away with a solution.

Therapist: Like Byron said earlier, most men haven't learned how to take in what someone else is experiencing, especially emotionally. They want to help, but end up disconnected and perhaps disappointing the person they love most.

In this short encounter, you have begun to form an alliance committed to relational safety and disrupting power imbalances, while attuning to each partner.

Create a Brief Sociocultural Genogram

After discussing the presenting issues, I always leave space in a first session to sketch a brief sociocultural genogram. This allows you to discuss the relationships and larger contexts connected with the presenting concerns. You won't get all the details, but it will enable you to expand the lens.

Therapist: To understand more about what you are dealing with, it will be helpful to gather some information about your family and cultural backgrounds. Would that be OK with you? [both agree] So, you said that you met in seminary about ten years ago and that you were both making a major life change. What stimulated these changes?

Byron: I was growing more and more disillusioned with a lifestyle where no matter what I did and accomplished, no matter how much money I made, it was not enough; it was not satisfying—and I was supposed do more. I'd been divorced about five years and hardly ever saw my son. My connection to the Unitarian Church was the only place I felt sane.

As Bryon and Madeline tell their stories, you inquire about the people involved such as former partners, how long they'd been married, what those relationships were like, etc. You also ask about their parents, where they live(d), the kind of communities they lived in—both past and present, the kind of work they did, migration, and cultural connections. You learn that there was a significant class difference in their backgrounds. Bryon grew up in an affluent, nearly all White neighborhood. He went to a private high school and college. His parents are still active and currently live in a gated community over a thousand miles away. He believes they do not approve of his career change.

Madeline grew up in a working-class family where both parents worked just to survive. Her father died of a heart attack when she was 15, which left the family financially destitute. She has been working ever since. Madeline left her first husband when he refused to address his alcoholism. She says she has always cared about him, but had to set clear boundaries. His inability to hold a job meant she was always the primary provider for her girls. He died alone during the COVID pandemic. Today her youngest daughter, Genevieve, lives with and cares for her elderly grandmother while completing graduate school, and Margot is struggling with her marriage. Byron's son, Denny, is putting in long hours in a prestigious law office and seldom has time to spend with his father. Byron's parents remain close to his former spouse.

You learn that the arguments in which Madeline persists are primarily around how to support her daughters, who seek her guidance often and also believe their mother could have done more to help their father. When you ask about the neighborhood in which they live, this turns out to be another current stressor. Byron ministers to a small mission-supported congregation dedicated to immigrants and the houseless. It is important to him to live in this neighborhood, to be part of this community. Madeline shares and appreciates his value stance, but describes considerable stress living there—the noise at night affects her sleep and she does not feel safe going for walks in the neighborhood or driving at night. Though she has expressed her worries about the neighborhood to Byron, moving has never been discussed as an option.

While none of this information is new to Madeline and Byron, they are so used to jumping from one situation and set of needs to another that they have not previously stepped back to take a meta-perspective on the many social and relational contexts impacting them. Doing so and naming them are validating. Though they share similar current values, this conversation helps them see that they approach their commitment to service and social justice from very different felt experiences.

Highlight Relational Ideals and Resources

SERT therapists assume everyone wants and needs relationships. You see and interpret clients' accounts through this perspective as they describe their presenting concerns. You listen for it in your exploration of clients' backgrounds. Even if you are not able to complete the whole genogram, you leave space in the first session to highlight the clients' relational ideals. Sometimes people's emotional pain (hurt, anger, hopelessness, self-deprecation, etc.)

masks their desires for relational connection and their care and love for others. In these cases, you may need to state what is implicit but not directly expressed in their accounts of suffering or disillusion; for example, "you are so hurt and angry by [person's name] betrayal, it's hard to let yourself get close right now; I sense that what you are longing for—what we all need—is to feel safe enough to let love in." Or, "What you have been through makes it hard for you to be the kind of parent you would like to be; how do you wish you could express your love for [name of child]?"

If clients cannot, at least momentarily, tap into their relational desires; or if despite your efforts, they appear committed to dominance over relationship, individual or group work may be necessary before engaging in clinical work directed toward mutual vulnerability, attunement, influence, and relational responsibility. In most cases, though, when you see and highlight the relational desires and hopes embedded in your clients' concerns, they respond positively and feel valued and understood, despite current behavior that may work against attaining those relational aspirations. In other cases, as with Madeline and Bryon, their relational dreams are not hard to see. In all cases, naming them is a key component of collaborative assessment and alliance building. Since Madeline has been more vocal about her desire for improved emotional connection with Byron, you turn to him to bring forth and expand upon his relational goals. Note that your question is focused to elicit a relational response:

Therapist: Byron, you said Madeline's heart attack was really scary for you. What was it like to imagine that you might lose her?

Byron: I didn't even want to think about it. I can't imagine my life without Madeline. Meeting her and marrying her is the best thing that has ever happened to me! She sees the best in me—makes me see the best in me.

Therapist: I can see how important Madeline is to you; how she sees the "you" you want to be. [pause] And you said you want her to be happy. [Byron agrees] Madeline expressed a strong need to feel closer to you, to be able to share more emotionally. Is that something you are looking for too—or open to?

Byron: (pause) Of course. I always want our relationship to be better, to be close. It troubles me that she was unhappy and I didn't know.

Offer a Shared Path Forward

At the end of the first session, you pull the threads of the socio-emotional assessment together to offer a tentative relational understanding of the clients' situation and an expectation that by working together there is a way forward. You do not pretend to have all the answers, but you are able to genuinely envision possibility, which catalyzes hope. As always, your assessment and thoughts about how to proceed are presented in a sincerely collaborative spirit. You want to inspire confidence that you are able to facilitate a process directed toward a shared understanding of what you are working toward; one in which they feel that you are interested in them as unique persons, open to their experience, and honest in your feedback.

◊ *To summarize, use clients' words and your experience*

In your summary, you serve somewhat as a reporter, referring to what the clients have shared and drawing on words and experiences that stood out to you. At the same time, you are not neutral; you are an editor intentionally crafting a contextual account of their situation that suggests new relational possibilities and engages them in the therapeutic process. With Madeline and Byron, you conclude by placing their response to the heart attack in context of their relational aspirations and sociocultural environment:

Therapist: I'm so glad to have had the opportunity to meet with you today. Let me share some of my reflections, and then we can decide how you would like to proceed. [clients agree]. First, I am struck by what a huge—and courageous—step it was for each of you to make such a major life change when you decided to move into the ministry. [clients nod] From what you've said, your life together is about making things better—not only for your own lives but for others. Madeline, you spoke about "being there" for others and how important that is to you—and I also felt so strongly your desire, now after the heart attack, to feel even closer to Byron, to connect in new ways. [Madeline agrees] Byron, I heard you speak of struggles over the years regarding the role you want to play in the world; that relationships and making a difference in the lives of others have become more important to you over time. [Byron agrees] I'm just getting to know you, but as I listened to the many commitments and connections that are important to each of you—your children and their problems, your congregations, what it means to be part of a neighborhood—I began to sense some of the pressures and responsibilities you must face. [both indicate that it is a lot]. And, though you're a team in so many ways, your backgrounds are very different. There may be a lot to learn about how you respond to each other and how your socialization and life experiences may be getting in the way of the connection you would like to feel. Perhaps if we focus on that, how you connect with one another, that will help you be better able to support each other in dealing with the other issues you face. What do you think?

◊ *Solicit client take-aways*

Byron and Madeline agree with your summary, and each indicates that they'd like to continue working with you as a couple. You probe to make sure each is genuinely in agreement and invite them to share what they are taking away from the session today. Madeline says she already feels less anxious; that it was a relief to discuss what she has been feeling with Byron. Byron says that he's still thinking about the differences between them; that he had always focused so much on what they share in common. You remind them that you're just getting started and that you look forward to learning with them. You preview that since they are interested in working on their relationship, in the next session you'll be focusing more on how they relate to each other.

Expand in Second and Following Sessions

In the first session you and the clients established an overarching picture of what the presenting issues mean to them and how these concerns connect to their social worlds and relationships. You've kept the discussion about these issues close to the clients' experience while also beginning to frame them through a wider lens. Assessment and alliance building will continue throughout the therapy, with interventions also always providing new information. In the second session, you use the SERT Assessment Guide

(Table 7.1) to guide clinical actions that begin to intervene in and provide additional feedback regarding the four elements of the Circle of Care and how these connect to felt identities and societal power processes. I usually begin by focusing on the process between partners (or with an individual client, on their interactions with others). I then explore the societal discourses and contexts that inform their relational process, drawing on and expanding the sociocultural genogram/history.

For example, when you check in with Madeline and Byron in the second session, Madeline reports feeling distressed and agitated by an incident between her and one of the church committee chairs. As you process this with Madeline, you note that Byron seems disinterested and use this as an opportunity to focus on relational process:

Therapist: Byron, Madeline is describing an experience that is important to her. You don't seem very interested. I'm wondering what's happening for you inside as she speaks?

Byron: (pauses, appears to be reflecting) It doesn't have anything to do with me.

Therapist: It doesn't have anything to do with you. How so?

Byron: This kind of thing happens often. There's nothing I can do about it.

This is important information about how disconnection between Byron and Madeline happens. You stick with Byron to help him reflect on the meaning and consequence of his response—a level of assessment more possible when partners are interacting.

Therapist: I know you care about Madeline. This sense that there is nothing you can do to help her and so you disengage, what do you think that is about?

Byron: (pauses to think) I feel incompetent . . . almost ashamed, like I should know how to help her.

Therapist: That voice that you're incompetent—should know what to do—whose voice is that? Where does that message come from?

Byron: (reflectively) You know, I think it is other boys, boys from my childhood. I was always little, uncoordinated. Kids made fun of me.

[speaks with more energy] all my life I've been trying to prove I am competent—that I'm [finger quotes] manly.

Therapist: (thoughtfully) so when Madeline is distressed and expresses her feelings, you feel incompetent and disconnect . . .

Byron: Yeah . . . it makes me feel uncomfortable.

Therapist: You feel incompetent. [pause] How do you think disconnecting like that affects Madeline?

This brief conversation leads you and Byron to explore in more detail what he learned about being a man growing up and in his work environments. This consciousness-raising is important to Byron because he has struggled with it all his life, and he wants to be comfortable and connected in his relationship with Madeline. Witnessing Byron take this step toward self-awareness and accountability is reassuring to Madeline. In this and subsequent sessions, you support Byron in staying present with Madeline when she expresses troubling emotion. As you do, you and the couple continue to make connections between what is happening in the moment and the social contexts around them.

Therapist Checklist: First Session

☐ Set the stage in intake and pre-session self-reflection
☐ Welcome clients and ask about presenting concerns and hopes for therapy
☐ Be transparent about your approach and thoughts
☐ Attune to the contextual meaning of presenting issues and felt identities
☐ Assess the flow of power and relational safety
☐ Create a brief sociocultural genogram
☐ Highlight relational ideals and resources
☐ Offer a shared path forward

8

SERT TREATMENT PLANNING AND CLINICAL DECISION-MAKING

Socio-Emotional Relationship Therapy targets development of mutually supportive relationships based on reciprocity in the Circle of Care. This relational foundation helps people overcome the effects of social inequities and envision possibilities beyond the dominant discourse. Change happens experientially as clients engage in a socioculturally attuned process that validates, and potentially revises, each person's felt identities and they relate in new, health-affirming ways. Change is embodied as emotionally salient interpersonal experience relationally and neurologically embodied, and clients navigate the social world with increased awareness and options.

As our clinical research team developed SERT (see Chapter 13), we focused on what worked—what therapists did, how clients responded, and the impact of these on power and the Circle of Care. Four key mechanisms are involved (Knudson-Martin & Kim, 2023, p. 284):

Mechanisms of Change

□ Sociocultural attunement to each person's felt identities and experience that promotes relational engagement

□ A shift in power imbalances that supports mutual engagement in the Circle of Care

---

DOI: 10.4324/9781003270232-8

☐ Experience engaging from positions of mutual support
☐ A vision of alternatives to inequitable societal power processes

As in most models of therapy, we found some actions need to precede others and detailed the clinical competencies involved to create the SERT clinical sequence depicted in Figure 8.1.

To apply the SERT model of change across a variety of presenting issues and contexts, imagine that the following are among your recent clientele.

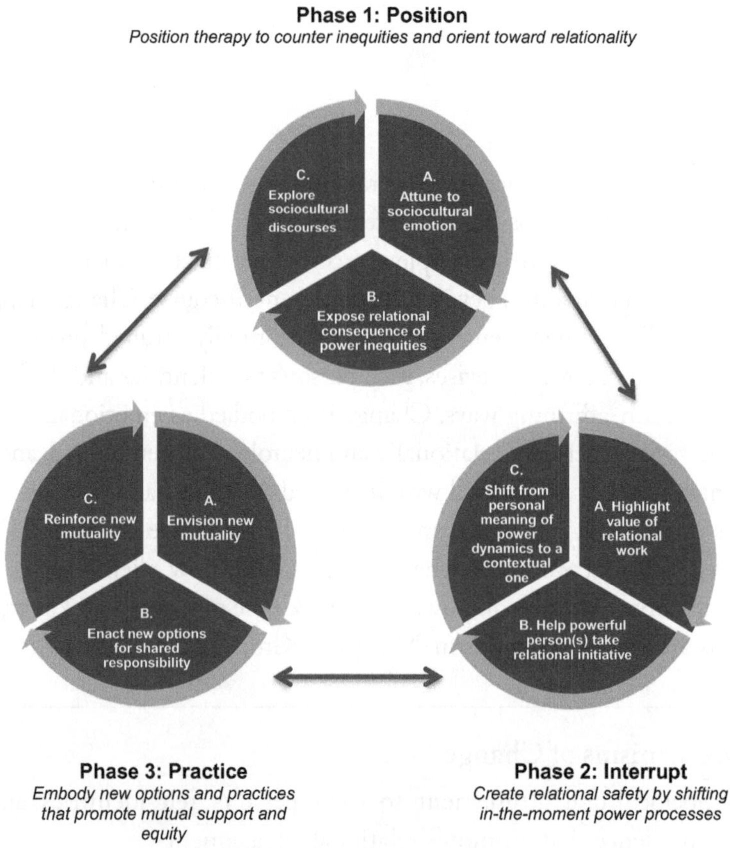

Phase 1: Position
Position therapy to counter inequities and orient toward relationality

Phase 3: Practice
Embody new options and practices that promote mutual support and equity

Phase 2: Interrupt
Create relational safety by shifting in-the-moment power processes

Figure 8.1 Socio-Emotional Relationship Therapy Clinical Sequence

Source: Knudson-Martin, C., & Kim, L. (2023). Socioculturally attuned couple therapy. In J. L. Lebow & D. K. Snyder (Eds.). *Clinical Handbook of Couple Therapy* (6th ed., p. 279). Guildford (used with permission)

Dave and Lula

Dave (56) and Lula (47) seek couple therapy. Dave, a physically large White man with a lengthy prison record, says he is seeking a "smooth" relationship; he is tired of all the drama. Lula, a petite Mexican American woman, reports severe abuse as a child and lists multiple psychiatric diagnoses from dissociative disorder to paranoia. She is fearful the relationship will end and wants to improve their communication. Each has had numerous prior relationships and views this as a "last chance to get it right."

Jayden

Jayden (age 28, White) identifies as queer. They are making a career change and seek your help dealing with anxiety. Jayden is puzzled because they are excited about the new career and usually feel capable and competent. As you discuss the impending change, you find that though Jayden has been out and comfortable in their identity for many years, they are uncertain how to come out as queer in this new setting. They are unsure of standards in the new work community and how their new colleagues will respond. They report a supportive queer community network and intimate partner, Dani, and a comfortable, though not close, relationship with their family of origin.

Leah

Leah (age 51, White and culturally Jewish) seeks your help for anxiety. She made the appointment because she has been "written up" for inciting conflict with younger multiracial colleagues at work. She reports that she has always been "high strung" but that it is getting worse. She is "at her wit's end" and can't sleep. In her first session she reports that she "can't stand" her partner Al's marijuana use, that it stinks and makes her stress worse. Al reportedly tells her she needs to "relax" and stop making waves at work. She worries about losing their health care if she loses her job.

Asiri

Asiri (age 40) sees you at his wife Sadia's suggestion. A second-generation Sri Lankan American, Asiri is an elementary school teacher; Sadia, a second-generation Pakistani American, is a nurse practitioner. Asiri says he has served as the primary caregiver for their two sons (ages 11 and 13) since they started kindergarten. Recently he has been experiencing what he calls "a midlife crisis." Though he "loves" teaching and coaching his sons' soccer teams, he is feeling "depressed" and "out of sorts." He wants more in life. He says his marriage is strong but would like "more energy" in it. He says Sadia does not want to attend the first session.

Samuel and Lena

Samuel (31) and Lena (33), an African American couple with a four-year-old daughter, see you because Samuel recently lost $20,000 gambling. Prior to disclosing this loss, Samuel—who works long hours developing his increasingly profitable business—had kept his gambling a secret from Lena. In the first session, you are surprised that Lena expresses little anger. When you explore their histories, you learn that Samuel grew up with very limited economic resources; his mother sacrificed "everything" for him to go to college. Lena, a software engineer, grew up in a more affluent family in which her mother was a professor and her father was a successful businessman.

How do you apply SERT to such diverse issues? This chapter helps translate the SERT theory of change into clinical goals and previews the SERT clinical sequence. You will also consider choices regarding who to involve in therapy and how to address individual symptoms/diagnoses and the tensions that arise when addressing power. I also offer suggestions for how to incorporate clinical strategies and skills from other therapy models.

Goal Setting

The overall goal of SERT is to facilitate new relational experience that promotes mutual support and enables possibilities beyond the limits of the dominant discourse. As you engage in a relational assessment process and form a therapeutic alliance with your clients (see Chapter 7), you will translate these abstract principles into personally meaningful goals. Following are examples of common SERT goals:

- Develop communication patterns that respect and value each partner's voice
- Build relationship bonds that enable mutual support
- Develop trust through reciprocal fairness and accountability

- Increase safety to be vulnerable with one another
- Increase awareness of the impact of larger societal contexts on personal biographies and choices
- Demonstrate shared relational responsibility

As in assessment and alliance-building, it is critical that goals evolve collaboratively. They need to connect with and grow out of the clients' experience and hopes.

◊ *Explore personal meaning of relational goals*

For example, in your first session with Dave and Lula, you begin to socioculturally attune to the tenuous nature of trust and vulnerability for each and observe a substantial difference in the flow of power. Lula and Dave agree that they seek a relationship that mutually supports each of them, so you explore what this means to them.

Dave: I'm always having to pick up after her—tell her what to do. All my life, because I was always "the big one," I had to be the boss. Everything I do, I end up being the boss. I don't like it!

Therapist: You're tired of being the boss. What would a more equal relationship with Lula look like to you?

Dave: We'd be "road dogs." [therapist looks puzzled] In prison, you need a road dog, someone who watches your back and you watch theirs. Someone who stands up for you and doesn't give up your secrets.

Lula says being equal would mean she is a "woman," not a girl. In the sessions that follow, you use the terms "road dog" and "being a woman" to discuss their process of mutuality. Over time, these images evolve and become integrated into what enacting the Circle of Care means to them and how they communicate and handle trust, vulnerability, and conflict.

◊ *Include relational goals when working with individuals*

If you are working with individual clients, goals should include a relational focus that takes the power context into account. Such goals highlight the relational consequences of the outcomes they are working toward. Examples include:

- Recognize and engage in mutually supportive relationships
- Step down from the need to be in control and always right (with clients in a power position)
- Recognize the value of contributions to the well-being of others (with clients in one-down power positions)

The relational goals you and Jayden develop help counteract the epistemic injustice (Fricker, 2007) gender and sexual minorities face because their experience is typically not part of "shared" social meaning. For example,

- Share experiences of invalidation and discrimination in the new work environment with trusted others
- Develop a sense of belongingness within the new work setting

SERT Clinical Sequence

Clinical goals such as developing mutual support or dealing with conflict in ways that respect multiple voices will not be attained unless the flow of power is equitable. SERT differs from other clinical models in that the clinical sequence first attends to the power context of the therapy and clients' relationships. Phase one positions therapy relative to relational and societal power issues. Phase two creates relational safety by actively interrupting power imbalances as they present in therapy sessions. The work of the first two phases creates a foundation for phase three, in which clients develop and practice new options based on reciprocal vulnerability, attunement, influence, and relational responsibility and are increasingly able to address difficult issues and societal pressures from a position of mutual support.

This overall sequence helps you link what happens from one session to another and determine how best to proceed at any given moment in time. Following is a summary of the important tasks and outcomes in each of these phases of treatment planning. In the chapters that follow, you will explore in depth the work involved in each phase.

Phase One Tasks—Position

In phase one, therapists position therapy to counter inequities and orient toward relationality. Key tasks and client outcomes include:

1. *Attune to sociocultural emotion.* Therapists must connect with clients' felt experience and the social meaning of their emotion. This makes abstract socio-contextual concepts personal. Outcome: clients feel felt, and the boundary between the personal and the societal begins to dissolve.

2. *Expose the relational consequences of power imbalances.* It is important to name power processes while also engaging powerful persons. This requires identifying their relational values and framing personal/interpersonal power processes within the larger societal context. Outcome: powerful clients begin to be aware of their position and demonstrate openness to accountability for their impact on others and shared relational responsibility.

3. *Explore sociocultural discourses.* This works best when focusing on current processes in session. Therapists must look for and recognize larger societal discourses in personal accounts and actions, helping clients connect them with felt experience and sociocultural vulnerabilities. Outcome: clients begin to see themselves and their relationships from a new sociocultural angle and open themselves to relational possibilities based on equity and mutual support.

Phase Two Tasks—Interrupt

In phase 2, therapists facilitate relational safety by shifting in-the-moment power processes. This usually means asking different things of each person based on their power positions and relational engagement. Key tasks and client outcomes include:

1. *Highlight the value of relational work.* This is important because the dominant culture tends to minimize it. As a result, clients tend to overlook caring work; some view care-taking or needing others as a problem. The less powerful person has usually been

doing most of the relational work without credit or acknowledgement. The therapist must make these positive contributions
visible and help clients credit themselves and others for it. Outcome: relationally oriented persons, who are usually also in less
powerful positions, experience validation.

2. *Help more powerful persons take the relational initiative.* This
involves helping powerful persons express vulnerability and take
accountability for relational engagement by attuning to and
being responsive to others. Outcome: powerful persons experience the positive consequences of relational engagement; less
powerful persons begin to feel safer and cared about.

3. *Connect interruptions in the flow of power to contextual meaning.*
When you do this, powerful partners feel less blamed or unfairly
targeted and are more receptive to risking vulnerability and
power sharing. Outcome: less powerful, more vulnerable persons
are likely to be heard, and clients join together to resist negative
societal effects.

Phase Three Tasks–Practice

In phase three, therapists help clients develop and embody new options
and practices for mutual support, which makes it easier to address hard
issues. Key tasks and client outcomes include:

1. *Envision a new mutuality.* Develop more fully detailed, personalized pictures of what is involved in mutual support. Therapists
invite clients to envision what their relationships will look like
when the relational load is shared, and each voice is genuinely
respected. When clients are off-track, you bring them back to
their relational ideals. Outcome: clients use images of mutual
support to describe and evaluate how they relate.

2. *Enact new options for shared relational responsibility.* Encourage
enactments that increase reciprocal engagement. This promotes
a neurologically accessible felt experience of shared relational
responsibility. Therapists also support clients in engaging in issues
that were previously too painful or conflictual to address. Outcome: clients incorporate images of mutual support into their felt

identities and experience confidence that they can safely communicate on hard topics.

3. *Identify, amplify, and reinforce positive relational options.* Therapists watch clients' progress in exhibiting relational ideals and recognize when clients enact an element of mutual support. They are on the lookout for small demonstrations that promote reciprocal relational engagement and help clients increase awareness of what they did that worked and see its positive relational impact. Outcome: clients are able to intentionally break from dominant discourse to consider and enact new options. New models of relating are interpersonally and neurologically embodied.

As illustrated by the two-way arrows in Figure 8.1, each phase of SERT is interconnected; they build on and reinforce each other. You start with positioning based on sociocultural attunement but never stop applying this lens. Similarly, you always design clinical decisions to interrupt power imbalances and look for ways to highlight and build upon people's relational ideals. Nonetheless, there will be movement from an active process of positioning at the beginning and interventions that create safety by interrupting power inequities as clients start to work on their issues to a process primarily about practicing mutuality and embodying the experiences that have begun to take root.

Consciousness-raising is an important element throughout SERT. Awareness of the effects of societal context evolves through clinical dialogue that both explicitly and implicitly expands the lens through the questions you ask and how you frame people's experience. At times, you may find it helpful to offer short moments of "social education" that raise awareness of societal discourses and inequitable social patterns and structures. These work best when directly connected to the immediate clinical issues and are offered as a possibility for clients' consideration. Group work, such as Rhea Almeida's healing circles that bring a variety of people together to consciously connect their problems to social realities (Almeida, 2018), can also help increase awareness and accountability. Fatma Arıcı Şahin (McDowell et al., 2023, pp. 131–319) uses experiential techniques such as art and presentation of equality manifestos in couples groups to raise awareness of sociocultural influences and develop social support for relational practices that challenge traditional discourse.

Treatment Decisions

The tasks in the three-phase SERT clinical sequence help organize the structure and flow of therapy. The five cases highlighted at the beginning of the chapter raise additional questions, such as who to involve in the therapy, whether to have individual sessions, how to interpret and respond to individual symptoms, and how to deal with ethical tensions when intervening in power processes. Rather than a one-size-fits-all response, SERT therapists consider how each option will impact the balance of power in clients' relationships and contribute to overall treatment goals.

Who to Involve in Therapy and How?

Since SERT works through development of mutually supportive relational bonds, in-session work among significant others is ideal. When intimate partners identify relationship improvement as their goal and each shows openness to engage in the process, the choice to work with them together is relatively straightforward. Their goals are better served by keeping partners together, which allows you to work directly with the relational process and make connections between individual, relational, and societal levels of experience. If you decide to meet separately with one or both persons, you do so with clarity regarding how the individual piece contributes to the overall relational goals.

◊ *Determine safety constraints*

In the case of Dave and Lula, you recognize some potential safety concerns. Their intake forms indicate that each of them has reacted at times with hitting and shoving. Dave is much larger than Lula. When you meet them, they talk openly about the violence that has sometimes erupted. Both are clear they do not want this and have come to you to find better ways to communicate. Dave says he will not stay in a relationship where either of them uses violence, that he is not "one of those men who needs to dominate women." Dave is assertive in his opinions; Lula is more measured. You observe a substantial power difference in their interaction patterns.

Given their reports of physical violence and the observed power difference, you see Dave and Lula separately before suggesting a plan for how to proceed. In the individual meeting, Lula is more forthcoming about what she wants—which is a more secure relationship with Dave—and says she is not afraid of him. She repeats that the violence is minimal and that she and Dave have agreed that if things "get hot," he will stay with a friend. When you meet with Dave, he says he learned a lot in prison; that it was a "good university." One of the things he learned is that most guys there "have a chip on their shoulder" and "dig themselves deeper with anger." He says he is now a sociology major at the local community college and on a new path. He declares that he loves Lula and wants to make a good life with her, but would rather end the relationship than live in a volatile one.

You decide it is safe to see Dave and Lula together. Following the research of Sandra Stith and colleagues (Spencer et al., 2020; Stith et al., 2011), you know that couple therapy focused on developing equitable relational bonds with attention to gender and power issues can be helpful when violence is low and not used to control or intimidate and when partners want to stay together and are willing to change their behavior. If Dave had demonstrated commitment to dominance and unwillingness to take any responsibility for the violence and/ or if Lula had appeared fearful of him, you would have considered alternatives such as referrals to individual therapy for each of them or a treatment program that focuses on intimate partner violence (see George & Stith, 2014).

◊ *Consider the impact of clinical choices on equity and mutual support*

When clients present individually, it is important to determine how your individual work will impact the flow of power in their relationships and whether individual work is fitting. Recall that Asiri came to therapy individually at his wife's suggestion. As you get to know him and his midlife concerns, he is clear that he wants more emotional connection in his life and feels disengaged from the community. There are few other Sri Lankans where he lives, and as a first-grade teacher and caregiver, he "doesn't have much in common" with most of the other men he meets. Sadia has always been his primary support person. As they and the children have gotten older, and with the stress of the recent pandemic on teachers and health care providers, he has become increasingly aware of his disconnection and "wants something more." You know this is not unusual at his stage of life and that the pandemic stress made relational needs more visible (Bucciarelli et al., 2022; Watson et al., 2020). When you explore Asiri's relational aspirations, you find he is quite passive; that he is in the habit of expecting Sadia to take the lead:

Therapist: What have you done to engage Sadia?
Asiri: Well, I tell her I'd like more time together; that I'd like us to talk more.
Therapist: And what do you do to make that happen? To have more time with Sadia?
Asiri: (looks puzzled) What do you mean? I tell her often. She suggested regular date nights, but that never seems to happen.
Therapist: It sounds like you are expecting—hoping—that Sadia will somehow connect more with you. Am I getting that right? That the responsibility for emotional connection has been her responsibility?

Asiri reflects a moment and agrees with your observation. You move the focus to what Sadia might need and his attunement to her:

Therapist: Hmm. I'm wondering what Sadia is experiencing. How can you be there for her emotionally?

Since Sadia does not appear interested in participating in the therapy (and possibly experiences it as a demand for more attention from Asiri), you proceed with individual therapy centered on helping him to take relational responsibility. You work with Asiri to take initiative in focusing on Sadia and help him experiment with reaching out to other fathers.

Asiri follows through, and after eight sessions reports that Sadia notices and appreciates the difference in his mood and relationship with her. She agrees to participate in some couple sessions.

◊ *Individual therapy can promote shared relational responsibility—if the therapist is mindful of the flow of power*

In contrast, it is important to engage Al in Leah's therapy, if possible. Though her anxiety regarding the interpersonal conflict and reprimand in the workplace needs immediate attention, an imbalance in the Circle of Care between Leah and Al exacerbates the problem:

Therapist: How does Al help you deal with all this stress?
Leah: He just sits there in his chair and tells me to calm down—like I'm disturbing his day!
Therapist: You want Al to show that he cares?
Leah: Yeah! Take me seriously. [angrily] He cares more about his pot!!

You and Leah decide to meet individually for a few sessions to focus on the trouble at work and then invite Al to participate. Al comes, but takes a very nonrelational stance.

Al: This is well and good what you're doing here. I think it's helping Leah. But it's not on me. She needs to work out her own issues.

Leah tries to calm him and then raises his marijuana use as a problem to her:

Leah: I know I have a lot to work on. I know I'm hard to deal with. [pauses] If you would just stop smoking, it would help me so much. The stink makes me sick.
Al: (emphatically) Whether or not I smoke is up to me.
Therapist: It sounds like your using pot is hard on her. How do you think it affects her?
Al: Look, I love Leah, but I won't choose between her and smoking!

◊ *Be careful that individual sessions do not perpetuate an imbalance in relational responsibility*

Though Al only attended two sessions, his participation clarifies the power imbalance. Differently than with Asiri, in your continuing individual work, you help Leah recognize what she has a right to expect in relationships—both at work and at home—and how she chooses to respond. When Leah asks if you can help her keep from upsetting Al, you are clear about your stance regarding shared relational responsibility:

Therapist: I understand how important Al is to you. And from what you've been telling me and what Al said when he was here, it seems pretty clear that you have been doing most of the work to keep the relationship going. You and I can work on how you want to be in the relationship, how you want to respond. But relationships are a two-way street; it will be important to me that what we do here doesn't place more burden on you at the expense of your health and well-being.

◊ *Access positive relational bonds*

Jayden is also experiencing anxiety, but their relational situation is much different than Leah's. In the assessment, Jayden describes a mutually supportive relationship with their partner Dani. The couple had worked to intentionally create a reciprocal relationship that reflects their non-binary identities and values. The power imbalance that needs to be addressed lies in the larger society. Jayden cannot realistically trust that colleagues in their new career will apprehend and affirm their identity, and this reactivates insidious trauma related to marginalization and childhood bullying (Brown, 2008). You invite Dani to the second session, primarily to actuate their support of Jayden in dealing with the anxiety stirred up by the job transition. Leaning on Jayden and others in their friendship network is appropriate because the relationship is balanced overall. In times that Dani needs support, Jayden is usually there. All agree that Jayden will continue in therapy individually, with Dani as a concerned and supportive partner.

How to Address Individual Symptoms

As we have seen throughout the book, the meaning and impact of individual symptoms (e.g., substance use, addictions, depression, anxiety, anger, child behavior problems) depends on the social and relational context. Sometimes, symptoms may be a form of resistance to power imbalances (McDowell et al., 2023). Treatment will need to attend to these symptoms while framing them contextually and not implicitly placing blame on the individual. What this means in practice will depend on your assessment of how the symptoms contribute to the flow of power and treatment considerations unique to the individual problem. A critical challenge is how to address the symptom without maintaining a power imbalance.

◊ How do individual symptoms resist and/or perpetuate a power imbalance?

For example, Lula suffered extreme childhood abuse. Over the years she saw many individual therapists, carried multiple psychiatric diagnoses, and took several psychotropic medications. Couple therapy and the possibility of a mutually supportive relationship has potential for healing some of those old wounds (Johnson, 2005; Wells & Kuhn, 2015; Wells et al., 2017). Excited about the couple therapy and wanting to make positive changes, Lula consults a psychiatrist to re-evaluate her medications and begins to see a favorite individual therapist to work on her reactivity. You support these efforts and consult with the individual therapist to align treatment plans. An ongoing task in the couple therapy is to avoid viewing Lula's victimization and mental health diagnoses as "the" problem. When things become "agitated," Dave often asks Lula if she had taken her meds. It is important to help Dave also examine and change *his* behavior. With Lula so willing to own her problems and take responsibility for her part in the relationship, it would be very easy for the therapy to organize around it.

Samuel's gambling is another example. Power and socio-contextual issues are important to understanding the gambling and what it represents in his relationship with Lena. When you ask what gambling means in his life, he says:

Samuel: It helps me get away from it all. And, until I lost the $20,000, feel good about myself.
Therapist: You get away from it all . . . all what?
Samuel: All the pressure—the pressure to perform, I guess. To make it. To be away from all that.

As you continue to discuss this, you begin to see how his experience around money and success is informed by his experience that as a Black man "you need to work twice as hard." You see how his socialization doesn't allow him to express the vulnerability he feels—to his wife Lena or even to himself. When you ask him to share some of this vulnerability with Lena, he stops cold, fearful that he, the son of an economically poor farmer, "has no right to be with her"—the daughter of a successful businessman. And when you comment to Lena that she doesn't seem angry, she says she understands the pressure he is under. You learn that her socialization as a Black woman says that you "stick together" as family to make it in an unfair world (see Cowdery et al., 2009). She doesn't want to add to his burden by sharing her concerns. The gambling is happening in a context where Samuel has no safe place to process his experience. Lena wants to be supportive, but it is almost impossible for the couple to engage in the Circle of Care. And Lena's relational needs and interests are overlooked.

Based on this assessment, you refer them to a problem gambling program with whom you collaborate. Both Samuel and Lena learn how gambling takes hold in the brain. Samuel participates in a group to take accountability for the gambling. You work with Lena and Samuel to develop their capacity to support each other through the Circle of Care, so they can confront the immediate gambling issue and face discrimination and pressures to perform together. While both partners need to risk more emotional engagement with each other, you are careful that the focus on Samuel's issues and sociocultural vulnerability does not come at the expense of Lena. His well-being, and hers, will be facilitated by also helping him focus on Lena and their young daughter.

Integrating Other Approaches

Good treatment planning is centered in an epistemological framework that situates how therapy is positioned and guides the development of goals. I think of it like the trunk of a tree—therapy is grounded in a clear vision of what therapy is about and what you are trying to accomplish. From this epistemological center, many clinical practices (branches) may be employed in service of the clinical goals (Dickerson, 2010). SERT is grounded in third order thinking that connects the personal and socio-contextual. It applies practices from many approaches, especially attachment, narrative, experiential, structural, and contextual. Techniques from any approach can be used in service of clients' goals, so long as they are used with intention regarding the overall treatment plan and their impact on relational process and the flow of power. Conversely, SERT can be applied as an umbrella or lens guiding clinical choices within another model.

In Leah's case, you use many experiential and mindfulness practices to help calm anxiety, but frame their use through awareness of the social context in which anxiety takes over (Strong, 2017). Instead of thinking of the anxiety as "in" Leah, you explore the context in which it arises. You expand the lens beyond the particular co-workers to whom she was "hostile" to look at the larger organizational system within which they all work. A picture emerges of pressures to do more in less time and with cutbacks in staffing due to administrative cost-savings measures and resignations because of the stressful work environment. Leah, an older worker who takes procedure very seriously, believes the younger workers on her team cut dangerous corners and are not conscientious enough. She finds their jokes unprofessional and off-putting and feels targeted as the butt of their jokes. When she was written up because of her hostile reaction, it felt unfair. And her supervisor did not support her.

With your guidance, Leah is able to step back and envision the tension in the workplace. You use experiential techniques to help her give it color and form through which she can picture the socio-emotional context. She can then also look inward to recognize her internal physiological response to the situation and visualize its color and shape. You are able to talk about what happened and how she prefers to respond using interactions among these metaphorical images. Together with narrative language that externalizes the anxiety—i.e., "when anxiety takes charge"—this imagery enables Leah to feel less "crazy" and "out of control" and able to imagine other stories regarding her colleagues' jokes and what it means to be professional. You are able to validate the unfairness, while helping Leah take accountability for her part in workplace relationships and consider her options going forward.

Leah is now also aware that Al is not willing to participate in developing an equitable, mutually supportive relationship. This informs her decisions about that relationship and, perhaps somewhat paradoxically, calms her. You and she decide to focus instead on family of origin work. Though her parents are not alive, a sense of unfairness from her childhood carries forward into current relationships and contributes to her "anxious, high-strung" nature (Boszormenyi-Nagy & Krasner, 1986).

How Long Does Treatment Last?

How long therapy lasts and when to terminate is quite variable. Following is how I describe the expected timeframe on my professional disclosure statement.

Professional disclosure statement

The number of sessions necessary to achieve your goals varies considerably from person to person, depending on the issues. Some people see substantial progress in 5 or 6 sessions; 12–15 is average. Some take 20 or more. Individual therapy often takes more sessions than couple or family therapy. Sessions are usually scheduled weekly until concerns stabilize, then less frequently as changes become more firmly established.

Sometimes only a few sessions provide clients the perspective they need to respond more positively to their concerns. This is especially true of younger people struggling early in their relationships or with situational issues. It can often be difficult to tell in the first sessions how long the therapy will take. I typically suggest that we get started and reassess after four or five meetings. I tell clients that therapy usually doesn't take a straight line forward; that what may seem like ups and downs are part of the process. I emphasize that as we work toward our goals, we may find sticking points that take some time to address. When childhood abuse or other traumatic experiences such as PTSD from war and political oppression are involved, therapy may be ongoing for several years. Usually, it is helpful to gradually space sessions further apart over time.

As clients are more able to mutually support each other and develop supportive networks, therapy is less needed. I often suggest clients take a break from therapy and return when new issues arise, just as they regularly check in with a dentist or physician. In Jayden's case, after five sessions, the two of you conclude that Jayden is once again able to access the strategies and relational support they need to cope with the anxiety stimulated by marginalization. You invite them to check back in as needed. Two years later Jayden and Dani make an appointment to see you regarding their decision to become parents.

Similarly, when Sadia joins the therapy with Asiri, their work is relatively short-term. They are able to enhance relational bonds that had been side-tracked by their immersion in dominant cultural discourses that prioritized individuality and accomplishment at the expense of relationships. The therapy raises awareness of how this happened in the context of their experience as second-generation immigrants in which time for personal connectedness was sacrificed by their parents so that their children could successfully claim dominant culture membership (see Kim et al., 2019). Since they do not live near either of their parents, after five couple sessions, Sadia and Asiri decide to include the boys in a virtual family session with each set of grandparents. Following social constructionist practices, the purpose of these sessions is to help solidify their evolving narratives that link the relational focus they wish to embody and transmit to their children with their cultural heritages and the sacrifices of the previous generation.

Therapy with Leah, Samuel and Lena, and Dave and Lula takes longer. The intersections of sociocultural vulnerability, power, and relational histories are complex and require that you are able to maintain hope and focus in the face of what can appear as setbacks and when pulls to prior power imbalances are strong. When this happens, it is helpful to think of the phases of therapy as ongoing and return to positioning and sociocultural attunement to vulnerability (Knudson-Martin et al., 2021).

Tensions Related to Power and Context

Clinical guides and examples can seem to oversimplify the complexity and challenges of actual practice. One of the important findings from our study of how our team learned to recognize and address the flow of power in couple therapy is that it was very helpful to view multiple sessions over time; to see the ups and downs and observe that even when therapy seemed to be going off-track, therapists (and clients) were often able to bring it back later in the session or another time (Morrison et al., 2022). When this happens, or you are unsure where to go next, I have two suggestions:

- Focus on process
- Socioculturally attune

Name and summarize what is happening, what you see. For example, after five months in which Samuel and Lena seemed to be making good progress toward more emotional connection and awareness of the contextual factors that had held Samuel back from expressing his vulnerability and Lena from expressing her wishes, the couple comes in upset. Lena says they are back to where they started; Samuel says he was simply acting on what he'd been learning in therapy and his gambling treatment and reduced the pressure in his life by putting the business up for sale and looking for a less demanding job. Lena is angrier than you have ever seen her. At first you are stunned. You hardly know what to say. For a moment, you feel back to square one too. Instead, you focus on process, beginning with what is happening in the room:

Therapist: Samuel, you decided to sell the business. Lena, you are more upset than I've ever seen you. It looks like a big division between the two of you.

Lena: How could you do this?! After all we've been through! After all
the work you put into it!

Samuel: I thought you'd support me in this. I thought we are trying to
reduce the pressure in our life.

You expand the focus on process to include a socioculturally attuned lens
and attention to power:

Therapist: So, Samuel, you thought you were responding to a shared understanding that running the business creates a lot of pressure on you.
And if I'm understanding correctly, it seems that Lena is surprised by
the decision. How did that happen?

Samuel: I don't know. I thought she'd be happy.

Therapist: You made the decision yourself and then told Lena?

Samuel: (hesitates) Well, yes.

Lena: There he goes—keeping secrets from me again. I can't do this
anymore! I can't!!!

You notice your own frustration popping up, but stay focused on process
and seek to apprehend what is happening for each. As you do, you learn
that Samuel is in many ways still operating from masculine discourses
that say he can and should make decisions on his own. He is trying to
incorporate a vision of what is best for their relationship and family and
to accommodate Lena's interests in daily decisions. But he is still approaching decision-making autonomously.

Lena is reacting to his unilateralism in a more expressive voice than
in the past, which is actually a positive change. However, as you continue
to explore her sociocultural experience, you find that she is still attached
to aspects of the dominant discourse that equate financial success with
social worth and value. In previous sessions, she told Samuel she cares
more about honesty with each other and time together than how financially successful he is. But these dominant discourses are powerful. It's
not just that he made the decision on his own; she also does not like the
financial implications.

As the session proceeds, you become aware that their argument is an
important part of the clinical process. In fact, it is necessary. Like many

couples, Lena and Samuel responded to therapy by making some initial changes that made them feel hopeful and loved. But shifting entrenched sociocultural power dynamics is not so easy. This new argument raises previously hidden issues. Now that there are two voices, they can address sensitive subjects, but they won't always agree. You frame the positive implications for their continuing work together:

Therapist: This is hard today. But it's an important part of your progress. You're trying to figure out how to make decisions together and base them on your priorities. In the old days, women were supposed to just follow what their husbands said, and Samuel, you'd make the decisions you thought were best for everyone. But you're working toward something different—to a path where each of you takes the other into account. And when you do, you learn new things about yourselves and each other. You're more able to resist some of the social pressures and injustices. It means you have to risk hearing what each has to say.

- *Recognize vulnerabilities as power shifts*

Change for Dave and Lula is also challenging. So long as Lula expresses vulnerability, Dave can make relational changes and feel good about himself. He does many things for her that she never experienced before. But when Dave faces circumstances that make him vulnerable, such as knee replacement surgery and his mother's death, he responds negatively to Lula's efforts to care for him. Even bringing him a sandwich when he has not asked for it makes him angry. He tells her to back off and leave him alone—which escalates Lula's insecurity. You try to socioculturally attune to Dave's fears, but he resists. You name this process, which helps calm Lula and leaves open the question of whether Dave will be able to risk emotional closeness when he is "not on top."

Therapist: Lula, it's hard for you when Dave's not able to receive what you offer. But that seems to be where Dave is.
Lula: I know. I wish I could show him how much I love him.
Dave: I know you love me; I just need you to give me some space!

You meet with the couple regularly for over two years. Lula also continues her individual therapy. Over time, the power dynamic shifts, such that Lula begins to expect more from Dave. Whether or not he will open himself to this level of vulnerability remains to be seen. Lula is less anxious when Dave distances, but may not be willing to remain in the relationship if he is not more open to her.

◊ *Prepare for contradictions, competing values, and limits to agency*

Even when therapy goes well, clients may struggle with competing or contradictory values (not only with each other, but internally). Social structures and circumstances may limit the kinds of change that are possible. Successful therapy can mean hard choices. SERT helps clients make these choices with contextual awareness and enables them to better navigate the social world within which they live.

For example, Leah needs to decide how to respond to the conditions put on her at work. On the one hand, she believes they are unfair and views continuing to work in that environment as a threat to her integrity. On the other, she has worked for this organization for 19 years and values the stability, good pay, and excellent retirement and health care benefits. She has limited influence to change that workplace. She decides to comply with the requirement to apologize to her work group and participate in conflict resolution training.

Similarly, she is hurt and disappointed by Al's emotional distance and apparent disinterest in her concerns. But she also values Al as a stable force in her life and loves the house they built together in a peaceful countryside setting. She decides "not to rock the boat." Leah continues to see you periodically, focusing on healing the unfairness she experienced in her family of origin. As a result, she develops more genuine relationships with her sisters and their families and feels the pain around her relationship with Al less intensely. A year later, she tells you she has found a new job where she believes her experience will be valued. Al has also agreed not to smoke in the house.

The goals to develop supportive relationship bonds based on mutuality and reciprocity in the Circle of Care are met in these cases in different ways, taking into account their varied circumstances, the limits to what the clients can control, and competing values that may impact relationality. You guide clinical decisions based on their impact on the flow of power and contribution to the overall treatment plan. When therapy seems off-track or stuck, you return to positioning based on sociocultural attunement to the connections between power and vulnerability.

Therapist Checklist: Treatment Planning

☐ Consider how each treatment option will impact the balance of power

☐ Identify the sociocultural vulnerability associated with behavior

☐ When in doubt, focus on process and attune to the sociocultural context

☐ Integrate techniques from other approaches with attention to clinical goals

☐ Expect contradictions and tensions when power shifts

PART III

SERT CLINICAL SEQUENCE STEP BY STEP

9

PHASE 1—POSITION TOWARD RELATIONALITY AND EQUITY

In this chapter and the two that follow, you will explore the competencies associated with each phase of Socio-Emotional Relationship Therapy and track a case from beginning to end. If you are currently working as a therapist, I hope you will consider how these practices apply to your cases and your evolution as a clinician. If you are just beginning to learn about relational therapy, picture yourself as the therapist. Imagine what you will think and do. My goal is to provide sufficient "how to" detail that you can envision what is involved in each of the competencies. Though we will take them one at a time here, note that in the diagram of the SERT clinical sequence (Chapter 8; Appendix C) there are two-way arrows between each of the three phases of therapy, and each of the competencies within each phase also build on and support the other. In real practice, the competencies won't necessarily unfold in linear fashion; you will move back and forth among them as you respond to your clients and follow and guide the evolving clinical threads.

DOI: 10.4324/9781003270232-9

The Case

Laurelle Carter calls the family center where you work, citing child behavior and marital troubles. She is referred by the school psychologist because their sons Brandon (9) and Logan (10) are "argumentative and disruptive." Laurelle is also concerned that their oldest son, Tyler (15), is "noncommunicative" and "keeps to himself." Laurelle (35) identifies as a Black African American, heterosexual, cisgender female. She is a certified nursing assistant (CNA) and works as a home health caregiver. Laurelle's husband, Nick (35), identifies as a White, heterosexual, cisgender male. The couple has been together since high school and married for 15 years. As a result of an injury on a residential construction job almost two years ago, Nick is not employed. After what he describes as an extended struggle, he was recently approved for Supplemental Security Income (SSI) disability benefits. Laurelle says that Nick is a "good man," but since the injury he is "unhappy" and "easily upset." She hopes therapy will improve their communication.

As a SERT therapist, you are aware that larger social systems (including mental health systems) do not automatically foster justice and relationality and that these contexts are important to what is happening for the Carter family. The first phase of your work is thus to position the therapeutic encounter to counter prevailing inequities and be accountable for how the therapy positions family members in relation to each other and their larger social worlds.

What Is Positioning?

As discussed in Chapter 6, SERT therapists are intentional and accountable regarding how they use their influence. Claudia Lini and Paolo Bertrando, systemic-dialogical therapists in Italy, call this responsible positioning. It applies to how therapists orient their roles in relation to all the contextual elements that impact the case, but also to how therapy helps clients position. As Lini and Bertrando (2022) say regarding a client named Diana,

> Diana is not responsible for the position she is put in, by her family members and by social and cultural rules, but she is responsible for the position she takes in regard to them. The therapeutic

process brings this to her awareness, and therefore enables the taking of responsibility.

(p. 349)

◊ *Positioning is an essential therapeutic activity*

Positioning connects cognition and action (Harré et al., 2009); people locate themselves in relation to social ideas and beliefs, which calls forth actions that support these "story-lines" (p. 8). People may also position themselves to counter these discourses, refuting them through word and action. For example, people may reject the idea of two opposite genders and define themselves as non-binary; their thoughts and actions counter prevailing gender constructs, yet also represent a position in relation to them. Positioning occurs at all social levels, from nation to nation to person to person, and even within an individual's internal dialogue. It is not static, and is thus a process that allows fluidity and change. Positioning in SERT orients toward relationality and equity.

◊ *Contextual emotional awareness helps map your place in the system*

SERT expands the notion of positioning to include emotion and power. Like Lini and Bertrando (2020),

> we see emotions as messages exchanged within a human system, rather than inner properties of individuals . . . emotions are influenced by and in turn influence context and reciprocal positioning. In other words, our position in the system is inextricably connected to our feelings.

(p. 210)

As a connection between the larger environment and the body (see Chapter 3), emotion is a salient force toward action and window to the personal meaning of context. Responsible positioning on your part— and facilitating it for your clients—requires awareness of the contextual nature of felt experience and identity and includes apprehending and naming salient power processes. This contextual emotional awareness provides a map of the intersecting complexities and enables you to know your place in the system (Lini & Bertrando, 2020).

◊ *Position toward relationality*

Like Saliha Bava and Sheila McNamee, SERT therapists consider justice a relational process embedded in and evolving out of human interaction (Bava & McNamee, 2019). As you approach the Carter family, you position your language, your questions, your ways of engaging to invite a relational process that encourages equity through contextual awareness and mutual care and responsibility. This includes exposing the relational consequences of power inequities. With the Circle of Care as a guide, you help clients position toward their relational values and equity. As illustrated in Figure 9.1, three competencies are involved: (A) attune to sociocultural emotion, (B) expose relational consequences of power inequities, and (C) explore sociocultural discourse.

As you demonstrate these three positioning tasks, watch for the following client outcomes.

Phase 1: Position
Position therapy to counter inequities and orient toward relationality

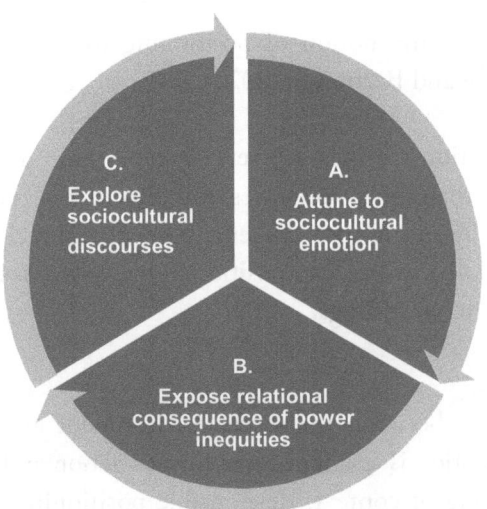

Figure 9.1 SERT Phase 1

Source: Adapted from Knudson-Martin, C., & Kim, L. (2023). Socioculturally attuned couple therapy. In J. L. Lebow & D. K. Snyder (Eds.). Clinical Handbook of Couple Therapy (6th ed., p. 279). Guildford (used with permission).

Phase 1 Client Outcomes

A. Clients feel felt, and the boundary between the personal and the societal begins to dissolve
B. Powerful clients begin to be aware of their position and demonstrate openness to accountability for their impact on others and shared relational responsibility
C. Clients begin to see themselves and their relationships from a new, sociocultural angle and open themselves to relational possibilities based on equity and mutual support

---

Competency 1A—Attune to Sociocultural Emotion

Your goal in this aspect of therapeutic positioning is to attune to each client's socio-emotional experience, as well as your own. Though it is impossible to ever fully know what it is like to be in another's situation, therapists must seek to connect with clients' felt experience and the social meaning of their emotion. This makes abstract socio-contextual concepts personal. Clients feel felt, which inspires trust and a therapeutic alliance in which participants feel validated and supported. Our research (Knudson-Martin et al., 2021) found that sociocultural attunement to clients' felt experience was the foundation for successful shifts in the flow of power and that effective therapists maintained this stance across sessions.

Because it arises from curiosity about the larger cultural meaning and power contexts of the client's emotion, sociocultural attunement to emotion is different than simply reflecting feelings. For example, in the first session Laurelle introduced each of the children by describing their diagnoses and the behavioral problems related by the school psychologist. You hear her expressions in context of her role as mother and the one who took the responsibility to schedule the appointment and convey the negative feedback from the school. This contextual awareness guides you to ask how *she* is doing.

Laurelle: (Laurelle looks a little surprised). Me? I'm OK . . . hanging in there.
Therapist: (You sense the tiredness in her voice and demeanor) You've got a lot on your hands. It sounds exhausting.

Laurelle: Yes. [sighs] I do the best I can. I told the boys coming here would help.

Therapist: You're hopeful that this therapy will make things better—for all of you.

Reflecting Laurelle's exhaustion and hope suggests attunement to her feelings, but sociocultural attunement goes beyond this to attend to the social meaning she experiences around their referral and the emotion in her statement "I do the best I can." Your response makes space for contextual meaning that is not yet fully expressed but is "inextricably connected" to her position in society (Lini & Bertrando, 2020, p. 210).

Therapist: (empathically) You're doing the best you can. [pause] When I talk to mothers, nearly all of them are exhausted and doing the best they can . . . but it never feels like enough—like they are somehow always expected to do more.

Laurelle: They're good boys. But I worry.

Therapist: (you again expand from emotion to the larger context) You worry that they are being labeled as behavior problems? That people don't see the good in them?

Laurelle: Of course. Anything can happen out there!

Laurelle may think it is not appropriate to raise the topic of race in a therapy session, especially if you are not a Person of Color. Your contextual exploration makes this possible.

Therapist: Anything can happen—especially if you are Black?

Laurelle: (begins to tear up) They are so young. And already the school says they are trouble-makers!

Therapist: You're doing your best to keep your boys safe—and enable them to grow into their full selves—in a world that doesn't treat everyone fairly, may not see the innate goodness in them.

In this example, you attune to the implicit sociocultural nature of the emotion in Laurelle's expressions. General societal concepts such as gender, race, and behavioral diagnoses are beginning to be identified and empathically reflected as personally felt experience. You have started to contextually position how you know Laurelle and the rest of the family, and they are beginning to feel felt as sociocultural persons, which is a shift from positioning toward diagnoses and behavioral problems.

Attunement to sociocultural emotion involves five steps:

1. Know your place in the system
2. Identify emotionally salient words or actions
3. Engage emotionally to resonate with the client's contextual situation
4. Mirror, sharpen, and focus the felt contextual experience
5. Voice the sociocultural context of relational hopes and fears

Know Your Place in the System

Sociocultural attunement is, first and foremost, an intentional stance. You approach the Carter family curious about the workings of sociocultural processes in their lives; ready to see and name them while genuinely, and respectfully, not assuming "truth." You are aware that whiteness is ubiquitous and central in your world and theirs (Hardy, 2022). Practices such as dichotomous thinking, a hierarchical view of the world, proclamations of objectivity, valuing stoicism and thinking over feeling, and an emphasis on product rather than process and relationality may not immediately be recognized as related to race, but reinforce whiteness as an organizing social principle—and typically define notions of professionalism (Hardy, 2022). You counter this notion of professionalism through emotional engagement and an orientation toward "being with" (Bava, 2023; D'Aniello et al., 2016). You are not afraid to give voice to race, and do so in a way that welcomes conversation and lets the family know you are willing to listen.

Since white patriarchy significantly defines how we know each other in the United States (Baima, 2022), it takes ongoing contextual awareness to recognize how it may subtly shape values and clinical processes, regardless of your race and gender identity or your client's. For example, my colleagues and I described elsewhere how consciousness of whiteness was important when working with an affluent White family with marital struggles and teens with poor school performance and substance use

(McDowell et al., 2023). Unlike Laurelle, who lives with awareness of race every day, the impact of race was new to the White family:

> [Therapist] helped the family validate their relational desires, while observing that societal messages prioritizing money and social appearances seemed to get in the way of their well-being and the connections they would like to have with each other. [Therapist] shared that many people who come to the Center struggle with these concerns, and that these pressures could be especially challenging for White families. This racial statement, which created curiosity and additional discussion among the family members, made sense to them since this observation followed [therapist's] careful attunement to their felt experience and connections to their sociocultural contexts.
>
> (p. 322)

The therapist recognized whiteness as integral to the values and contextual experience that organized the White family but worked against their relational desires.

Sociocultural attunement can be difficult when in a powerful position. Justice requires "proactive, socially aware listening . . . that listens as much to what is *not* said as to what is said" (Fricker, 2007, pp. 171–172) and is open to hearing grounded in contextual awareness. Even if you do not feel powerful as a therapist, it is important to be aware of how therapists can (re)traumatize and oppress though "professional" practice and assessment. As we will discuss in more detail in Chapter 12, it is critical to be aware of your own contextual emotion, which will influence how you perceive and judge clients and may prevent you from moving toward them.

If you doubt your own competence or (perhaps correctly) fear that your clients question your credibility because of your race, age, gender, newness to the field, etc., you could [inappropriately] respond to this sociocultural vulnerability by taking a "knowing" stance that blocks your curiosity and prevents you from attuning with the sociocultural emotion that underlies clients' symptoms. Ongoing attentiveness to contextual self-awareness is vital. If you think you are not having a socio-emotional response to a client and are simply "objective," you need to pause to take in your own place in the system. Use supervision or peer consultation to help raise your awareness and responsibly position.

Identify Emotionally Salient Words or Actions

Sociocultural emotion is present in words or actions that seem to carry significant meaning, whether or not they are expressed as "feelings." The clues may be subtle—a person's voice may change volume or tone; they may pause, sit up straighter, look down. Listen for and observe these signs of emotional salience, and move your focus toward them. For example, when Laurelle begins to tear up, Brandon and Logan start to playfully kick at each other. Their father, Nick—who appeared disengaged up until now—tells the boys to "quit fooling around and sit up." Though you had been about to turn to Nick anyway, his sudden assertion suggests to you that the boys' behavior carries significant meaning to him. Your question moves toward emotion, especially those connected to identities, social expectations, fears, and vulnerability.

Therapist: What are your worries for the boys, Nick?

Nick: I tell them they should stay under the radar, not bring so much attention to themselves. [pause] I know I should spend more time with the boys, shoot hoops with them, wrestle on the floor, but I'm in too much pain since this [explicative] accident.

As is not unusual, there are multiple salient moments in Nick's response. You decide to "pin" his desire to spend more time with the boys as important to return to later and go toward the sense of staying "under the radar." You are curious about the socio-emotional context of his advice:

Therapist: You tell the boys to stay under the radar. Could you say more about what that means to you?

Nick: I used to get in trouble at school. I had a hard time focusing and being quiet in class. My dad's thing was "when you get in trouble at school, you get double trouble at home!" I learned to keep it down—to stay under the radar.

Therapist: (gently) School was painful for you. You don't want that for your boys.

Nick: They're smart kids. If I could make it through, they can too—if they quit acting like screwups!

Engage Emotionally to Resonate With the Client's Contextual Situation

You are beginning to get a sense of some of the socio-emotional contexts around how each parent responds to their children's problems at school, which raises additional questions for you. It is important that this is not primarily a cognitive information-seeking process. As you gather more information, you orient toward "getting" what it is like to "be" each family member in their particular contexts. For example, what it is like for Nick, a cisgender, heterosexual, White man, husband, father, to not be able bodied, not employed, and worried for his children and marriage?

The key is for you as the therapist to take an emotional tone, to as much as possible allow your mirror neurons to take in your client's socio-emotional experience. For me, this means softening my tone of voice, perhaps leaning in or getting at the client's level (literally or subjectively). Though sociocultural attunement is a process that will grow over time as you continue to engage with the clients and get to know their backgrounds, hopes, and vulnerabilities, opening yourself to let in the experience of each family member is essential in this early stage of therapy.

The word "screwups" touches you. Nick says it with intensity and looks at the boys. Your body viscerally registers that being a screwup is not good. Rather than a question from your head, your response stays at the affective level and reflects the underlying emotion you sense:

Therapist: (slowly, softly) Being a screwup, (you breathe in and out) that hurts.

Nick: (softens his voice, too) Yeah. [sighs] I felt that way a lot . . . I was a screwup—still am, I guess. [looks down]

Therapy: (still with an emotional tone) You worry you're not the kind of man—husband, father—you should be? Want to be? [Nick slowly nods] And you don't want that for Brandon and Logan. [Nick agrees]

There is a lot of sociocultural identity–related emotion around "screwup" that you will return to, probably many times, as the therapy continues.

As you get to know Brandon, Logan, and Tyler, you are wondering what it is like to be them. What is school like for them? The neighborhood? What is their place of belonging? Who do they identify with? What is it like being biracial? How are they dealing with gender and sexuality? What is it like being at home? How connected to and supported do they feel with their parents? You notice that Brandon and Logan's skin is chocolate brown, similar to their mother's. Tyler's skin is much lighter. You are curious about what this means in the family and beyond.

You notice that when Dad told Brandon and Logan to "quit fooling around," Tyler began to gently rub Brandon's back and are curious about the socio-relational meaning of this action. You stay with experience around "screwup:"

Therapist: (turning to the boys who are all sitting on the couch) Did you know Dad sometimes felt like a screwup when he was a kid?
Brandon: I think it's cool.
Therapist: (thoughtfully) Cool?
Brandon: (smiles, glances up at Dad) Yeah. He got in trouble . . . I like it!

You tentatively reflect the emotional current you feel in the room:

Therapist: You feel better knowing that you're not so different from him?
Brandon: Yeah. [giggles] We're both screwups!
Nick: No, Brandon. You're not a screwup. I never want you to think that!

You feel Brandon's longing for connection with his father and emotionally recognize Nick's feelings of failure in the eyes of the world and as a father.

Therapist: (to Nick) Yet Brandon finds it comforting to know that he's not alone in this—and to feel like he has something in common with you. How is that for you? To know that he likes being like you?

As you get to know all the family members and the socio-emotional context of their problems, you not only listen for and attune to other emotionally salient words, you open yourself to let their experience in.

Mirror, Sharpen, and Focus the Felt Contextual Experience

Clients tend to feel experience that is significant to them but of which they are not fully aware. They feel pain or disappointment but may not have words to bring their experience into consciousness or their hopes into focus. The links between their emotion and contextual situations are probably under the surface. As you attempt to internally mirror their sociocultural emotion, to be with it, you are in a position to begin to voice it. Like Sue Johnson (2004, 2019) regarding Emotionally Focused Therapy (EFT), the SERT therapist's response is emotionally evocative to capture and crystalize what is implied and help clients connect with and make sense of their experience. In the example of "screwup," your response helps to focus and intensify the sociocultural emotion:

Therapist: (softly) If Brandon sees himself as a screwup—or if others see him that way—that would say he's . . . ?

Nick: That he's not good enough, not as good as everyone else—that he'll not make it.

The therapist guides clients to "the leading edge of their experience" (Johnson, 2004, p. 80) and—differently than EFT—invites them to see themselves and their reactions contextually. You do this tentatively, allowing space for clients to reformulate:

Therapist: You feel like you've not made it? That others look down on you?

Nick: And judge me—like I'm a second-class citizen because I can't work.

Empathically resonating with "screwup" provides the foundation for further exploration of experiences around masculinity, race, and relationships with school and other social expectations that emotionally connect Nick and his sons.

Voice the Sociocultural Context of Relational Hopes and Fears

As you attune to sociocultural emotion, people to begin to feel the connection between the world around them and their personal struggles. It is helpful to remember that implicit in painful or negative feelings are values and hopes for more positive connections and experiences. While Brandon and Logan speak freely about themselves and what they want, even in front of their parents, Tyler seems attentive to what everyone is saying but holds back from revealing much about himself. When you ask about high school, he shrugs and says it is OK. The look in his eyes says it is not. Rather than push him to expose himself before it feels safe, you attune to the relational hopes implicit in his responses during the session:

Therapist: Tyler, you care a lot about your brothers—yeah? [Tyler nods] And there's a lot of unfairness in the world. [Tyler nods] What keeps your family going?

Tyler: Well, we've never had much money, but Mom and Dad used to like each other. They'd laugh and tease each other and play with us. Now, everyone just does their own thing.

Therapist: You worry that the love in your family is getting lost—that it can be hard to see?

Tyler: Yeah. The love can be hard to see.

You expand the conversation about seeing love to everyone. In so doing, you are helping to position the family toward relationality and to counter social forces that make it difficult.

Therapist: I sense that too, Tyler—that there's a lot of love in this family. With all the things coming in—school, the accident, needing money, racial injustice—love can be hard to see sometimes. I'd like to hear from everyone, how do each of you still see love?

In sum, attunement to sociocultural emotion involves:

- Knowing your place in the system
- Identifying emotionally salient words or actions
- Emotionally resonating with the client's contextual situation
- Mirroring, sharpening, and focusing the felt contextual experience
- Voicing the sociocultural context of relational hopes and fears

Competency 1B—Expose the Relational Consequences of Power Imbalances

With this competency, therapists not only identify power processes, they also make visible how power imbalances interfere with clients' relational goals. This includes identifying clients' relational values and framing personal/interpersonal power processes within the larger societal context. A goal is to engage those in powerful positions to recognize the relational consequences of their position—what they lose or miss out on or how they may be hurting someone they love—and to demonstrate openness to being accountable for their impact on others and willingness to share relational responsibility.

Identifying power imbalances without making the connection to relational consequences and ideals does not help clients position toward relationality, and those in powerful positions are likely to feel blamed or misunderstood. On the other hand, focusing on their feelings and relational interests without naming power contexts may reinforce the power imbalance and could intensify the burden of responsibility on less powerful persons. Our research shows that connecting powerful persons to the relational consequences of their actions is critical (Samman & Knudson-Martin, 2015).

Exposing the relational consequences of power imbalances involves four steps:

1. Consider the power contexts of client issues
2. Track the flow of power
3. Explore the relational impact of the flow of power
4. Name the consequences of power imbalance on relational goals

Consider the Power Contexts of Client Issues

As discussed in earlier chapters, it is important to identify the sociocultural power contexts that have an impact on the issues clients face, how they are framed, and the options available to them. Clients may not describe these contexts unless you ask about them. When you do, you begin to position client issues and the therapy itself within this bigger picture. Discussing the power contexts is especially validating for those in less powerful positions. When you asked about race, Laurelle was relieved. As an "experienced" client, she came prepared to discuss the boys and their marriage from a deficit position that placed their problems within family dysfunction. She and Nick feel like parenting failures because of how their boys are labeled. In other words, they approached therapy in a one-down position relative to dominant mental health and individualizing discourses. Your interest in the world around them begins to help them re-position. You ask about the school and their neighborhood:

Therapist: What is the school like? Is it mixed-race? Mostly White? Affluent?

Laurelle: The elementary school is pretty mixed—more White, but a lot of everything. It's in a pretty well-off neighborhood. Our house is one of the smallest ones—on the edge of the district.

Therapist: So a lot of the other kids come from families with more money?

Logan: Yeah! They all have Kyries or LeBrons [basketball shoes]. That's what I want.

Laurelle: I know, I know. [raises voice] We can't afford them—you know that!

Therapist: (softly) It's hard when Logan sees what the other kids have.

Laurelle: (nods) You want them to feel good about themselves.

Questions about neighborhoods, access to green space, socioeconomic status, ethnic/cultural and religious communities, and how clients experience them provide an initial sense of the social power context and should be a regular part of getting to know clients' worlds. Building these questions into discussions of family background, genograms, sociograms, eco-maps, and sculpting or drawing activities can be especially helpful in bringing power contexts to light.

In the second session you engage the Carters in creating a family cartography (McDowell, 2015) that helps them make connections between physical space, power, social interactions, safety, and belonging. You give them a big piece of paper (or poster board or chalk board) and markers and ask them to work together on it with your guidance. You invite them to draw a map of their town—where do different kinds of communities or groups live? Where is their house? Where do people with more money live, with less money? What is the physical environment like (how close people live to each other, location of parks, train tracks, stores)? Where are their schools? Where do friends and family live? You ask where they feel safe/unsafe and how easy it is to get from one place to another.

Through this conversation, you learn that earlier in their marriage, when housing prices took a sharp decline, Nick's father helped them by a small three-bedroom "fixer-upper" at a very low price because it was in foreclosure (i.e., Nick had access to social and financial capital). With skills learned on his job with a builder, he was able to do the work to make their home livable. It is in a quiet and "safe" neighborhood, but the family does not feel accepted by their neighbors, who tend to be more affluent and White. Since the accident, they have one car that Laurelle uses to get to her home care sites, unless Nick needs it for an appointment; the boys take buses to school. Laurelle's mother and sisters live in a "poorer" neighborhood a 15-minute drive away and stop by regularly. They avoid visiting Nick's family, who live in a "good" community about an hour away, because his mother is "racist" and treats Laurelle and the boys differently than her other grandchildren. You summarize the felt experience of this power context:

Therapist: You all feel a little [air quotes] less than in this neighborhood—and in Nick's family. Mom and Dad, you feel judged as . . . what? Less competent? Less valuable? Not good parents?

Laurelle: It's hard to put words to, it's just a feeling, I guess—that we should be doing better. That we're not as good as them. [pauses] Nick always worked so hard, but not the "right" kind of work, you know. [pauses] Our boys are just as good as the other kids, but it's hard to keep up!

Therapist: (to Laurelle) And you? How safe and accepted do you feel?

Laurelle: (wry chuckle) I never expected to fit in. But this house was a good choice for our family, something I never expected. I'm grateful.

Track the Flow of Power

In SERT, power is not intrinsic to the individual, but rather the outcome of social/interpersonal processes (see Chapter 4). As you get to know the family, you are watching for the flow of power and make it a priority to track this so they can see it as well. For example, in relation to his family of origin and in the more affluent White community, Nick feels "less than." But as a White, cishet man, he feels entitled to respect and is angry about his position, which has been intensified because he is no longer able-bodied or employed. In contrast, Laurelle, who also has a medical condition that causes her considerable pain, feels grateful to Nick, and her socialization as a Black woman tells her not to expect respect and to keep going no matter what. This creates a disparity in how the partners are positioned in relation to each other, with Nick expecting respect and appreciation and Laurelle expecting little.

As another indicator of power, in the first session you notice a lot of back and forth between Laurelle and the boys, but unless you are focusing on Nick's interests, he does not seem very attentive. You describe this process without making an interpretation:

Therapist: (to the family) As we're talking, I notice that you all seem engaged and interested in what each other is saying, except Dad seems less involved. Is this how it is at home?

Logan: Dad mostly stays in his room.

Brandon: He just comes out to yell at us—he's mad all the time.

Nick: You'd be mad too if you were in this much pain. I need you to keep it down.

You name the process they are describing, which makes it visible and open for reflection:

Therapist: So, Dad's in his room, not feeling so good, [turns to boys] and he wants you to be quiet. And what's going on for you? What about Mom?

Brandon: Mom's at work—or working in the kitchen. We're in the living room—just watching TV or playing our games. [smiles impishly] Sometimes we have homework to do.

To track power, you explore the two-way nature of their relationships. Who is attending to whom? Whose interests seem to matter?

Therapist: Mom's working. [pause] Dad says he wants some quiet. What are you wanting from Dad?

Logan: He could play with us.

Brandon: He could help us with homework. Tyler does that sometimes. And Mom when she has time.

Therapist: So you'd like Dad to be more interested in what you're doing? More involved? [Brandon and Logan enthusiastically agree]

In the described pattern, Nick expects his children to attend to his interests but does not attune to them. This power imbalance limits his relationship with them.

Explore the Relational Impact of the Flow of Power

Questions about relationships bring forth relational awareness but may require persistence. You position your responses to acknowledge Nick's love for his children and also focus on the impact on them of his anger and distancing.

Therapist: Nick, Brandon and Logan see you as off on your own and angry; they don't see you being interested in them and what they're doing. What do you think that is like for them?

Nick: They should know I love them.

Therapist: (maintains focus on relational impact) What do you suppose happens for them when your love is buried under anger?

Nick: I suppose it's upsetting.

Therapist: Upsetting? How?

Nick: Like they want attention from me and don't get it.

Therapist: You think they'd like attention from you and that it's upsetting—hurtful maybe—when you don't seem to care?

Nick: I don't always feel like they care whether I'm there or not.

Parent-child relationships are inherently hierarchical. When parents attune to and are responsive to their children's experience and also help them attune to their impact on others, including their parents, a developmentally appropriate reciprocal flow of power helps build relational bonds. So as not to reinforce the power disparity here, you are careful not to put the burden of vulnerability on the boys, and instead invite Nick to consider his impact on them. When he shifts the focus back to his needs, you name what the boys just said about wanting his involvement (the current process is hard to argue with) and bring the focus back to his impact on them. Later you *will* want the boys to also consider their impact on their parents, but you begin with the more powerful person.

Therapist: Just a moment ago, Brandon and Logan were very enthu-
siastic about the idea of your doing things with them. [pause] You
said they probably want attention from you. How do you think your
showing interest in what they're doing would have an impact on
them?

Nick: I suppose it would feel like they are important—that I care.

Name Consequences of Power Imbalance on Relational Goals

Since power imbalances interfere with relational connections, it is important to help clients bring their relational goals to the forefront. Seeing the impact of the just-exposed power imbalances on their rela-tional goals is a motivation for a shift in power, and especially critical for those in powerful positions. It is important to highlight these relational goals together with how the flow of power just described limits their ability to attain them.

Therapist: (to Nick) It's clear from what you've said that you love your
children and are here, in large part, because you are concerned for
them. You want to help them feel good about themselves. You also
said you'd like to spend more time with them.

Nick: Of course. All three of my boys are very important to me.

Therapist: It sounds like anger about the pain takes over and keeps you
from being attentive to what the boys are doing and how you could
engage with them.

Nick: Yeah, I guess. I've been pretty miserable since then—useless.

Therapist: (you maintain focus on the impact of anger on his relational
goals) When you focus on anger and misery, it's hard to show how
much you care about them or pay attention to what they need.

Nick: Yeah. [sighs] Yeah. But I *do* care.

You reinforce how the power disparity impacts Nick's relational goals by inviting reflections from Laurelle and the children.

Therapist: Laurelle, when pain and anger keep Nick from focusing on the children, how does that affect you?

Laurelle describes her awareness that the boys are hurt by Nick's withdrawal and anger and how she tries to suggest ways he could better communicate and engage with them, but this seems to make Nick even angrier. She feels alone as a parent and wife. When you ask the boys what they miss from their dad, Brandon and Logan reiterate that they miss having a dad who likes to be with them. You turn to Tyler, who has been quieter and less animated throughout the session:

Therapist: Tyler, we have been talking about how since the accident, Dad ends up focusing mostly on his pain and anger and misses focusing on all of you; that keeps him separate from everyone and not able to show how much he cares. What is this like for you?
Tyler: (pauses) I think maybe I'm becoming like Dad—just keeping to myself. [pause] I try to look out for Brandon and Logan when I can, but . . .
Therapist: You feel a burden to look out for your younger brothers? [Tyler nods] And I'm guessing what you're experiencing, what you need, is hard to bring into the picture?
Tyler: I'm OK. I don't want to upset anyone.

These reflections from the rest of the family help concretize the power disparity in whose needs are addressed and who gives care. They make the relational impact real to Nick and begin to activate his caring and accountability. Your role tracking the flow of power, naming the power disparity, and highlighting the relational consequences makes these processes visible and enables him to position toward a more equitable, mutually supportive future.

Nick: I didn't realize . . . I can be selfish sometimes. [looks at Tyler] It's not your job to take care of your brothers. If something's bothering you, I want you to come to me, talk to me.

In sum, exposing the relational consequences of power imbalances involves:

- Consider the power contexts of client issues
- Track the flow of power
- Explore the relational impact of power
- Name the consequences of power imbalance on relational goals

Competency 1C—Explore Sociocultural Discourses

Societal discourse, emotion, and power are all interconnected. Making the links between what is happening and talked about in therapy and larger social discourses reduces blame and enables clients to begin to see themselves and their relationships from a new, sociocultural perspective and begin to consider relational possibilities based on equity and mutual support. Rather than thinking about the stories people tell about themselves and others as individual ones, listen for the social discourses incorporated into these accounts.

Pay special attention to societal messages regarding expectations of self and others, what constitutes success, how one should enact their roles, ideas about autonomy and togetherness, right and wrong, good or bad. As described in Chapter 3, these societal discourses serve as building blocks of felt identity and are thus central to therapy and the process of change. Sometimes you can access societal discourse by moving outward from emotion, as discussed earlier in the chapter. Other times, you will begin with client words that imply a "should" or "ought," guilt, judgment, or disappointment.

Four steps are involved in exploring sociocultural discourses:

1. Move from the personal to the contextual
2. Name the expectation/discourse
3. Explore the personal/relational effect of the discourse
4. Invite possibility of alternative or marginalized discourse

Move From the Personal to the Contextual

Exploring social discourse works best when you begin with the personal, with what is already being discussed, and expand the conversation outward. Questions such as "What have you learned about . . . ?" "What do people say about . . . ?" "How does the idea that . . . affect you?" or "What have you noticed about how people in your culture (or community) deal with . . . ?" all begin to shift from a personal story to a larger one and set the stage for more direct conversations about culture, race, gender, religion, social class, etc. Using words clients have already used and staying close to their lived experience usually works better than broad questions such as "tell me about your culture" or "how does gender influence you?"

Laurelle and Nick also want to work on their marriage, and their children are worried their parents might divorce, so you decide to alternate between couple sessions and family sessions. You also agree to meet separately with Tyler, who seems to be struggling as a high school freshman and—unlike Brandon and Logan—is not receiving other support from school or a counselor and seems to welcome the chance to speak with you privately. You are curious how societal discourses are part of their stories.

In the first couple session, you ask Nick and Laurelle what attracted them to each other and listen for social messages and expectations in their accounts:

Nick: We met in high school—were friends. I remember she sat next to me in biology. She was so smart and kept cracking these really funny jokes. [looks at Laurelle] She helped me write up the lab assignments. I'd probably have failed without her.

Therapist: You were attracted to her intelligence and wit.

Nick: Still am! It was like nothing could get her down. She always had a smile. [thinks] School wasn't much fun for me. Laurelle made it better and didn't judge me.

Therapist: Laurelle, Nick says you made school better for him— supported him, didn't judge him. What attracted you to him?

Laurelle: Honestly, I wasn't at first. But then I started to appreciate that he wasn't so cocky like most of the guys. He wasn't a smartass. He treated me with respect.

You expand outward:

Therapist: You said earlier that as a Black woman you didn't necessarily expect respect.

Laurelle: No. I didn't. And among teenage guys, I didn't see much respect for girls, period.

Therapist: So Nick didn't fit the stereotype—he didn't act like a [air
quotes] typical teenage guy. [pause] Was it unusual in your school to
date across racial lines?

Laurelle: There was some crossover. But we didn't really start out dating.
It was more like support for each other. [looks at her body] I was
kinda chubby. Boys weren't very interested in me.

Therapist: So you didn't feel very attractive to boys. Those ideas that
to be attractive, girls shouldn't be "chubby"—and I'm guessing also
maybe not smart—how did those ideas affect you?

You are now engaged in a conversation about the larger context. Laurelle
describes believing she was not attractive as a potential girlfriend; that
her Black body should look more like a White body. When Nick started
to show physical attraction to her, she was surprised and grateful.

Therapist: You were surprised that any guy, especially a White guy,
would find you attractive? [Laurelle nods] And Nick, you're a White
guy—from a more affluent family—how do you think it happened
that you resisted those stereotypes about women?

Nick: Honestly [turns to Laurelle] don't get me wrong, I've always been
lucky to have you—but I think it was partly an "up yours." I didn't
like school, I didn't like authority, I didn't like my parents' snobbish-
ness. I was looking to rebel.

Therapist: And from what you said, when you stepped outside those stereotypes, you had fun together and appreciated and supported each
other.

Name the Expectation/Discourse

Despite attraction based on mutuality that challenged prevailing social
discourses, many dominant discourses have taken hold of their current
relationship. Beneath the surface expectations based on old social stereotypes guide their marriage in ways neither intended. Listening for and
naming these expectations brings them to the surface so they can be addressed. When Laurelle raises their fights and Nick's anger, you track the

process and probe for sociocultural expectations regarding anger, which you know is prescribed for men, but not usually for women.

Laurelle: I'm so tired of the fights. Nick is angry all the time. It seems like no matter what I say to him, he takes offense. Either I say nothing or endure a fight.

Therapist: You'd like to be able to address issues without so many fights, with less anger?

Laurelle: Yes. The anger just wears me down.

Therapist: You expect that when you have disagreements, you should be able to talk about them—without anger?

Laurelle: I know there will be anger. We are human, but it's like anger is all Nick's got. He won't let me get close to him.

Therapist: (to Nick) Laurelle experiences anger from you getting in the way of the two of you dealing with things together, being together. How do you experience the anger?

Nick: I can't help it if I feel angry. Picking on me makes me angry. That's how it is.

Therapist: You expect that when someone—when Laurelle—has a concern she'd like to discuss, that she should expect you to respond with anger?

Nick: (pauses, shakes his head) I don't know! I think she should know I'm having a hard time.

Therapist: So you expect that when you're having a hard time, anger is appropriate and others should put up with it? Where do you suppose that idea comes from?

Nick says his father was often angry and that the family knew to leave him alone. You explore this a little and then expand to the broader society and masculine socialization.

Therapist: I don't think your father is the only man who uses anger like that. It's pretty common. How do you suppose so many men learn to use anger, rather than sharing what's really going on for them or being willing to hear what others have to say?

Nick: I don't know. It seems like anger is all there is. It's all I've got.

You are now able to have a brief conversation about how men often learn that anger is the only emotion it is appropriate to express and what is lost by this.

Explore the Personal/Relational Effect of the Discourse

In this case, as in most, societal discourse limits personal options for identity and expression and also restricts what is possible relationally. You address both the vulnerabilities Nick feels when positioned toward this "men can only express anger" discourse and the impact it has on communication and connection with Laurelle.

Therapist: When you picture yourself not expressing anger—Laurelle raises something that makes you anxious or you don't want to talk about—what would that be like for you? What might be hard about that?

Nick: I don't know—that I don't have an answer; that I don't know what to do.

Therapist: You are supposed to have the answers? And when you don't, you feel . . . ?

Nick: Useless! [explicative] I feel useless all the time!

Therapist: And when you feel useless and use anger to keep that part of you from Laurelle, how do you think that affects your relationship with her?

Nick: Well, obviously it's not working very well.

There is a lot more regarding Nick's vulnerability around feeling useless and the social discourses and power processes related to that expression. For now, identifying this salient discourse, and some of the emotion around it, helps position the couple and the therapy toward their relational goals and alternatives to masculine discourses such as "anger is the only acceptable emotion" and "I should always have the answers."

Invite Possibility of Alternative or Marginalized Discourse

Our research (Williams et al., 2013) showed that naming problematic societal discourses is not sufficient to create mutually supportive change; therapists must take the lead in inviting alternative discourses.

Usually, these alternatives are not new to clients, but have been marginalized and not validated in the dominant discourse. Like many couples, Nick and Laurelle's attraction to each other was based, at least in part, on egalitarian discourse (Rusovick & Knudson-Martin, 2009). You highlight these ideals and open conversation about alternatives to the "men should have the answers" discourse as part of their goals going forward.

Therapist: When you were talking about your initial attraction to each other, I was struck that it was based on mutuality and being there for each other [both partners nod]. You were drawn to each other, in large part, because you broke away from gender and racial stereotypes. I'm guessing that's still important to you?

Laurelle: Absolutely! I wouldn't want a relationship any other way. I want to be partners with Nick.

Therapist: Is that what you want too, Nick? To be partners with Laurelle—in it together, finding answers together.

Nick: Sure. Of course. This accident has gotten us off track.

Therapist: Part of what we can do together is to figure out how to get back on track—so that you each share in working out the challenges and support each other through them.

Part of Nick and Laurelle's motivation is to model different ways to relate and express masculinity for their sons. When you meet individually with Tyler, you learn how central this is to his life as well. When you talk with Tyler about school and his relationships, you learn that Tyler does not know where he fits. He feels like he doesn't belong anywhere. You hear him describe how racialized identities intersect with heterosexist assertions of masculinity (Pascoe, 2007).

Tyler: It's not like middle school where everyone pretty much got along. Kids hang out in groups and I don't fit in any of them.

Therapist: Is it more difficult to be biracial in this school?

Tyler: (shakes his head) What am I supposed to do? My dad is White; my mom is Black. I can't pick one or the other!

Therapist: And it feels like you have to? You have to be either White or Black?

Tyler describes how the Black guys tease him for being a "White Dude." The White guys joke about condoms and call him "fag," which refers to his not exhibiting hypermasculine behaviors. Tyler is not comfortable with the way masculine gender is sexualized among the guys at school; he says he keeps mostly to himself and hangs out with a couple of girls. He is beginning to question whether he is straight. Expanding the conversation to alternative gender discourse engages Tyler more than you have witnessed from him before:

Therapist: From what you said, when guys call you "fag," it seems they are saying "you aren't masculine enough," not necessarily that they think you are gay. Is that right?
Tyler: Yeah. But I don't want to be a man like that. It makes me wonder if I am gay. [pause] It's OK if I am, but I just don't know.
Therapist: You'd like other options for how to be male—whether or not you are gay.
Tyler: Exactly!

You and Tyler have a rather animated conversation about gender fluidity, gender expression, and how that differs from sexual orientation. Tyler says he looks forward to talking more about this with you; however, he believes that his parents are too stressed to deal with this issue. You suggest that his parents are worried about him and would want to know what he is dealing with and how to help. You agree not to tell his parents about the confusion he's experiencing until the two of you have discussed it some more and he feels ready.

In sum, exploring sociocultural discourses involves:
- Move from the personal to the contextual
- Name the expectation/discourse
- Explore the personal/relational effect of the discourse
- Invite the possibility of alternative or marginalized discourse

Conclusion

During the first phase of therapy, you have helped the Carter family position toward their relational ideals and counter social forces that interfere with them through three interrelated competencies:

Competency 1A—Attune to sociocultural emotion
Competency 1B—Expose relational consequences of power inequities
Competency 1C—Explore sociocultural discourse

You have positioned the assessment process to establish a therapeutic alliance in which family members are less focused on blaming each other and their own inadequacies (see Chapter 7). By attuning to each family member's sociocultural emotion, they feel felt by you, and the ways you see them and how they view themselves are beginning to connect the personal and the societal.

Nick, whose use of anger and distancing maintains a powerful position in the family despite—or as a result of—his feeling vulnerable, is beginning to be aware of his position and his impact on Laurelle and his sons. By recognizing Nick's relational values and helping him connect with them, he has expressed openness to a shift in this power dynamic and willingness to be accountable for sharing relational responsibility. While seeing the hurt he has caused, he has also seen that his sons and Laurelle want to engage with him. Helping Dad relationally engage with the family becomes a primary clinical goal.

The family, who in various ways each came in to therapy feeling like failures and expecting their "bad" behavior/parenting to be corrected, are beginning to see themselves and their relationships through a new, sociocultural lens that validates their socio-emotional experience and enables them to see relational possibilities based on love, equity, and mutual support. They have previously resisted dominant culture discourses in ways that have been masked, problematized, or show up as symptoms. Therapy is positioned to highlight these more inclusive values and help the family recognize and affirm them and join together to address the multiple stressors in their lives.

Therapist Checklist: Phase 1—Positioning

- ☐ Be aware of your own position and sociocultural emotion
- ☐ Redefine professionalism to include "being with"
- ☐ Identify clients' emotionally salient words and actions
- ☐ Connect sociocultural identities, expectations, and vulnerabilities to social discourse and power
- ☐ Identify the relational consequences of power imbalances
- ☐ Highlight discourses that support relational values and equity

10

PHASE 2—INTERRUPT THE FLOW OF POWER

In phase 1, the Carter family began to see their lives and the nature of their problems through a broader sociocultural lens and to reposition from problem/failure discourses to relational ones. All the family members—including Nick—affirmed their desire to make the love in their family more visible and engage more with Dad. However, the flow of power among them and in relation to their larger environment remains inequitable, which makes it difficult to support each other and resolve the problems that brought them to therapy. Brandon and Logan still have "problems" at school, despite their efforts to "do better." Tyler is less anxious, but keeps his distress regarding his identity and fitting in at school to himself. Though Nick is attempting to tamp down his expressions of anger, he remains in considerable socio-emotional pain (as well as physical), and his role in the family is unclear. Laurelle is hopeful, but worn out with the burden of care she gives both at home and at work. Financial realities are stressful. While Nick and Laurelle are trying to fight less, the closeness between them is tenuous.

◊ *Shift in-session power processes*

The family's overall goals are to strengthen mutually supportive relational bonds and to better negotiate their social environment. As

DOI: 10.4324/9781003270232-10

you and the family move into phase 2 and the content of sessions center on their day-to-day process of enacting these goals, it is important to interrupt the inequitable flow of power so that the family can experience reciprocity in the Circle of Care. This shift in moment-to-moment power processes facilitates relational safety and makes it possible for family members to risk engaging with each other. Interrupting usually means asking different things of each person based on their power positions and is intentional regarding which discourses you propagate.

Why Interrupt?

One of the factors that distinguishes Socio-Emotional Relationship Therapy is the therapist's active attention to power processes when making clinical choices. As described in Chapter 6, recognizing and interrupting the flow of power is key to ethical, socially responsible use of the therapist's influence. When therapists take a less intentional role in relation to power, inequitable power processes are likely to be reproduced in the therapy. For example, you decide that it is important to speak with Brandon's and Logan's teachers to get their perspectives. When you take the societal flow of power into account, you do not want your participation to reinforce the problem talk; you want these conversations to interrupt the process of labeling Brandon and Logan as "problems." Though interrupting problem-focused discourse is important with any child, you are aware that being perceived as Black and lower income increases the risk that Brandon and Logan will continue to be viewed as "problems."

◊ *Prevent societal power processes from replicating*

On a Zoom call with Brandon's teacher about his experience of Brandon in the classroom, you interrupt the dominant problem discourse by asking about strengths and inviting more supportive possibilities.

Teacher: Brandon is always up to something—egging another kid on, fighting . . . anything but focusing on his lesson!
Therapist: It sounds like he has a lot of energy.

Teacher: He does! If only he could channel it into something productive.

Therapist: I'm curious what you've noticed about the positive aspect of that energy.

Teacher: (reflective pause) The positive aspect of his energy? Well, it's disruptive, of course, but it never seems malicious. He has a good spirit about him. It's like he just wants to stir things up.

You join with the teacher around Brandon's "good spirit" and positive intentions.

Therapist: (thoughtfully) Hm. A good spirit? I'm trying to picture that—how he's trying to make something happen. What does that good spirit look like?

Teacher (smiles) Brandon has this sparkle in his eye. Like he's up to something—or sees something that's outside the box.

Therapist: I've noticed that sparkle in his eye too.

After you talk a little more about the sparkle in Brandon's eye and his good spirit, you ask the teacher to help you by keeping an eye out for how Brandon uses his good spirit in a positive way.

◊ *Interrupting power makes space for alternatives*

In this example, you shift the in-the-moment power of the dominant discourse to make room for an alternative one. Other ways to interrupt may include who you direct a question toward or focus on; what you ask each person to do; what your questions focus on; and what kinds of explanations, actions, or outcomes you orient toward. Interrupting the flow of power requires attentive third-order experiential awareness regarding what and who are being privileged or disregarded in-session. Three interrelated competencies are involved: (A) Highlight the value of relational work, (B) help powerful persons take relational initiative, and (C) connect interruptions in the flow of power to contextual meaning (see Figure 10.1).

As you demonstrate these three interrupting tasks, watch for the following client outcomes.

Phase 2: Interrupt
*Create relational safety by shifting
in-the-moment power processes*

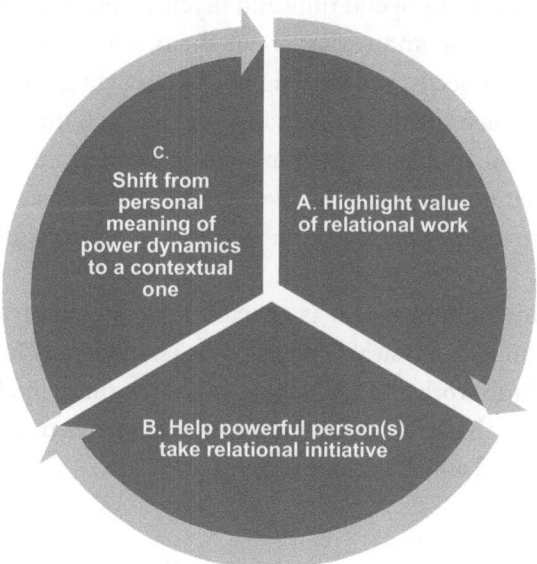

Figure 10.1 SERT Phase 2

Source: Adapted from Knudson-Martin, C., & Kim, L. (2023). Socioculturally attuned couple therapy. In J. L. Lebow & D. K. Snyder (Eds.). Clinical Handbook of Couple Therapy (6th ed., p. 279). Guildford (used with permission).

Phase 2 Client Outcomes

A. Relationally oriented persons, who are usually also in less powerful positions, experience validation

B. Powerful persons experience the positive consequences of relational engagement; less powerful persons begin to feel safer and cared about

C. Less powerful, more vulnerable persons are likely to be heard and clients join together to resist negative societal effects

---

Competency 2A—Highlight the Value of Relational Work

The dominant culture tends to minimize and overlook the value of relational work. This means that what people do to give care to others and build and sustain relationships gets lost and those who do this work are easily marginalized. What people value about themselves and others often discounts important relational qualities such as kindness, empathy, listening, and tending to the needs of others. People who carry substantial relational responsibility spend time and psychic energy anticipating what others need, thinking and caring about them, planning and organizing how to meet their needs, and tending to and managing their feelings and moods. While such giving can be satisfying and rewarding to the giver, when imbalanced, it can also result in an unacknowledged load that is potentially deleterious to health and well-being (Dean et al., 2022). In addition to being socially devalued, care work is also unrecognized because:

> (1) it is invisible in that it is enacted internally yet results in a range of unpaid, physical labor; (2) it is boundaryless in that can be brought to work and into leisure and sleep time; and (3) [it is] enduring in that it is never complete because it is tied to caring for loved ones which is constant.
>
> (p. 13)

The less powerful person in the family or couple is usually doing most of the relational work without credit or acknowledgement. Like much of society, clients may also frame carrying the relational load as a personal deficiency, pathologizing it as being too focused on others or caring about them too much.

SERT therapists interrupt this stressful and marginalizing process by watching for relational contributions, making them visible, and helping clients appreciate their value. Three steps are involved:

1. Look for and uncover examples of unrecognized relational work
2. Detail what is involved in doing relational work
3. Identify the positive consequences of relational work

Look for and Uncover Unrecognized Relational Work

Recognition of relational work happens as it comes up in session. In this example, because attunement to others also involves awareness of self (Siegel, 2007, 2019), as part of addressing the concerns about Brandon's and Logan's behavior at school, you are helping the family practice mindfulness regarding what is happening in their bodies in the present moment (Beaudoin & MacLennan, 2021). You have discussed that this will calm them and help them develop awareness of the emotions that are coming in and be more intentional about their response. You are aware that family members are not participating from equal power positions and attend not only to the mindfulness activity but also to how they engage together in the process. As you discuss how their practicing is going at home, you notice that Laurelle is carrying the burden of ensuring that everyone remembers to practice the breathing and focusing. You move the conversation to create awareness of this relational work:

Therapist: (to boys) So you've all been practicing. Wow! How did you make that happen?

Logan: Mom makes us. (rolls his eyes)

Brandon: She's like the practice police!

While shifting the power imbalance means you want family members to each share responsibility for relational processes, including self-awareness, you do not want to pathologize Mom as too involved (or overlook her role altogether). Validating relational work goes beyond positively reframing her "police work" to caring; it is an opportunity to credit the importance of this care work:

Therapist: Mom takes the time to make sure you do your practicing?

Tyler: She even makes sure Dad practices.

Therapist: How does she do that? How, in addition to everything else she is doing, does she make it possible that all of you practice mindfulness?

Nick: I tell her to butt out—that the kids need to learn to be responsible for themselves.

You notice Nick's use of common discourse prioritizing individualism but do not join with it and stick with recognizing the more hidden caring activity:

Therapist: How does Mom's attentiveness help all of you with your practice?

Brandon: (giggles) We wouldn't do it otherwise!

Therapist: You depend on Mom to organize your practice, to make sure you do it? [everyone agrees]. How is that helpful to you—that she remembers and makes sure everyone practices?

Tyler: We don't think about practicing. We'd probably be wasting our time coming here. You know, "in one ear—out the other."

Therapist: So you think Mom does the [air quotes] hearing and remembering for you? That without her you might not learn to calm yourself?

Tyler: Probably not.

Therapist: It sounds like you all depend on Mom to watch out for you. Is that right?

The family agrees. You encourage them to reflect on what it takes for Laurelle to be responsible for their mindfulness practice and for their well-being overall. This acknowledgement and validation of Laurelle's relational work serves as a foundation for considering how they might all share this responsibility.

Detail What Is Involved in Doing Relational Work

Because much of relational work is done outside the awareness of others, what is involved is not noticed or taken into account. Asking about these details helps clients develop this otherwise invisible story. For the unmasked story to stick, it helps to create detailed images that connect to evocative personal experience (Zimmerman, 2018). For example, in the course of discussing what happens at school with Brandon and Logan, you learn that Laurelle is knowledgeable about their experience:

Therapist: How's it going at school? What have you noticed about yourself?

Brandon: (shrugs his shoulders) It's better, I guess.

Therapist: Better? How?

Brandon: Maybe . . . I don't get in trouble as much?

Laurelle: You are keeping calmer and staying more focused.

Brandon: Yeah. I don't get so distracted.

Therapist: What is it like for you to be calmer, less distracted?

Brandon: Good. School's more fun when I'm not in trouble.

You help Brandon identify what he does to calm himself and enjoy school. Then you return to your observation that Laurelle knew what Brandon was experiencing and could help him name it. You want to detail what is involved in this caring work:

Therapist: Laurelle, a little while back, I noticed you seemed in touch with what is happening for Brandon at school. How were you able to know that?

Laurelle: Well, I check in with Brandon and Logan every day. And I talk with their teachers—I try to check in with Tyler, too, but he doesn't have much to say.

Therapist: You check in with them every day. How do you that? What's it take for you to connect with them that way?

Laurelle: (chuckles) I have to find space between their games. [pause] I always think about them, of course, and how their days go. But before, I didn't push as hard to get them to talk.

Therapist: You always think about them? How so? What are you thinking about?

Laurelle: When I'm at work, I pay attention to the time. You know, when they have lunch, when they get out—I picture them and wonder how they are doing.

Therapist: You think about them during the day—even when you're at work.

Laurelle: Yes. Especially since all this trouble happened. I want to make sure they're applying what we're learning here at school.

Therapist: So you think about them during the day, picture them, and then talk with them about it at home? [turns to boys] Did you know your mom thinks about you so much? That you're nearly always on her mind?

Logan: Not really. She does always want to talk to us about our days—a Mom Thing, I guess.

The family is used to Laurelle's "Mom Thing," but have not consciously valued it. It has not been internalized as important and has been "feminized" as sort of silly. As the conversation unfolds, you help them create an image of what Mom actually does to engage them and know about them.

Therapist: OK. I'm trying to picture this. Mom comes home, she's been working all day and she's tired . . . and she comes to check in with you. How does she do that? What would I see?

As you probe to flesh out the picture, the boys describe Mom "appearing" where they are playing games or right before bed. She makes a game of focusing on their breathing and then asks when they tried it at school and how it worked. Your summary captures both the "how" of what she does and the "feel" of her caring.

Therapist: (softly, with feeling) Mom comes to you. She breathes with you. She's interested in your day. She talks with you about it. [boys agree] I can feel her caring so much about you—wanting to help make it good for you. [pause] Do you feel it?

Identify the Positive Consequences of Relational Work

In terms of the flow of power, the issue is not that Mom cares too much or does too much relational work; it is that the rest of the family needs to do more. Engaging other family members in recognizing the positive contributions of relational work validates (rather than pathologizes) Laurelle and invites other family members to become more aware of what they can do to support each other. In another session, as the family comes in, they seem testier with each other than usual. You ask what is going on. This spurs conversation about the value of what Mom does and how all of them can step in to reduce her load:

Therapist: What's up? You all seem a little on the grumpy side today.
Brandon: Mom's mad at us.
Laurelle: (shakes her head) I've had it! I really have! You all knew we had to come here tonight. I had to work late because my replacement didn't come on time, and I get home and the house is a total mess—dishes everywhere. No one's done their homework. My body is aching, and no one lifts a finger!

Nick: (to the boys) I tell you to help your mother.

Tyler: Why should we? You don't!

You use curiosity to explore and name what Laurelle usually does and how everyone benefits:

Therapist: I'm curious. You are all waiting for her to come home to clean up after you? [pause] How is tidying up or doing your homework helping her? I'm not sure I understand.

Tyler: (to Nick) You don't do anything anymore. You think we should all tiptoe around you! You leave everything to Mom! She has a sore back, too, you know.

Therapist: So you're all aware of how much you depend on Mom. That she keeps you and the house—everything—in order. Are you aware of that, too, Nick?

Nick: (looks down). Yeah. Laurelle has always been the strong one. I'm not worth much, I guess.

You resist the societal pattern of protecting men from shame (Chen-Feng & Galick, 2015) and remain focused on identifying the positive consequences of Laurelle's relational work:

Therapist: Sometimes we take for granted what others—especially mothers—do for us. Let's make a list of all the things Mom does for you.

The boys get interested in making the list. Nick appears to watch from the side.

Therapist: Nick, what would you add? What does Laurelle do to make your life better?

Nick: It's too much to count. [pause] She stays with me, even though I'm a screwup. She takes care of me and my boys. I'm not sure I'd even be here without her.

You invite Nick to have a conversation with the boys about how to let Mom know they appreciate her and how he and the boys can share the load—take the burden off Laurelle. You prompt Nick as he takes the lead through this enactment and ask Laurelle to simply watch. When they are finished, you ask them to turn to her and tell her how what she does makes their lives better and what they will do to contribute.

In subsequent sessions, you notice not only how what Laurelle does benefits the rest of the family; you recognize when Nick and the boys do relational work and help them see the positive consequences. For example, though Tyler stays in his room a lot, he also frequently calms Brandon and Logan when they are "going off the walls" or are "at each other." You highlight how this relational work is helpful.

Therapist: (to Brandon and Logan) So sometimes you feel all worked up inside, and all that energy comes out in ways that are not so good. How does it help when Tyler calms you down?

Logan: He doesn't yell at us—at least not much. He kinda comes and puts his hands on our shoulders and says "hey–'zup?"

Therapist: So when he comes to you and touches you like that, it feels . . .? That he's there with you?

Brandon: Yeah. [smiles] Like he's our brother.

Therapist: And feeling your brother like that calms your body inside? [Brandon and Logan agree]. You know, our bodies are made that way—we're designed to need each other and do better when those who love us are around or we can feel their presence in our hearts.

In sum, highlighting the value of relational work includes:

- Looking for and uncovering it
- Detailing what is involved
- Identifying the positive consequences

Competency 2B—Help More Powerful Persons Take Relational Initiative

In SERT, social power refers to the ability to be understood and influence one's world. Mutuality in the flow of power enables each person to "feel felt" (Siegel, 2007, 2012) and supports the well-being, needs, and interests of everyone. Interrupting an imbalance in the flow of power requires you to prioritize encouraging those in powerful positions to express vulnerability and take accountability for relational engagement by attuning to and being responsive to others. This takes intentionality and persistence on the therapist's part, because, like responsibility for mindfulness practice falling on Laurelle, clients will otherwise replicate the power imbalance in how they respond to therapy.

Being in a powerful position usually makes it harder to express vulnerability or take in the experience of others. Practicing relational attunement increases awareness of the other, which typically invites responsibility toward that person's well-being and accountability for the impact of one's actions. An important outcome at this stage is that the more powerful person, in this case Nick, recognizes the positive consequences of relational engagement, and less powerful persons begin to feel safer, more cared about, and better able to fully and honestly engage in the therapeutic process.

Five steps are involved in helping powerful persons take relational initiative:

1. Consider the flow of power when inviting clients to express vulnerability or attune
2. Address accountability for the impact of a nonrelational position
3. Name the powerful person's relational interest in engaging in the Circle of Care
4. Support the powerful person in carrying out relational acts
5. Identify the positive consequences of the relational act

Consider the Flow of Power When Inviting Vulnerability or Attunement

Couple and family therapists regularly ask clients to share feelings or personal experience with their significant others. A goal is usually to increase awareness of each other's perspectives. In SERT, you put this process in the context of power, actively working with those in power positions to relationally engage and to not let the most vulnerable person (the one with less social power) carry additional vulnerability and the burden of relational repair. When in a couple session Laurelle expresses anger that Nick bought an iPad without considering the rest of the family, you focus on the power position embedded in this action:

Therapist: Let's see if I am getting this right. Nick, you received a back payment for your disability benefits and then went ahead on your own to spend some of that money on an iPad for yourself. Is that right?

Nick: Yeah. After all this time, I deserved it! [pause] I didn't spend all the money.

Therapist: You felt that you had the right to decide how to spend the money?

When power processes are identified, those in powerful positions are often uncomfortable.

Nick (hesitates) Well. Yeah. I guess so.

Therapist: (to Nick) How did that go for you? Are you accustomed to making financial decisions on your own?

Nick: No. But I was pretty sure Laurelle would think the iPad wasn't necessary, and I deserved it.

You recognize that, in part, buying the iPad is a way to restore some of the social power Nick has lost due to his disability. It could be easy to "explain away" Nick's nonrelational action because of his feelings of diminishment. In so doing, you would perpetuate the process by which Nick's pain and unhappiness combine with masculine entitlement to maintain him in a power position in the family. Instead, you acknowledge his experience but keep the impact of his power move foremost as you determine how to proceed.

Therapist: In that moment, those feelings of "I have a right to what I want" got in the way of what the family needed—what you expected Laurelle would say?

Nick: We have so many debts to repay—her mother has been helping us out—it would be a long time before we could afford the iPad . . .

Therapist: So you thought it through on your own and made the decision yourself, which if I'm understanding right, is not how you expect your relationship with Laurelle to work.

Nick: We were always a team, making decisions together.

Nick believes in egalitarian ideals. As you continue to process this purchase decision with him, you take care to balance attunement to his socio-emotional experience with clarity about the power involved and its impact on Laurelle and the family. To interrupt the power dynamic, you invite him to attune to Laurelle:

Therapist: You've spoken a lot about how important Laurelle is to you. How do you think it affected her when you decided on your own to buy the iPad?

Nick: She's mad, obviously.

Therapist: Underneath the anger, what do you think Laurelle experienced when you didn't consult her regarding how to spend the money the family so badly needs?

When he stops to think about it, and with your encouragement to keep reflecting on it, Nick is able to describe that Laurelle would feel not cared about; that it would seem like he cared more about himself than the family and that it would be hurtful. You check in with Laurelle to see if Nick is accurately understanding her experience:

Therapist: (to Laurelle) Nick says that it must have been hurtful; that it must have seemed that he didn't care about you or the family. Did he get that right?

Laurelle: (softly) Yes. [sighs]

Address Accountability for a Nonrelational Position

Willingness to take accountability for the effect of one's actions on another is a substantial aspect of relational justice (Boszormenyi-Nagy & Krasner, 1986). It is important to not just assume that accountability is implied. Once Nick focuses on Laurelle's experience regarding the iPad, you name the hurt and invite him to address his accountability for the effect of his action on her and the family, knowing that it is also a vulnerable position for him to take—one he needs to be able to hold:

Therapist: (softly) Spending the money on your own without consulting her violated what you expect from each other. It hurt Laurelle deeply.

[pause] I know you care about her and your marriage. What do you want to say to her about the hurt you caused?

Nick: (to Laurelle). I'm sorry. I should have talked with you about it. [looks down]

You encourage Nick to stay with the spirit of vulnerability and say more about his relational desires:

Therapist: Can you tell her what it means to you to be sorry? What it means to you to have hurt the woman you love?

Nick: (Looks at Laurelle) I love you—I do! I don't want to hurt you. [pause] I'm not me these days. It's hard—I know it's hard for you, too, for all of us.

Therapist: (softly) Tell her what you hope—for how to treat her, connect with her, as you go through this time together.

Your coaching intentionally supports Nick in staying in a relational place. When he does, he expresses that he wants to be a team again but that he doesn't always know how to do that or feel worthy of it. You observe that Laurelle—who is tearful and has moved closer to Nick—seems to have responded positively to his honesty:

Therapist: (to Laurelle) It seems that Nick's words—his apology, his honesty—mean a lot to you.

Laurelle: They do. [to Nick] I'm sorry I was so angry. I know how hard it is for you. I just want us to be loving to each other again.

Nick's relational response invited a relational response back from Laurelle—a step toward mutuality in the Circle of Care. This is common; when the powerful person takes relational initiative and accountability, the less powerful person follows. But sometimes it takes time. It could have happened that Nick's apology and expression of relational desire made it safe for Laurelle to express resentment that she had been holding back. This may especially happen when one has not previously felt safe to risk anger. If that happens, it is important that you help the powerful person stay in a vulnerable position and take in the other's anger and the more vulnerable feelings underneath it.

Name Powerful Person's Interest in the Circle of Care

Decisions about who to engage in initiating elements of the Circle of Care need to take into account the flow of power over the history of the relationship. Laurelle and Nick began their relationship with a power imbalance in which Laurelle, a low-income, "chubby," Black, young woman who did not feel attractive to guys, felt grateful for Nick's attention. Though Nick rejected the "hard" masculinity demonstrated by his father, he had access to social, racial, and economic capital and took pride in being able to provide a home for their young family. Like many couples, despite their egalitarian values, they fell into stereotypical gender patterns without being aware they were doing so (Knudson-Martin & Mahoney, 2009). Over time, their relationship was not as satisfying and emotionally close as they preferred, but as Nick said, "they made a good team." Nick's response to his injury, however, has been to disengage relationally, focus on his loss and unhappiness, and expect his wife and family to attend to him—which magnifies his power position within the family even as he has lost power in the wider society.

The motivation for more powerful persons to engage will be awareness of their relational interests and how their actions support or inhibit them. Relational interests include both one's own need and desire for the relationship and empathy, concern, and care for those we love. Working to relationally engage Nick in the Circle of Care also illustrates the important idea in SERT that everyone has something to give and needs to give. Even if he were bed-ridden or chronically ill (which he is not), it would be critical for Nick to take relational initiative, as well as receive care (D'Arrigo-Patrick et al., 2020). To facilitate this, you help Nick recognize and articulate his relational interests.

For example, Nick and Laurelle are discussing his progress in dealing with pain. Since completing physical therapy about a year ago, Nick has been committed to getting along without opioids, but until your referral to a chronic pain education group, he felt helpless to do anything about the pain, which only seemed to be increasing and made him feel useless. The group helped Nick be more optimistic that he can impact how his brain responds to pain through mindfulness, stress reduction, increased exercise, and diet (Butler & Moseley, 2013). You help him be in touch with how his focus on pain has kept him from his family and from giving to them, making his desire for relational engagement part of more effective responses to pain.

Laurelle: (to Nick) I'm so glad you're feeling more positive about managing the pain. I know it's been hard for you—I hate to see you in so much pain.

Therapist: (to Laurelle) What has it been like for you to witness Nick's pain?

Laurelle: It's been awful. I can't stand to see him hurt like that—and it doesn't seem to matter what I do; there's not much I can do to make him feel better.

Therapist: It's hard to see the man you love be in so much pain and not be able to help him—to emotionally touch and support him.

You shift the focus from what Laurelle could give to what Nick would want to give:

Therapist: (to Nick) It's hard for Laurelle. She'd like to be able to make your pain go away, to make it better. What is it that you wish you could give to her?

Nick: (pause) I wish I could be more loving—be the man I used to be.

Therapist: More loving. What would that mean?

Nick: Well, I've never stopped loving her, so I guess it would mean showing her, talking with her, doing things with her, [looks at Laurelle] putting my arm around her.

Therapist: What would it mean to you, Laurelle, if Nick could move beyond the pain and show his love?

Laurelle: I always need his love—even if he's in pain. I don't want to be shut out.

You emphasize the relational impact of Nick's response to pain:

Therapist: So one of the things pain has done is shut you off from each other and not let the love get through. [to Nick] How does your response to pain keep you away from Laurelle?

Nick: It makes me be the kind of person I don't want to be. [pause] It keeps me from being part of the family, from being a good husband.

Therapist: When you respond to pain as a part of the family, as a loving husband, what will you do? What will that look like?

Nick describes coming out of his room, joining the family more often, and using his breathing to be aware of his body and aware of his family. You summarize by emphasizing his awareness that he has something to give:

Therapist: What I'm hearing you say, Nick, is that when you focus on the pain and your anger about the pain, you lose sight of how much Laurelle and your family need you, love you. And today, you're saying "I do have something to give—and I want to be there for them." Am I getting that right?
Nick: (nods) Yeah. I want to be there for them. [pause] I just don't know if I know how.

Support Powerful Person in Relational Acts

By admitting he's not sure he knows how to be there for his family, Nick has taken a step toward vulnerability and resisting stereotypic discourses for masculinity. He is not likely to maintain this relational position without your help and would probably respond to the vulnerable feeling by pulling away or shutting down. If Laurelle suggests what he can do or tries to engage him, he may take it as criticism or a sign of his inadequacy. You use your sociocultural attunement to his vulnerability around competency to support Nick in staying with his experience of vulnerability and speaking with Laurelle from that position:

Therapist: (softly, empathically) You've been taught that you're supposed to have the answers. It must be hard to feel that you don't know what to do.
Nick: Laurelle always looked up to me. I mean, I wasn't good at school, but I could make her feel good. I fixed up the house, had a good job . . .
Therapist: And when you can't do those same things, you feel like you're letting her down?
Nick: Letting everybody down!
Therapist: You feel like you're letting everybody down, and . . . ?
Nick: (softly) And I don't know why they'd even want me around.

Therapist: That's a hard place to be. [pause] And hard to let others see. [Nick emphatically agrees] Where do you feel the vulnerability inside? That sense that you're not worth anything to others?

Nick: (puts his hands across his chest) It's like my chest is pulling in tight—like I can hardly breathe.

Note that in other times when Nick has said he's useless, he's said it in a way that kept others from him; in effect, it was an abnegation of his relational responsibilities and covertly put the onus on Laurelle or the boys to take care of him. Now that Nick is in touch with his vulnerable feeling of unworthiness, you interrupt the pattern of responding by withdrawing and support him in sharing this feeling with Laurelle.

Therapist: (keeping your voice soft) Tell Laurelle what it's like for you inside when you don't know what to do. Can you look at her and tell her?

Nick: (turns toward Laurelle). Like I said, I feel so stupid and inadequate. You're the people person.

You bring Nick back to his relational worries. He is able to stay there because he feels that you understand his experience:

Therapist: (encouragingly) And when you feel inadequate inside, what is your worry with Laurelle? Tell her what you're afraid of.

NICK: (to Laurelle) Well, when I'm feeling inadequate, it's hard to breathe; it's hard to know what to say. I'm afraid I'll do it wrong—that I'll disappoint you.

You continue to encourage Nick to approach Laurelle in this spirit of vulnerability and share more of his internal experience since the accident. It is a new relational experience for both of them.

Identify Positive Consequences of the Relational Act

Given his socialization to maintain a power position, it was emotionally risky for Nick to initiate a vulnerable position. It is helpful to bring the positive consequences of his relational act to awareness and reinforce them. You can see that Laurelle is moved by Nick's genuine expression and invite her to share her response:

Therapist: (to Laurelle, softly) Nick has shared a lot. What was it like for you to hear him, to take it in?

Laurelle: (a single tear rolls down her check, she looks at Nick) I feel so much closer to you. I've known that it's been so hard for you to not be able to do the things for us you used to do. What you said doesn't surprise me—I had a pretty good idea. But to hear you tell me about it [reaches toward Nick], that's what I've wanted—needed.

Therapist: You've needed Nick to share his worries and fears?

Laurelle: I've felt so alone. I want us to be in this together.

You turn to Nick to reinforce Laurelle's message that what he just did is, in fact, what she needs from him—what she has been looking for.

Therapist: (to Nick) What is it like to hear how much Laurelle appreciated what you just did in sharing your fears and uncertainty with her; that it made her feel closer to you?

Nick: I feel closer too. And I understand a little more what she wants from me.

You are now able to have a conversation about what Nick can do to relationally engage, both as part of managing his pain and to begin revising his image of what it means to be a good, competent husband and father. Nick's shift toward relationality is a significant interruption of their usual flow of power. Subsequent sessions can build on and reinforce this budding transformation.

In sum, helping powerful persons take relational initiative involves:

- Inviting powerful person to express vulnerability or attune
- Addressing accountability for impact on others
- Naming the powerful person's relational interest
- Supporting the powerful person in relational acts
- Identifying the positive consequences

Competency 2C—Connect Interruptions in the Flow of Power to *Contextual* Meaning

While you actively interrupt the flow of power by validating relational work and supporting Nick in initiating relational action, the focus is evocatively personal, exploring both internal and relational experience. However, if your work remains at this family level without contextualizing how Nick and his family are performing societal discourses, you run the risk of oversimplifying these interaction patterns. Sally St. George and Dan Wulff suggested enabling clients to "speak back to the discourses by questioning them, challenging them, altering them, or rejecting them" (St. George & Wulff, 2014, p. 133). When clients "become aware of the [societal] stories and discourses that support and justify the behaviors that become 'who we are' . . . [it is also possible] to see the path not (yet) taken" (p. 131), simultaneously facilitating opportunities for personal/interpersonal change and revisioning societal discourses.

As discussed in the previous chapter, there are a number of ways to expand from personal experience to conversation about the larger context. The key is that you listen for, explore, and integrate ideas related to unwritten and largely invisible social scripts for who matters, how one *should* behave, and the implicit social meaning associated with living within these constraints. For example, as Nick considers what he can do to relationally engage, your questions help him reflect on how male competency discourse is part of his process:

Therapist: It makes sense to me that sharing your worries—your fears—with Laurelle might not come easily. [pause] A lot of men learn being competent means they are not supposed to show doubt or "soft" feelings. Has that been part of your life?
Nick: Oh yeah! My dad always said, "Man up!"

Nick has a lot to say about "manning up." He tells stories about being told not to cry as a child and about his father who was always in control, who would never let anyone see him in doubt. You encourage Nick to take context a step further, beyond the family.

Therapist: So your father reinforced the idea that being a man meant being in control, never letting weakness show. Where do you think these ideas come from?

Nick describes the idea of never letting weakness show being everywhere and gives examples of his friends in high school. When you ask him how well he thinks this script for men works, Nick says "I never liked it—never wanted to be like my dad. I wanted to be closer to my children, to my boys." You pick up previous conversation as you probe for other models for masculinity in his experience:

Therapist: Laurelle said she was attracted to you because you weren't as "cocky" as the other guys. Where do you think you got those other models for how to be a guy?

Nick identifies several men that "were kind, put people first." This enables conversation about what Nick thinks would be different if what kids learned was that "manning up" meant putting people first. When Nick responds, "I think my life would have been a lot less stressful—maybe I'd be having an easier time now," you move the conversation toward developing the idea that kindness is part of Nick's image of a good man and not necessarily separate from competency and strength (Englar-Carlson & Kiselica, 2013). You work with Nick to detail this alternative masculinity discourse. Without this kind of contextualizing conversation, shifts in the flow of power are hard to maintain, with the most relevant discussions connected to vulnerabilities around sociocultural expectations and judgments (Knudson-Martin et al., 2021).

Four steps are involved in connecting interruptions in the flow of power to contextual meaning:

1. Frame behaviors or conflicts in terms of social position and/or competing societal discourses
2. Identify personal meaning around the societal discourse
3. Explore consequences of enacting the societal discourse
4. Discuss choices and preferences regarding enactments of societal discourse

Frame Issues in Terms of Social Position and/or Competing Societal Discourses

The first step in contextualizing interruptions in the flow of power is to position what is done and said within competing societal discourses. This is possible because there are always multiple potential discourses within a situation, and personal meaning depends on which discourses clients adopt (Combs & Freedman, 2012, 2016). Framing an issue within competing societal discourses externalizes the problem and makes it possible for clients to engage with it and consider alternatives. It can also help clarify why certain issues create an impasse (Fraenkel, 2023; Scheinkman & Fishbane, 2004).

For example, Laurelle recounted a fight with Nick that was still festering. When the family came home from watching Logan's and Brandon's basketball games in the community Hooper League they recently joined, they discovered that the gate to the backyard was open and garbage from the trash can was spilled all over the driveway. According to Laurelle, Nick jumped out of the car and immediately began yelling at all of them to pick up the trash and then yelled even more that Laurelle's sister had left the gate open when she came to use their washer and dryer while they were gone. Laurelle, distressed by Nick's loud expression of anger, told him to keep it down, to not yell outside. This made Nick yell more. They have been tense with each other since. Though not yet obvious how their reactions are related to societal context, you listen through a socio-contextual lens.

Therapist: (to Nick) It was irritating to see all that garbage in the driveway.

Nick: Yeah! [Laurelle's sister] is not very responsible. She comes and goes—which is OK, but she needs to be more respectful of us, our property. And I was tired. Sitting on those bleachers was hard on me, so I didn't need this! I don't see why Laurelle was so mad at me!! I'm not the one who knocked the garbage all over the place!

Therapist: It felt unfair that Laurelle was mad at you? You felt disrespected by her sister. And by Laurelle?

Nick: I don't see what the big deal was—I was just letting off a little steam. She didn't need to put me down like that. I'm not a kid!

Therapist: You felt Laurelle was belittling you—diminishing you.

You begin to see that Nick responded from a position of expecting respect. He experienced Laurelle's admonishment as a challenge to his White male identity. Laurelle reacted from a very different position:

Therapist: (to Laurelle) I imagine the garbage all over the driveway was upsetting to you, too. [Laurelle nods] Nick's not clear why you were mad at him. You said you wanted him to keep it down.

Laurelle: I was afraid of what the neighbors would think.

Therapist: What did you fear the neighbors might think?

Laurelle: That we're the Black family trashing up the neighborhood— that Nick's yelling would make them afraid; that they'd call the police.

Nick: You thought they'd call the police?! Why would they do that?

Nick is well aware that they are a biracial family. He worries his sons will be stopped by the police when they begin to drive, and he is angry with his parents for what he sees as their racist treatment of his wife and children. But as a White person, Nick does not fully apprehend Laurelle's experience of living as a Black person, especially in a predominantly White community. It never occurred to him to worry that his yelling would reflect on them as a Family of Color or that their White neighbors might call the police. You frame their conflict with each other through their conflicting social positions and discourse.

Therapist: It seems you each approached the spilled garbage from very different positions. Nick, you responded through the eyes of one whose property has been disrespected and as a man whose body is tired and feels a right to understanding from his wife. When she asked you to keep it down, it was like she was not treating you with proper respect. [Nick agrees] Laurelle, you approached the spilled garbage through the eyes of a Black person, aware that your neighbors may see you as representative of your race and conscious that they might respond to the disruption by calling the police. [Laurelle agrees]

Each partner experienced the other through the effect of the societal flow of power on their relationship. Nick experienced Laurelle as challenging his social position and entitlement to express his anger; Laurelle experienced Nick as adding to her one-down social position where the burden is on her to "prove" her respectability. In this emotional situation, neither attuned to the other. You seek to understand the personal meaning of their positioning around each of these societal discourses.

Identify Personal Meaning Around Societal Discourse

You move the conversation to the sociocultural vulnerabilities each partner faced in this situation. Because her experience of social degradation as a Black woman tends to be overlooked by Nick, you decide to start with Laurelle. You name the Black inferiority discourse (Watson, 2013) and ask about her experience with it:

Therapist: (to Laurelle) What is it like for you to live with the idea that Black people are less than, disreputable—even dangerous. How have you experienced it?

Laurelle: (sighs) It's always there in the back of my mind—like I have to prove myself over and over. And that my kids have to prove themselves.

Therapist: Can you tell Nick what it's like live with the sense that, as a Black person, you have to prove yourself over and over?

Laurelle: (looks at Nick) It keeps me on edge. I don't really know what other people are thinking, what our neighbors are thinking. I guess I want them to approve of us.

Nick: Why should it matter what they think? They're nothing to us.

Laurelle: Maybe you can say that. I don't have that luxury—people get hurt. We could get hurt.

Therapist: So, it's easier for you as a White person, Nick, to have the choice not to care what others think—something you more or less take for granted. [pause] In that moment, for you, Laurelle, what my colleague Marlene Watson calls the Black Shadow came down heavy; you felt judged as part of a group, and racist history said you needed to be quiet to survive.

As you continue this conversation, Laurelle describes specific instances when she has experienced that it is not safe to be Black and stories that her family and friends have told. You notice that Nick appears quite interested and highlight his experience of attunement.

Therapist: What is it like for you, Nick, to hear Laurelle's stories of judgement, fear, discrimination—of being seen as less than just because she is Black?

Nick: I didn't realize. I mean, I knew but I didn't *know*. It makes me angry because Laurelle is a good, hardworking woman. She deserves respect!

This, of course, also raises the question of how Nick respects Laurelle and whether he is willing to take influence from her. You have a similar conversation around the discourse that being a man means being respected; that being questioned or told what to do is an assault to dignity—something Nick has felt in short supply of since the accident. As you explore Nick's personal experience with this discourse, he has both positive and negative stories. Being able to feel heard as he openly discusses these experiences and considers the consequences of this ideology draws him toward his egalitarian ideals and expectation that both he and Laurelle should be able to influence the other.

Explore Consequences of the Societal Discourse

Another imbalance in the societal flow of power that affects the Carter family regards how discourses of gender and sexuality interfere with Tyler's ability to share his experience and receive attuned support. Like many households, expectations about growing up and the life course tend to assume a child is cisgender and heterosexual and that gender expression will follow dominant stereotypes. When children do not conform to these stereotypes, parents may not know how to respond (Malpas, 2011). You have met individually with Tyler several times to focus on his experience fitting in at school and how these relate to his intersecting racial, gender, and sexual identities. Though Tyler is clear that he identifies as male, stereotypic discourse equating sexuality and gender confuse him. He does not relate to ideas of masculine sexual aggressiveness and female domination expressed by guys at school and is relieved to discuss more fluid options.

Tyler found a group of students in the drama club whose ideas are more similar to his. At this point in time, he does not want to label his sexuality and prefers to remain open to what evolves. Finding clarity about the sources of his anxiety and unhappiness and a peer group where he experiences belonging has interrupted the effects of heterosexist power on his self-esteem and adaptation to school, at least for the time being. But he still feels apart from many, especially his family. After considering options for how to approach it, Tyler has decided to raise the topic in a family session. Your job is to facilitate and support this interruption in the flow of heteropatriarchal power by helping Tyler contextualize his experience in terms of the consequences for him of dominant sex/gender discourses.

Therapist: Tyler, your parents have been worried about you; they've seen you keep to yourself and wonder what is going on for you. You and I have been talking about this, and you said you'd like to share some of your experience and insights with them. Do you feel ready to do this now?

Tyler describes the way kids at the high school form groups and that he didn't know where he fit. He speaks first about being biracial, which his parents understand and offer their support. Then he switches to gender and sexuality issues. Because of your prior conversations, he has language to contextualize his experience. With your support, he tells them about not agreeing with the ways the straight guys talk about girls and sex. His parents agree with this as well. When he says he doesn't want to label his sexuality—that he doesn't know yet and wants to remain open, his parents struggle. Nick is most supportive:

Nick: It's hard for me to understand how you don't know. It's OK with me if you are gay. Is that what you are saying?

Tyler: Maybe. Or maybe bisexual. Or maybe pansexual. I don't see a need to label it. I don't even have anyone I want to date yet!

Therapist: (to Nick) So the part that's hardest for you is not knowing what words or language to use regarding Tyler's sexuality? What do you think are the consequences for Tyler of feeling he has to fit one model of sexuality or another?

After hearing some of Tyler's experience, particularly when framed as dealing with conflicting discourses regarding sex and gender, Nick is able to see why Tyler had been having a hard time. He gets interested in the benefits of a broader, more flexible view. It is more difficult for Laurelle:

Laurelle: I don't get it. Why would you want to be gay? Or bisexual! Being gay is a sin—your grandmother will never accept it!

You frame Laurelle's response in terms of multiple discourses and their consequences:

Therapist: (to Laurelle) It's hard to take in a more flexible way of how sexuality and gender work together. I'm curious what you heard Tyler say was hurtful to him about trying to fit into those socially pre-scribed categories.

Discuss Choices Regarding Societal Discourses

Contextualizing the issues that trouble them helps the Carter family be more open to each other and begin to see alternative ways of relating. Framing Tyler's confusion around gender and sexuality as questions regarding how to enact societal discourse makes it possible to have a nuanced conversation. After helping each parent reflect on their reactions to ideas of sexuality as less categorical—and checking with Brandon and Logan, who each think the ideas expressed by Tyler are "cool"—you invite them to consider how they prefer to respond to Tyler by helping them consider alternative relational positions:

Therapist: (to the family) You are having a different kind of conversation than you are used to. Like many parents, you've pictured your boys as boys who would probably grow up to be with a woman. And you are used to thinking of people being either gay or straight. [pause] Tyler, you learned these ideas too, but have been discovering they don't fit for you. You don't feel and respond to girls the way other guys talk about them. Trying to figure out who you are and where you fit in these social categories has been troubling, and you didn't know how to share your confusion with your parents. [Tyler agrees] So, we're in new territory here. Tyler needs support and space to work out this part of who he is. There can be a strong social push to decide—to fit one category or another. There can also be strong messages like what Tyler felt before, to be silent and not speak of something that might distress his parents. What matters to you going forward?

Nick: Well, what matters to me is that Tyler can talk with us—or at least not feel that he is doing something wrong that he has to hide.

Therapist: So your top priority is to make the family a safe place for Tyler to discover who he is?

Nick: Yeah. I never had that. I mean, I never thought I might like guys, but I didn't like how guys talked about girls—and my dad wasn't any better.

Therapist: You want your home to be a welcoming place for Tyler— where he can question what he needs to question? [Nick agrees] What about you, Laurelle? What kind of place do you want to create for Tyler?

Laurelle: This is hard for me. [looks at Tyler] I need space too. Be patient with me.

Therapist: (to Laurelle) What I hear you asking for—what you want most of all—is to keep in relationship with Tyler. You don't want to close off from one another. Is that right?

Laurelle: Absolutely. I need time—but I love you, Tyler. I've been so worried for you. I'm glad to finally understand what's been going on.

Discussing the impact of multiple sexuality discourses on Tyler and how they want to respond interrupts the power of heteronormativity on the family and helps them draw on relational ideals to frame how they want to react.

In sum, connecting shifts in power to contextual meaning involves:

- Framing experience within social positions and/or competing societal discourses
- Identifying the personal meaning of societal discourse
- Exploring consequences of the societal discourse
- Discussing choices regarding societal discourse

Summary

In phase 2, you helped the Carter family establish a foundation of relational safety by interrupting the flow of power in session as you began to work with them on the issues that brought them to therapy—the boys' disruptive behavior in school and the deteriorating relationship between Nick and Laurelle, both of which also relate to challenges in response to Nick's injury and his place in the family. You used three interrelated competencies to interrupt the flow of power:

> Competency 2A—Highlight the value of relational work
> Competency 2B—Help powerful persons take the relational initiative
> Competency 2C—Connect interruptions in the flow of power to contextual meaning

As a result, Laurelle, who has been carrying the bulk of the relational load without receiving reciprocal attunement and support from her family, experienced validation—not only from you as the therapist but also from Nick and the boys. Nick, for whom stereotypic masculine socialization interacted with physical and socio-emotional pain to keep him in a position of power despite the assault to his felt identity, discovered positive consequences of taking a more relational position by attuning to others and expressing vulnerability. With your guidance, space has been opened for Tyler to safely express uncertainty regarding his sexuality, and Brandon and Logan—and those around them—are beginning to experience positive aspects of their energy. Rather than directing their anger, confusion, and loss toward each other or inward, the family is learning to join together to resist the limits and negative impacts of discrimination and dominant societal discourses.

Movement toward these changes has required you to be mindful of the flow of power as you made choices regarding how to address the clinical issues and intervene. In so doing, you have repeatedly interrupted the usual unbalanced flow of power to create opportunity for new experience based on mutuality and to enable family members to recognize possible, more relational, alternatives and experience the positive impacts of relating through positions of mutual support. Facilitating an equitable flow of power is thus a fulcrum for other clinical change (Knudson-Martin & Huenergardt, 2010).

Therapist Checklist: Phase 2—interrupt power

☐ Recognize the in-the-moment flow of power
☐ Prevent replication of power imbalances in session
☐ Base clinical interventions on the balance of power
☐ Recognize and validate the importance of caring work
☐ Encourage powerful persons to initiate relational acts
☐ Use relational goals as motivation to move out of a position of power
☐ Connect shifts in power to a larger context
☐ Emphasize positive consequences of shifts in power

11

PHASE 3—PRACTICE MUTUALITY

In the final phase of Socio-Emotional Relationship Therapy, clients have begun to see themselves and their relationships through the Circle of Care and to envision relational options through a larger contextual lens (phase 1). They have experienced relational connection as a result of shifting the flow of power (phase 2). Embodying these new experiences takes practice and focus as clients experiment with, detail, and fine-tune their emerging mutuality (phase 3). You know you are in this phase of therapy with the Carter family because they don't need you to interrupt the flow of power as frequently, and they are more able to address difficult issues from positions of mutual vulnerability, attunement, influence, and relational responsibility. They need you to help them stay on track, bring them back to their relational goals, and see where they are headed as they focus on embodying new, equitable options and practices.

Embodying Third Order Change

According to Francisco Varela and colleagues (2016), such changes in what we know (and see) and how we respond are "the result of ongoing interpretation . . . inseparable from our bodies, our language, our social [and cultural] history" (p. 149). As we simultaneously interact, feel, and think "to enact a world" (p. 151), we create each other (and, to varying extents, our contexts). Transformation is made possible as we "embody a different way

Phase 3: Practice
*Embody new options and practices that
promote mutual support and equity*

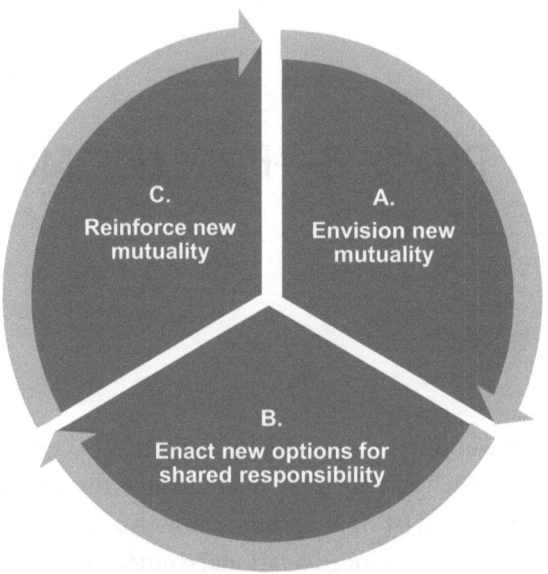

Figure 11.1 SERT Phase 3

Source: Adapted from Knudson-Martin, C., & Kim, L. (2023). Socioculturally attuned couple therapy. In J. L. Lebow & D. K. Snyder (Eds.). *Clinical Handbook of Couple Therapy* (6th ed., p. 279). Guildford (used with permission)

of being in the world" (Thompson, 2016, p. xxix). This third order change (see Chapter 2) involves transformations at multiple levels.

◊ *Shared focus facilitates transformation*

Making the Carter family's dreams real (i.e., embodiment) requires focused intention and engagement (Siegel, 2012, 2019; Zimmerman, 2018). With intentionality, over time they will embody new patterns in their communities and relationships, new stories about themselves, and new physiologies (Ewing et al., 2017; Mehl-Madrona & Mainguy, 2015; Zimmerman, 2018). To make desired change stick, the family needs to enact it; to practice mutuality and evocatively experience and embody it.

Three competencies are involved in this practicing phase of SERT: (A) envision a new mutuality, (B) enact new options for shared responsibility, and (C) reinforce the new mutuality.

As you demonstrate these three practicing tasks, watch for the following client outcomes.

Phase 3 Client Outcomes

A. Clients use images of mutual support to describe and evaluate how they relate

B. Clients incorporate images of mutual support into their felt identities

C. Clients experience confidence that they can safely communicate on hard topics

D. Clients are able to intentionally break from dominant discourse to consider and enact new options

E. Clients demonstrate and embody new models of relating

Competency 3A—Envision a New Mutuality

Throughout the preceding therapy, you helped the Carter family envision third order goals. What this looks like in the details of their lives is not yet clear and may seem illusive or frustratingly fragile. There are times when Laurelle feels they are "back to square one" or Nick doubts whether he'll ever feel good about himself again. Your task is to help them focus on developing more fully detailed, personalized pictures of what is involved in mutual support. When they are off-track, you bring them back to envisioning a rich picture of what they do when enacting their relational ideals and what it means to them. This comprehensive portrait of who they are in relationship with one another is not simply a cognitive representation; through intentionally shared focus, it is evocatively accessible and enables Nick, Laurelle, and their children to actualize their relational goals and trust that off-track moments are temporary and repairable. Increasingly, they will draw on specific images of mutual support to recognize, describe, and evaluate how they relate and to illuminate their path forward.

◊ *Develop personalized pictures of mutual support*

Four steps are involved in envisioning a new mutuality:

1. Invite relational/equitable ideals to the foreground
2. Create a detailed image of mutual support/equity in this circumstance
3. Identify what is involved in enacting the ideal
4. Envision the meaning and consequences of the ideal in clients' lives

Invite Relational/Equitable Ideals to the Foreground

Your role in bringing relational ideals to the foreground is proactive. As in earlier phases of therapy, you listen for and recognize when equitable expectations and ideals are implicit in clients' accounts or distress. You notice when—despite experiences of mutuality in previous sessions—the flow of power in the current situation is not equal or something is impeding the Circle of Care. Oftentimes dominant societal discourses and related power imbalances are still working to mask or interfere with clients' goals. For example, Laurelle and Nick want to respect, validate, and share caring work, but still fall into old stereotypes that perpetuate prior patterns. Or partners criticize and attack each other without recognizing how their socioemotional responses are connected to larger societal contexts in this instance.

At this stage of therapy, clients also typically begin to surface issues that may previously have been too charged to address or, though important in the long term, were not an acute source of pain at the start of therapy. Clients trust you, the therapeutic process, and each other sufficiently to raise them now. Sometimes you, as the therapist, bring forward a topic you noted in earlier sessions but did not address in depth. For example, in a couple session, you check in with Laurelle and Nick on how they are experiencing intimacy. Laurelle says she would like more sex. To envision mutuality in relation to sexuality, you first need to recognize the sociocultural meanings surrounding their sexual encounters.

Laurelle: Well, I would like more sex. Nick doesn't seem very interested in it anymore.

Therapist: When you say more sex, what do you mean?

Laurelle: Nick would approach me; he'd show that he desires me. [looks at Nick] Instead of turning his back to me.

Therapist: When Nick doesn't approach you, turns his back to you, what does that say to you?

Laurelle: That he doesn't love me.

Nick: That's not true—I love you! It doesn't have anything to do with not loving you.

You use questions about messages, ideas, and what they have learned to bring forth internalized sociocultural meaning regarding sexuality.

Therapist: (to Laurelle) How do you think you came to think of sex as a measure of love?

Laurelle: Well, sex is how men show love.

Therapist: You've learned that men show love through sex. [pause] So when Nick doesn't seem interested in sex, the message is that if he loved you, he'd want to have sex with you? [Laurelle agrees] Is that how it was when you got together? When Nick first showed sexual interest in you, you felt loved, that you were more than friends?

Laurelle: I'd never felt attractive like that before. And that made me feel loved.

Therapist: That's a pretty strong message you got as a girl; that you had to be attractive, to look good, to be loved by men? How do you think that affects you today—with Nick?

Laurelle describes Nick's sexual interest in her as her marker of her attractiveness; that when he does not seem interested in her sexually, it's hard for her to feel lovable and good about herself. You turn to Nick to understand his socio-emotional experience:

Therapist: Nick, Laurelle said she learned that men show their love through sex, that if you're not approaching her sexually, she must not be loveable. You said that's not what it means to you. How do you explain it?

Nick: It's not about love. It's about performance. [pause] I feel a lot of pressure to perform, and I don't have the energy for it. [looks at Laurelle] It's not about you. It's about me.

You discuss where the pressure to perform comes from and how it affects Nick now. He describes how sexual performance, the need to show himself as a "stud," is what it meant to be a guy growing up. He didn't like it then and he still doesn't like it, but he feels it. Though Nick and Laurelle had what each describe as a "good" sex life earlier in their marriage, Nick carried the burden to initiate sex and "perform well," something that's harder to do following the accident, when he's physically less strong and struggling with his worth and depressing thoughts.

The gender models that Laurelle and Nick absorbed confound gender and sexuality in ways that limit intimacy and sexual pleasure based on mutuality. As you explore these discourses, you invite alternative ideals that support relationality:

Therapist: Wow. You've gone through your sexual life together based in large part on ideas that so many people learn—that women's value is in being sexually attractive to a man and that to be a man you need to be a sexual performer. It doesn't sound very relational [you chuckle] or even fun.
Laurelle: (smiles) We did have some fun. . . . But I think what was fun, for me at least, was being together [pauses to reflect] making each other feel good.
Nick: I agree. Being together—physically. [chuckles] We were good together—really good.
Therapist: So what you appreciate about sex is feeling good together? Being together in this uniquely close and physical way?

Having brought the ideal of mutuality to the foreground, you are now set to envision a detailed picture of what their sexual relationship will look like through their ideal of togetherness and shared pleasure.

Create a Detailed Image of Mutual Support/Equity

Had you not first contextualized their experience of sexuality, asking each partner what they wanted sexually would likely have brought forth answers *within* the current sex-gender system, i.e., first order change. Now that discussion of sexuality is framed within an alternative system based on mutuality, Laurelle and Nick are free to envision what this will look like for them. You use both open-ended questions to get an overall picture and narrowing questions that help the couple develop a tentative but specific and focused image of sex as togetherness and mutual pleasure. Keeping the dialogue within the framework of possibilities encourages a spirit of curiosity and openness to previously marginalized or silenced ideas, while questions such as "what does that look like," "who is doing what," or "what happens next" move the conversation from something fantasized or dreamed of to something that can be experimented with and embodied.

Therapist: Let's imagine that you're not burdened by those old stereotypes of sex and gender, what will your sexual relationship look like? How will it go?

Nick: I could relax—the pressure will be off.

Laurelle: Nick will look at me, touch me.

Nick: Yeah. I can look at her and touch her without feeling like I have to perform. [pause] And she could touch me without all those expectations about what happens next.

Therapist: You'll have more options for how to be physically together—to connect sensually—without having to perform. [pause] What else? When sex is not performance, what can it be?

Laurelle: I think it could be a lot of different things, depending on the day.

The couple discusses that sex can sometimes be sharing with their bodies that they are not alone; sometimes it can be holding each other and expressing their love. Sometimes shared sexuality can be about play and fun; sometimes it will involve penetration, sometimes not. As the couple expands their picture of what sex can be, you include questions that focus on their relational process and how they will enact mutuality:

Therapist: How will you know whose sexual interests are determining what you do?

Nick: We'd have to talk about it, I guess. [looks at Laurelle] We've never done that. It's like sex was supposed to happen naturally.

Therapist: In the old model something was wrong if you had to talk about it? [Nick agrees]

Laurelle: In the old model I wouldn't say anything about what I wanted; [pauses to reflect] sort of like Nick was supposed to know what I wanted—if I said something, it was like I was questioning him, criticizing him.

Therapist: So in the new model you're describing now, it would be safe—and necessary—for each of you to feel comfortable talking about your sexual desires . . . without worrying about offending the other or that you should already know?

Similar to Michael White's (2007) guidance that developing a narrative includes a focus on both the landscape of action (as you have been doing thus far) and the landscape of identity, you ask what it will say about them and their relationship when they can speak comfortably and openly about their sexual life (landscape of identity).

Laurelle: It will say that we are truly partners—that we trust we are each interested in the other and want to know what's going on, what we need.

Nick: I never thought I would say this . . . I think it would say our love is strong enough that it's OK to ask and to not have to be perfect—to not have to have the answers.

These are responses that the couple would not have been able to make at the outset of therapy. Now in phase 3, once you opened mutuality as a context for discussing their sexual activity, Laurelle and Nick readily draw on their egalitarian and relational ideals to envision new possibilities. You conclude this envisioning session by helping them detail what it will take to make their image of mutual comfort with and flexibility around sex happen. You ask questions such as "what will help you relax when pressure to perform pops up" and "what do you think is a first step in expanding how you share love?"

The couple decides to set times when they will hold and touch each other without "going further." You help them detail their expectations about this experience, such as who will initiate and how much talking will be involved. As you wrap up, you ask what they think the consequences of their focus on sexuality as togetherness and mutual pleasure will be. Each envisions relating to sex from a new relational position:

Laurelle: Just having this conversation makes me feel closer to Nick, more optimistic. Whatever we do or don't do, I think I'll feel more loved.

Nick: Yeah, I don't know what's going to happen either—how often we'll [finger quotes] have sex, but I think I'll be less on edge about it. [chuckles] Making it happen won't be all on me. [looks at Laurelle] I'm looking forward to touching you—I've missed that.

Identify What Is Involved in Enacting the Ideal

As described earlier, the process of envisioning moves from abstract ideals to an image of meaningful action. From a SERT perspective, the purpose is less about developing a behavioral plan or contract (though that can occur as well) and more about clients experiencing the emerging vision viscerally. As they do, they take in and begin to embody new or preferred ways of knowing themselves and each other that include and inspire action (Zimmerman, 2018). Once you have foregrounded the equitable relational values associated with the issue and created a specific image of what mutuality and equity look like in the topic at hand, your questions focus on detailing what is involved. This includes who, what, when, where, and how. As well explained in narrative therapy (White, 2007), this may also include how others are involved, what others see and know, and connections to past and future.

Consider this example. Nick and Laurelle tell you his mother sent a group text announcing Thanksgiving dinner. They are unsure how to respond. Most years they have gone to Nick's parents on Thanksgiving Day and gotten together with Laurelle's mother and sisters at another time. In previous sessions they said they limit time with Nick's family because they believe his mother treats Laurelle and the boys as "less than" his siblings' families, which Nick attributes to racism. They attend "formal" family functions, but do not have a warm, ongoing relationship with

Nick's family, who live about an hour away in a more affluent community. Since the accident, and because of increased reflexivity as a result of therapy, they do not want to automatically repeat the old patterns.

You have not met Nick's parents, so do not know what relational ideals they may hold that are masked by the workings of white supremacy. You do know that resistance to racism has structured how Nick and Laurelle react to them. To help them determine how they want to respond to the Thanksgiving invitation, you engage them in envisioning what family patterns based on equity and mutuality would look like and what is involved in enacting this ideal.

Therapist: Let's step back a moment. When you picture your family being treated with as much respect and love as Nick's siblings' families, what does that look like? What will I see?

Nick: They'd spend time with us—be interested in the boys and Laurelle and how we are doing.

Laurelle: It will be OK to say no to their plans. They would ask what works for us.

You continue to develop the picture of a context in which Nick's parents are interested in his family and planning is reciprocal, then turn to detailing what would be involved in enacting this ideal. As in other situations in which clients have to deal with discrimination and inequities, your questions validate the injustice and also help them envision alternative responses based on relationality and equity.

Therapist: It's very hurtful to see Nick's parents more engaged with their other grandchildren and to not seem to care about your schedules. [both partners agree]

Your conversation addresses the kind of family connections they not only prefer but need for optimal development and what is involved in enacting more equitable patterns.

Therapist: In a more back-and-forth relationship with Nick's parents, what will you be doing? What will be involved in engaging them in your lives and the children's lives?

Nick: They'd come to Brandon's and Logan's basketball games—some of
    them, at least. And they'd come to our house sometimes.
Therapist: What would it take for them to come to the basketball games?
    Or for them to come to your house?

They discuss how they never ask Nick's parents to their home. They
expect Nick's mother will not want to come or will be critical. They don't
think Nick's parents even know that Brandon and Logan are playing
basketball. You don't assume it is easy to change inequitable patterns, but
third order thinking helps you explore possibilities that do not perpetuate
Nick and Laurelle's reactive position in relation to the racism they experience from his mother.

Therapist: When families love each other despite racial and social dif-
    ferences, what will you see yourself doing in regard to basketball, for
    example?
Nick: I'd tell them about the games.
Therapist: You'd tell them about the games. And what will you tell them
    about what you want or need? What you're feeling?
Nick: I guess I'd tell them that we want them to come; that we want
    them to know the boys better.
Laurelle: And I'd be able to say "no" to them sometimes and suggest a
    different time to get together.

You take the conversation a step further to explore what will be
involved for them to enact these responses.

Therapist: So Nick, you picture telling your mother that you would like
    her to know your boys better and would like her and your father to
    come to their games. What will it take for you to do this? What will
    you have to do?

You discuss the familiar feelings that are likely to emerge, their expectations that his mother will not be interested. You invite them to consider
how they will respond to these feelings and what it will take to share
their desire for family connection, even though they don't know how his
mother will react. You summarize the picture they are envisioning:

Therapist: (to Nick) What you picture is to not let the effects of racism continue to take over your relationship with your mother. You see yourself having a conversation with her and telling her that you want her to be more involved in your family's life—that coming to a basketball game would be a good place to start. You're not sure how she'll respond, but you can see yourself standing up for your family from a position of love rather than anger. Is that right?

Similarly, you summarize Laurelle's picture of not always playing the subservient role, of expecting she can offer alternative ways to get together without the Black Shadow (Watson, 2013) telling her she is less than, adding to the barriers between her and Nick's mother.

Envision the Meaning and Consequences of the Ideal

For a full picture of what mutuality will look like, it is helpful to also carry the picture forward into the future. When the ideal is enacted, what will be the effect? And what will that effect mean to the clients? Questions involve who will be affected and how, what the change will make possible in the future, and what this vision says about the clients and their relationships—about who they are and what matters to them. In the example of the relationship with Nick's family, you ask what the consequences will be when his mother knows that her relationships with his wife and sons are important to him:

Nick: We've never had a conversation like this—ever—so I don't know what to expect, but she'll know more about me. And I'll know more about her. She'll know we care about her.
Therapist: She'll know you care about her. And that will have an impact on . . . ?
Nick: I don't think my mother and Laurelle ever got to know each other. It was easier not to. [looks at Laurelle] I'd love for my mom to know what a great person you are. And the boys too.

As you continue discussing the consequences of getting to know each other, you help him tap into what he'll see that may have been masked:

Therapist: What do you know about your mother that you will see when racism and old history are not in the way?

Nick says family is everything to his mother; that she put aside her own dreams to support his father and him and his siblings. He thinks his whole family will do better when they can pull down some of the barriers. When you probe for the effect on him, he says he will no longer be torn between his two families, no longer the only connection between them. Envisioning these consequences helps both Nick and Laurelle determine how to approach his parents—not only regarding Thanksgiving but for the future. They decide that Nick will invite his mother to lunch to share his hopes with her and to tell her that they will be spending Thanksgiving Day with Laurelle's family and would like to find another time to celebrate together, perhaps in combination with one of the boys' basketball games. You discuss the possibility of inviting Nick's parents to a therapy session if that seems helpful down the road.

In sum, four steps are involved in envisioning a new mutuality:

- Invite relational/equitable ideals to the foreground
- Create a detailed image
- Identify what is involved in enacting the ideal
- Envision the meaning and consequences of ideal

Competency 3B—Enact New Options for Shared Responsibility

Enactments in which family members interact directly with each other while therapists pay attention to and coach the process are a cornerstone of family therapy (Minuchin et al., 2014; Seedall & Butler, 2006) and an experiential approach to change (Hargrave & Houltberg, 2020; Johnson, 2019). Enactments increase shared focus and intentionality, which supports relational and physiological embodiment (Ewing et al., 2017; Siegel, 2007; Varela et al., 2016). In SERT, enacting what is envisioned happens both at home and in session. While over time clients will spontaneously enact new ways of relating to each other and their larger worlds (see competency 3C), facilitated enactments provide more structured practice.

The preceding examples of working with Laurelle and Nick to envision plans for trying a new kind of sexuality based on mutuality, togetherness, and shared fun and for how to reflectively respond to the Thanksgiving invitation from Nick's mother led to facilitated enactments that will happen outside the session and then be processed when clients return. Like all enactments, these are developed in the spirit of experimenting with something new. Enactments facilitated in session are sometimes quite brief as you move from clients talking with you about an issue to inviting them to engage with each other. Other enactments are longer, and sometimes even scheduled in advance.

Enabling clients to enact new options for shared relational responsibility includes five steps:

1. Create the relational focus and goal
2. Clarify what clients will do
3. Coach behind the scenes
4. Process what happened and how
5. Carry learning forward

Create the Relational Focus and Goal

Clients need to know what they are focusing on and why. Since the enactment likely arises out of prior conversation, creating the relational focus may not take a long time, but it is critical. As in the examples noted earlier, enactments are structured to support clients in how they seek to position themselves relative to each other and dominant discourses and inequities. Your role as the therapist is to form the focus on mutuality, shared relational responsibility, and equity.

Goals may involve experimenting with a new way of relating and/or engaging with issues that clients have not previously been able to address. Your overall goal is to facilitate a process in which they are able to experience something new. Success does not necessarily mean resolution. It could simply mean being able to take the risk to engage around a challenging issue and/or to tolerate staying with a partner's or family member's anger. Ideally, clients feel closer or more connected to each other. Alternatively, they (and you) are more able to recognize the vulnerabilities that make dealing with the issue challenging, and thus have a better idea of where to focus. In other words, there is no way to fail so long as you process the experience and learn from it.

For example, as a result of the conversation regarding their interactions with Nick's family, you and the couple decide to explore their family and relationship histories in more detail. In the course of this, Laurelle says she is still hurt regarding how Nick responded when she was raped. Before she and Nick were dating, she went to a party with friends and was raped by someone at the party. Not knowing what else to do, she called Nick—her trusted friend—to take her home. Nick immediately came to get her. Laurelle has always been grateful to him, but also hurt because he was angry and seemed to blame her for the rape. They have never spoken of it since. When Laurelle shares this now, Nick says he never blamed her for the rape and is surprised she carries hurt regarding his role. You sense an opportunity for an enactment that allows Laurelle and Nick to experience discussing this emotional issue from a position of mutuality and with increased awareness of patriarchal practices that invite rape and blame victims. You use your "proxy voice" (Seedall & Butler, 2006) to name their relational interests and create a relational frame for the possibility of such a conversation:

Therapist: (gently, to Laurelle) You have carried the trauma and pain of the rape alone all these years. [Laurelle sighs and nods]. And in addition to the terrible assault to you by the rapist, the rape created a barrier between you and Nick—you did not feel safe to discuss it.

Laurelle: I was ashamed and hurt. I didn't think he'd understand—I couldn't risk that again.

Therapist: (to Nick) It seems you were in the dark about Laurelle's experience of the rape. She experienced you as angry and blaming her.

Nick: I was a stupid kid! I was so angry at that [expletive] guy. I couldn't bear to imagine what it was like for Laurelle.

Therapist: You're both in a different place now. Nick, you've been working on how to take in what Laurelle is experiencing. Laurelle, you had the courage today to open a topic that has felt unsafe for so long. Is the rape, and how Nick hurt you, something you'd like to share with him now?

Laurelle indicates that this is a conversation she would like to have and says she thinks they are ready for it. You begin by being clear about the relational focus and goal:

Therapist: OK. This is an opportunity to approach each other as trusted partners; Nick, for you to become aware of what Laurelle experienced and has carried with her—for you to make it safe for her to do that. [Nick agrees] Laurelle, you're wanting to share this most vulnerable part of yourself with Nick, to talk not only about the rape but about how his reaction hurt you. [Laurelle agrees] Is that the goal, to open space between you that the rape destroyed?

By naming the relational goal, you set the stage for Laurelle and Nick to engage with each other in a new way. You developed the frame for the enactment in context of the shifts in the flow of power the couple has already experienced, and you highlighted what practicing mutuality means in this situation.

Clarify What Clients Will Do

Building on the specific relational focus for their conversation, it is helpful to provide guidelines that clarify what clients will do and assist them in getting started. When enactments will happen outside the session, clarity about who will do what is especially important. You can ask them to repeat their understanding of what they will do, or even write it down. In session, as in this example, clarifying what each will do is important, but likely to be brief. The action is between Laurelle and Nick, while you step back. Clarification helps them develop a shared focus, which as we have learned, is important to change. In keeping with the larger goal of increasing Nick's relational initiative, you set it up for him to seek her experience and clarify that his actions will be guided by wanting to know and understand her and how he hurt her:

Therapist: OK. Turn toward each other [they do]. Nick, let's begin with you. Let Laurelle know that you are interested in her experience of the rape and how your response hurt her—make it safe for her to tell you. You'll probably be tempted to defend yourself, but this is not the time. Try to listen and understand. Does that make sense? [Nick agrees] Laurelle, you share whatever you want him to know about what happened and how he hurt you in the process. It's up to you to decide what you feel ready to share. Does this sound good? [Laurelle agrees]. OK, go ahead Nick. I'll be here to coach you if you get stuck.

Because this enactment is happening in session, you do not detail what will happen next. You get them started and watch the interaction between them. You may step in periodically to provide additional guidance as they engage.

Coach Behind the Scenes

One of the advantages of in-session enactments is that your presence contributes to safety and enables you to support clients by inviting them back on track and offering periodic suggestions. Your behind-the-scenes coaching is responsive to the immediate process and communicates your attunement and encouragement. Clients experience you from a position of being *with* them, rather than a distant observer or instructor. For example, Nick and Laurelle start well; Nick begins by expressing genuine interest in Laurelle's experience and she speaks freely. Nick mostly listens and asks a few questions that communicate his care and interest. They speak quietly, and you feel the emotion. This changes when Laurelle begins to describe how hurtful it was when Nick raised his voice and said, "What were you thinking! Why would you come to this party with older guys and booze!" Nick responds by defending himself, so you gently step in:

Nick: (his tone escalating) You were in trouble! You asked me to come and get you—of course I was upset!

Therapist: (reaching toward Nick) Just a moment. . . . This is hard to hear. Take a breath and focus on what it was like for her.

Nick: (takes a breath and looks at Laurelle) What I said sounded like I was blaming you.

Laurelle responds by explaining why Nick's response was hurtful. This time, Nick is able to take in her pain and respond from a position of care:

Nick: I am so sorry I hurt you. You were terrified, and I made it worse. You quietly step in again, maintaining the emotional tone of their shared pain:

Therapist: (softly) Tell her what you think she needed from you.

Nick: You needed me to comfort you, to be there for you. And instead, I judged you. [softly] I didn't know what to do. When you needed me, I took it out on you.

Laurelle: I wanted you to hold me . . . but I was ashamed and scared. I didn't feel worthy of you. [softly] You said the things I was saying to myself.

Nick's attunement to Laurelle, his vulnerability, and his willingness to be accountable invites Laurelle to reflect on the traumatic experience more broadly and begin to take in Nick's perspective. For their conversation to continue, it is important that your attuned input joins their affective level. If your stance had been more cognitive or distant, the emotional connection between the partners would have been disrupted.

Laurelle and Nick continue their conversation a few more minutes without needing coaching from you and are beginning to develop a new, shared understanding of the trauma, which promotes healing through connection (Herman, 2015). Had they not been able to respond to your guidance in a way that facilitated mutuality in the Circle of Care, you would have stopped the enactment and moved into processing their experience.

Process What Happened and How

The focused affective connection Laurelle and Nick experienced promotes reciprocal resonance around a new image of self and relationship; connecting this charged experience with reflective processing joins emotion to meaning. This creates coherence across systemic levels, which is integral to the embodiment of new narratives (Siegel, 2012; Zimmerman, 2018). To help Nick and Laurelle organize their experience and respond more intentionally, you process what happened in the enactment. Had the couple completed the enactment outside the session, you would process their experience in the next meeting.

You ask Laurelle what this experience was like for her, probing for what is meaningful. She describes feeling supported in a way new to her:

Laurelle: I always thought of Nick as supportive of me, but this is different. I felt his caring inside me, in a way that made me feel better about myself.

When you ask Nick, he says it was hard; that this way of relating is new to him and he felt out of his comfort zone. Then he adds,

Nick: But I feel good. I thought we knew each other, but we didn't. There is so much we brushed away. I feel like we understand each other better, that I'm not a bad person.

You help them become aware of what they did to create their new understanding.

Therapist: (to Laurelle) You opened a topic that the two of you had never been able to discuss before. What did you have to do to make that happen?
Laurelle: Coming here, I guess. I stopped being scared and I just said what I was thinking, what was on my mind.

You process what made her feel safe and how Nick contributed. You also explore the meaning to her of being able to say what was on her mind:

Laurelle: I can trust, I guess; trust that it's OK [pause] No, better than OK—important! If I want Nick to know me, I can't keep so much of me inside. [pause] I'm used to just pushing forward no matter what.

Similarly, you help Nick reflect on what he needed to do to step out of his comfort zone and what that means to him. He describes caring more about Laurelle than "looking foolish" and that when he did, he let his heart guide him.

Nick's overcoming "looking foolish" and Laurelle's trusting that her experience is important and she doesn't always have to keep going "no matter what" are each tied to sociocultural discourses that informed their felt identities. When you expand the lens by asking how they were able to resist these social messages, each now readily recognizes the impact of societal context:

Laurelle: That's what Black women do—we learn not to expect anyone to be there for us.

Nick: (smiles wryly) Well, we've talked about this before—men should never look foolish!

You explore the impact of these new ways of knowing and expressing themselves. You also reiterate that sexual assault is never the victim's fault, though society still tends to blame them; that it is not surprising that both Laurelle and Nick originally responded to the rape with some of those damaging dominant culture messages.

Processing Laurelle and Nick's immediate enacted experience contributes to embodying new images of gender and sexuality. To help them carry this new learning forward, you ask what they will take away from today. When Nick says that it was hard to be so vulnerable but worth it, that he wants to be a more positive model for his sons, you share Mark Green's (2018) short and highly readable *The Little #METOO Book for Men*, which compassionately invites men out of the rules of the brutal, but often unconscious, "man box" culture into daily actions that "flips it on its head . . . and calls up every relational capacity we were taught to deny" (p. 73). You suggest Nick take a look at the book and that in the next session you'll discuss what it means to him and how to carry these ideas forward.

Carry Learning Forward

In the next session, you ask Nick what spoke to him in *The Little #METOO Book for Men*. He points to two places. The first is Greene's (2018) statement, "Men do not want to be angry. Men do not want to be alone. Men are not naturally inclined toward the toxic confines of the man box. If we were, it wouldn't be killing us" (p. 75). Nick says he believes anger, the need to be right, and the resulting isolation have been killing him and hurting his family. Reading this gave him increased appreciation for Tyler's resistance to the man box culture and that he remembers his own struggle with masculinity when he was a teen. This is why he was especially struck by Greene's discussion of what boys learn:

> Go to any middle school or high school classroom in America. Ask the boys to tell you the rules for being a man. They'll all tell you the same things. Always be tough. Always be successful.

Always be confident. Always have the last word. Always be the leader. But one of the first rules of manhood these boys will tell you is that "real men" don't show their emotions . . . to this day we coach our sons to present a façade of emotional toughness and our daughters to admire this façade in men.

(p. 20)

You and Nick decide to develop another kind of enactment—one to help him have a discussion with his sons about masculinity. In consultation with Laurelle, you and Nick discuss his goals and what will happen. Together, you decide to have a father-son session in which Laurelle observes. You discuss that Nick wants to engage with the boys in a way that shares his own struggles and vulnerabilities and to listen with genuine interest in learning from them. He wants to model relational masculinity and communicate support for a more flexible understanding of what it means to be strong. Since you anticipate that this enactment will take most of the session, as the therapist, you will ask questions and provide guidance that will help structure the session, but will play only a supporting role, with the primary interaction being between Nick, Brandon, Logan, and Tyler.

In the next session, you tell the boys that Nick wants to have a conversation with them about what it means to be a man and that Mom will observe. You invite Laurelle to a comfortable chair in the corner (or, online, ask her to turn her temporarily turn her camera off) and pull your chair back so that Nick and the boys are focused on each other. You begin the conversation by inviting Nick to share why he wants to talk about this subject. Nick pauses, then leans in and in a soft tone (different than a teacher or leader) describes his struggle with anger and isolation and that he wants something different for them:

Nick: When we first started coming to these sessions, I was angry all the time and kept to myself—that hurt you and it hurt me too. I was behaving that way because of what I learned about being a man—that I wasn't supposed to feel out of control or show my emotions. I was hurting and I didn't know how to connect with you—to be the kind of dad you needed. [pause] I'm trying to learn a different way to be a man, to be your dad.

Therapist: (to Nick, helping to structure the session) What is your hope for today?

Nick: I hope we can just talk—about what it's like for you; what it's like for men in general. Maybe talking about what it means to be a man will help you have more options than I did. [looks at Tyler] I really want to know how you're dealing with it. And Brandon and Logan too.

Therapist: (to the boys) Does that sound OK? [boys all nod]. So, to start your conversation, what are the rules for being a man? Make a list.

They readily make the expected list. Drawing on Greene (2018), Nick calls them "the man box."

Therapist: Talk with each other about these rules. How do they show up at school? At home? On TV? Other places? How does the man box affect boys and men? How does it affect you? How does it affect others? Your relationships? I'll step back and listen to you talk.

Everyone has a lot to say. They are used to therapy by now, and Nick uses the list of rules to move the conversation forward. They discuss how each of the rules works and identify its problems and limits. You step in to suggest they each offer examples of how they're personally affected—at school, at home, with friends. Unlike earlier sessions, Tyler speaks comfortably about the isolation he experienced; that at first most of his friends were girls, but now he has a wider group of friends who resist male dominance and some who identify outside the gender binary. Nick asks respectful questions and resists telling Tyler "how it is." If he moves into an "I have the answers" stance, you coach him to share his thoughts from a more curious position.

To help them carry learning from this enactment forward, you suggest they make alternatives to each of the man box rules. This raises considerable conversation. Brandon and Logan especially enjoy the playfulness of developing possibilities. When this discussion appears finished, you rejoin them to process what is meaningful about this conversation. Nick describes it as a "relief," that's he's never had a conversation like this before and he feels more optimistic for himself and his sons. He says he liked not having to have all the answers. Tyler says he has conversations about gender with his friends, but is happy to be able to share these ideas with his dad and brothers.

To conclude, you bring Laurelle into the conversation and ask her what it was like to see the rest of the family engaged with each other in this way. Like Nick, she describes relief and optimism:

Laurelle: I never thought I would see Nick be able to talk with the boys like this. It makes me happy to see them together like that—hopeful that he can a fuller part of the family.
Therapist: And what would that mean to you?
Laurelle: (laughs) That it's not all on me. [more somberly] That man box—it's not easy to live with.

Carrying learning forward from this enactment involves many possibilities for shared relational responsibility, mutuality, and options for the well-being of each family member. The Carter family is incorporating these images into their evolving identities and experiencing confidence that they can safely communicate on hard topics.

In sum, five steps are involved in enacting shared relational responsibility:

- Create the relational focus and goal
- Clarify what clients will do
- Coach behind the scenes
- Process what happened and how
- Carry learning forward

Competency 3C—Reinforce New Mutuality

Throughout the therapy, you have been actively encouraging the Carter family's relational values, noticing and highlighting when they demonstrate them and underscoring the positive effects. In this final stage of therapy, reinforcing clients' emergent relational practices facilitates long-term embodiment. As the therapist, you watch clients' progress in exhibiting relational ideals and recognize when they enact an aspect of mutual support. Your reinforcement helps link emotion and meaning to intentional action outside otherwise taken-for-granted dominant discourses and social patterns that reproduce inequities. This is how new models of relating are neurologically and relationally embodied (Ewing et al., 2017; Siegel, 2007, 2019; Zimmerman, 2018).

Four steps are involved in reinforcing enactments of mutuality and equity:

1. Identify demonstrations of transformative action
2. Amplify what was involved
3. Reinforce positive relational outcomes
4. Encourage commitment to reflective action

Identify Demonstrations of Transformative Action

Focusing on client actions that transform inequities in the flow of relational and social power or resist problematic social discourses—however small—is important to the process of change. This element of SERT draws on the distinction between problem talk and solution talk (Berg & DeJong, 1996; de Shazer, 1991). So long as conversation is focused only on problems, change is not likely. Talking about what works, what clients are already doing, illuminates the path forward. For example, in a conversation about how Brandon and Logan are doing in school, Nick says that when he spoke to their teachers, both reported that the disruptive behavior had mostly stopped. In addition to exploring and reinforcing what the boys are doing that is positive, you notice that Nick is the one who spoke to the teachers. You interrupt the discussion of the boys' transformative action (to which you'll return) to highlight this variation from the prior pattern in which Laurelle did all the communication with the school:

Therapist: If we could pause for just one moment. Nick, you said you spoke to their teachers. [Nick nods] I'm curious how that happened—that you, rather than Laurelle, were the one to make the contact.

Nick says that Laurelle has so much on her plate and he had the time, so he told her that he would check in with their teachers. You highlight that this is a development you'll be interested to know more about:

Therapist: You saw that Laurelle had more than her share of responsibility with the boys and took on checking in with the teachers. I'll
be interested in hearing more about how that happened and what it
means to you and Laurelle—and to Brandon and Logan.

Nick: I never liked school, so talking to teachers wasn't easy, but I'm glad
I did.

You reiterate the importance of this step on his part and indicate that
you'll return to it, then engage Nick and the family in noticing what
Brandon and Logan are doing positively, rather than simply emphasizing
what they are not doing (i.e., not disrupting).

Therapist: It's a meaningful step for you. Let's be sure to talk about it
some more. [to Brandon and Logan] What do you think your teachers see you doing in class that's positive? What do you see yourself
doing?

The boys describe a variety of things—practicing their breathing, asking the teacher questions, helping other kids—all of which you amplify
and explore the positive consequences.

You could also wait until the discussion of the boys' behavior is finished and then draw attention to Nick's transformative act of speaking
with the teachers. What is important is that you noticed this emergent,
in-the-moment action and do not let it pass without highlighting it and
making it available to amplify.

Amplify What Was Involved

You are aware of many shifts in the way the Carter family relates to each
other and engages with the world. Amplifying what is involved helps
embody these new ways of thinking and behaving. As a result of the
therapy with you and his involvement with the pain management support group (see Chapter 10), Nick has been taking intentional steps to
respond to the pain and to think about his identity and family roles differently. Everyone agrees that he is less angry and more engaged with the
family. You notice that instead of feeling useless, he seems to be finding
new ways to contribute, new ways to recognize his value. In one session

he mentions that Logan and Brandon are helping him build a cradle for the baby Laurelle's sister is expecting. You amplify what is involved in this transformative action—both in terms of his physical activity and in engaging with Logan and Brandon:

Therapist: You're building a cradle. How did that come about? What moved you to do this?

In response to your prompts, Nick tells you that he always liked to build furniture and cabinets. Though he did not have much time to do this before the accident because his construction job kept him busy, he had occasionally done special-order projects for some of the customers. When he heard that Laurelle's sister was pregnant, he remembered a cradle he had made. The injury limits how high he can raise his arms and how much he can lift, but Nick thought it might be fun to "fool around" with the tools still in his garage. You continue to amplify by asking questions that detail and expand his experience of renewed engagement:

Therapist: That's quite a change for you to have the energy and interest to "fool around" with building something. Where did you feel that energy?
Nick: (pauses to reflect) The memory of the other cradle touched something in me—like I saw myself again and it made me wonder if I could still do it. If I could still build.
Therapist: You recognized a part of yourself that you value and that gave you energy to try?
Nick: Yes. I think it was the first time I realized that maybe I hadn't lost everything. [pause] Well, I knew I hadn't lost everything, but pain and anger took up most of my energy.
Therapist: When you're working on the cradle, you see more than pain and anger. What do you see?
Nick: I see a competent man—that I have something to give. And I focus less on the pain.

You continue exploring this revised image of himself as competent and able to give, emphasizing what he did to see himself this way and how his image of what it means to be a man has evolved. Then you move to how he came to include Brandon and Logan.

Therapist: What did you do to engage Brandon and Logan in the project?

Nick: That session when they said they wanted to do more with me really hit me. I've been trying to do more with them—homework and such—but when I was out there in the garage, I realized I was lonely. I wondered if they'd be interested.

Therapist: Was that awareness of being lonely new to you?

Nick: Yeah. I suppose I was lonely before, but I didn't let myself feel it, you know. Just tried to power through.

Therapist: You let yourself feel your desire to connect with the boys, and then . . .

Nick: I thought about how to approach them. I knew they would resist me if it sounded like an order. So, I brought it up after school one day—asked if they'd like to see what I was working on.

Therapist: (amplifying the relational action) You stopped to put yourself in their place. How did that work?

Nick describes that Brandon and Logan seemed a little reluctant at first, but slowly made their way to the garage with him. You ask how he responded to what seemed like reluctance on their part:

Nick: I didn't let it bother me. I get it. I showed them the plans [pauses] and then I actually told them I was lonely out here; that I'd love their help.

Therapist: You understood them and then were honest with them—and that worked? They wanted to help?

Reinforce Positive Relational Outcomes

Identifying positive relational outcomes is a theme throughout SERT. Reinforcing these is especially important in embodying relational actions that counter dominant discourse and change the flow of power. In this case, Nick took a less authoritative stance toward his sons and instead shared some of his felt experience, including vulnerable feelings of loneliness. You reinforce that though this shift felt uncomfortable at first, he did it. Then you name and explore the positive relational outcomes. Since Brandon and Logan are in the room, you are able to ask them directly:

Therapist: (to Brandon and Logan) What was it like to have your dad say he was lonely, that he would like your help?

Logan: I was kinda surprised. I never thought about him being lonely.

Brandon: Yeah. He seemed a little sad—and happy about the cradle. So, I wanted to help him.

Therapist: You wanted to help him?

Brandon: Yeah. It made me feel good. [looks at Nick] My dad is good at building stuff. He never let me help before—maybe I was too little.

Therapist: (to Nick) Brandon and Logan seemed to see you more like a person and wanted to help you. [pause] They seemed honored. [boys agree]

Reinforcing the positive relational outcomes encourages Nick to continue to risk similar shifts, which contributes to his evolving relational identity. It is important to note that Nick does not have to give up all that he valued about his White male roles; rather, he is able to edit and expand them. He and the rest of the family are now more able to confront challenges together and create new options based on awareness of their context and what they want to value.

Encourage Commitment to Reflective Action

One of the outcomes of this therapy is that each family member is less defined by restrictive social norms and discourses and judges themselves more positively. They are all engaging in the Circle of Care rather than seeing this as only Laurelle's domain. Experiencing a more mutual Circle of Care gives Laurelle a sense of support from Nick and the children. Increased awareness of the sociopolitical context in which they live has improved their capacity to be "in it together" and take reflective action, which enables new possibilities.

For years, Laurelle has been going, going, going; taking responsibility for everyone with little thought, but sometimes with resentment and anger. Several years ago, she turned down a possible promotion to field supervisor because she couldn't imagine carrying a larger burden of responsibility and because she doubted other employees would respect her. Now she is able to rethink her options. One of the significant shifts that has happened is that Laurelle and Nick are beginning to have conversations about how they want their relationship to work and how to solve their personal and economic challenges. While discussing Laurelle's work-related goals, you reinforce how Laurelle and Nick are approaching the issue through commitment to reflective action:

Therapist: (to Laurelle) You mentioned that you and Nick have been talking about what it would mean for the family if you apply for a field supervisor position. How does that talk happen? Is the way you talk different than before?

Laurelle: (thoughtfully) Well, we always did talk. But this is different. Before when I was offered the supervisor job, Nick said I should do it; that I'd be good at it. It was like he was saying "do what you want." But we didn't talk about what I'd need from him to be able to take on that responsibility—what would be different at home. It was like he wouldn't be affected—except by having more money. Now we're thinking things through together and discussing our roles and expectations of each other.

Therapist: You are approaching this as "we're in this together" [both nod] And you're looking at all the aspects of how this choice affects everyone—including you, Laurelle, and what you need.

Nick: Yeah. I don't just assume that she's going to do all the work around the house. And I want to be a real support for her—not just say "go for it," but to support her emotionally.

Therapist: The two of you are consciously talking about what it means to support each other, not only financially but also emotionally and in day-to-day life at home and at work. You're being more intentional.

The couple describes having conversations about their values and how they want to live. Nick says he is taking steps to begin developing a furniture-making business. You note that as he talks about this, he is evaluating himself not only by his ability to provide for his family but to also be available to them:

Nick: SSI allows me to take time to start over—to do what I need to be able to do work my body allows. And the good thing about that—it's been hard that's for sure, on all of us—but I think we're headed to something better. I can be a more involved dad and husband. It's like we're making our life the way we want it to be.

In sum, four steps reinforce enactments of mutuality and equity:

- Identify demonstrations of transformative action
- Amplify what was involved
- Reinforce positive relational outcomes
- Encourage commitment to reflective action

Summary

In the final phase of therapy, you demonstrated three competencies that helped the Carter family draw on their relational resources and values and intentionally enact them:

Competency 3A—Envision new mutuality
Competency 3B—Enact new options for shared relational responsibility
Competency 3C—Reinforce new mutuality

You used your role to help the family keep their values of mutuality and equity at the forefront and to increase their awareness of what they do to embody them. They still live in a society that privileges White male heterosexuality and economic success over relational well-being, but they are better equipped to recognize the impact of these contexts and reflectively respond to each other and decide how to position themselves in the larger world. Their enhanced mutual support will enable them to better handle new troubles or crises.

Though there are many ways therapy can be successful (see Chapter 8), the positive outcomes for the Carter family illustrate the connection between individual well-being, reciprocal relational engagement, and equitable power processes. Throughout the therapy, your persistent ethical and responsive positioning created an environment in which Nick, Laurelle, Tyler, Logan, and Brandon could envision and embody a wider range of options for themselves as individuals, family members, and part of the larger community.

Therapist Checklist: Phase 3—Practicing

☐ Keep relational ideals at the forefront
☐ Envision specific images of mutual support and equity
☐ Move from abstract concepts to embodied action
☐ Detail who, what, when, and how
☐ Encourage enactments focused on mutuality
☐ Reinforce relational actions
☐ Identify positive relational consequences
☐ Carry learning forward through reflective action

PART IV
LEARN THROUGH RESEARCH AND REFLEXIVITY

12
ENGAGE CONTEXTUAL SELF-OF-THE-THERAPIST

Socio-Emotional Relationship Therapy (SERT) requires an engaged, contextually conscious therapist. The work is "inevitably personal as well as professional" (Knudson-Martin et al., 2015, p. 145). It involves awareness of the socio-emotional nature of our own responses to clients and the clinical moment. Sociocultural engagement *with* clients is more than cognitive understanding (D'Aniello et al., 2016). It demands courage to step toward our own vulnerabilities as we move with clients toward theirs—especially in the face of power and sociocultural differences (Vargas & Wilson, 2011).

This chapter includes activities to increase your contextual emotional awareness, research on how to develop and embody a contextual socio-emotional lens, and guidelines for using contextual self-of-the-therapist in service of client well-being, with implications for clinical supervision and peer group accountability across the professional lifespan. The experiences of the following four therapists will help you examine your own contextual self-of-the-therapist and responsibly use it to further therapeutic goals.

- Shade (age 48) is a pre-licensed, White, queer-identified, divorced, and repartnered parent of an autistic teen and former manager of

DOI: 10.4324/9781003270232-12

a nonprofit agency. They recently completed a couple and family therapy master's program as part of a career change.

- Anna (age 24) is a cisgender, heterosexual, single Taiwanese American in her second year of a mental health counseling program and in clinical practicum. Prior to graduate school, all her education and experience have been within primarily Asian communities.
- Charles (age 36) is a licensed psychologist. He identifies as a Black, cisgender, gay Christian and is married and father of a two-year-old. With relatively light skin, his race is not necessarily visible.
- Max (age 29) is a recently licensed marriage and family therapist (LMFT) in his first year in a family therapy doctoral program. He identifies as a White, heterosexual, cisgender, feminist male and attends a progressive Jewish synagogue. His mother is a licensed social worker.

Increase Socio-Emotional Awareness

To begin my course on equity in family therapy, I ask students to introduce themselves by sharing about the context in which they learned what is normal, valued, and good. I suggest they speak for a few minutes about the communities they grew up in and messages and expectations they absorbed. I invite them to think about these in relation to social locations such race, gender, socioeconomic status, sexuality, religion, migration, etc. I offer my own example of being a smart girl on a farm in North Dakota where the only professional options I saw for women were to be a teacher, nurse, or home extension agent. I share the confusion I felt when I walked by a Black person in a grocery store in our White community and sensed I should do something special to be welcoming and that I still feel the strong cultural/family messages to work before play, never waste money, and always "be nice."

These initial introductions are necessarily brief, but consistently bring forth a multitude of sociocultural experiences among the 20 or so persons gathered to start their family therapy training. Beginning in this way—by expanding the contextual lens—is a valuable frame for how to approach each other and our work as clinicians. Always, some say they never before considered how the circumstances of their lives informed what they "knew" and understood as "normal." Others may already have a degree in gender or cultural studies or been involved in consciousness-raising activities or movements such as Black Lives Matter or #MeToo.

Regardless of starting point, the self-learning involved as you connect your contextual experience to emotional awareness is intense. No matter how many years I facilitate these kinds of activities and engage in this exploration with others, I always learn something new. While private reflection is helpful, contextual self-awareness grows out of shared inter-action and focused attention to your internal and relational responses. This includes intentional activities integrated into a program of study, supervision or peer consultation regarding your clinical reactions, and awareness generated through reflexivity regarding daily interactions with others, including efforts to expand your social experience by engaging with others beyond your usual comfort zone.

What Is Socio-Emotional Awareness?

There are many similar terms: cultural awareness, critical consciousness, contextual consciousness, critical self-of-the therapist, and cultural sensi-tivity, to name a few. Some emphasize the impact of ethnicity and culture (including religion); some (but not all) include the processes of power, privilege, and domination. Socio-emotional awareness incorporates and builds upon all of these to include attention to your own felt awareness; how socioculturally situated emotion intertwines with perception to pat-tern your experience as you simultaneously evaluate yourself and others (Mehl-Madrona, 2010; Wetherell, 2012). Rather than seeking to become "objective" by overcoming bias, developing socio-emotional awareness means attuning to the sociocultural context of your felt internal responses and responsibly using this emotional awareness in service of therapeutic goals.

For example, Glade is becoming aware that they learned to cope with the pain of gender and sexual marginalization and challenges of par-enting a neurodivergent child by applying dominant culture values of goal-directedness and independence. They find themselves feeling impa-tient with classmates or clients who seem stuck in helplessness or "overly" focused on what others think. Charles, who is highly aware of the nuances and complexities in his life as a Black, White-passing, gay Christian par-ent, is surprised to discover that he reacts to nearly all straight White men similarly—with restrained resentment and fear, which he responds to by maintaining social distance through a pleasant demeanor.

The emotions generated for Glade and Charles have the potential to be either helpful or harmful (Garcia et al., 2015). They have helped each navigate social injustice in their lives and can serve as warning that inequities are part of the personal and clinical picture. Awareness of these feelings and knowledge about how one usually responds can help therapists identify the personal salience of client issues and use themselves appropriately and effectively to connect with clients and facilitate change (Aponte & Carlsen, 2009).

Activities to Develop Contextual Awareness

There are many activities that can help you and/or your supervisees explore your sociocultural identities and increase awareness of the impact of systems of power, privilege, and oppression in your life. *Finding Your Voice as a Beginning Marriage and Family Therapist* by Dana Stone and Jessica ChenFeng is an excellent source, with detailed descriptions and suggestions for using a number of them (Stone & ChenFeng, 2020). One is the ADDRESSING framework (Hays, 2008), which is a good way to reflect on the impact of your varying identities (Age, Developmental Disabilities, Religion and spiritual orientation, Ethnic and racial identity, Socioeconomic status, Sexual orientation/identity, Indigenous heritage, Nation of origin, and Gender identity). Start by putting a star on those in which you have privilege. Questions such as which part of your identity do you think people notice first about you, which parts of your identity are you most/least comfortable sharing with others, and which did you struggle with most growing up help raise awareness of your belongingness and associated emotional responses.

Stone and ChenFeng (2020) also describe how to use cultural and critical genograms. Begin with a cultural genogram (Hardy & Laszloffy, 1995) to show your family's cultural/religious organization across generations and identify migration patterns, identities, and associated beliefs and behaviors, with colors and symbols to highlight societal messages and areas of pride and shame. Add a critical genogram (Kosutic et al., 2009) that expands the cultural genogram with overlays representing the operation of power through social forces such as nationism, sexism, racism, classism, and other forms of oppression. Use arrows and boxes to depict the flow of power and access to resources, both within the family and between the family and larger social systems. Consider examples of how you and your family have benefitted as a result of these societal disparities and how you have been disadvantaged. How did these societal inequities influence how you've come to think about yourself and others?

Developing contextual emotional awareness is challenging (and a lifetime project) because all of us—privileged and dominated—internalize societal discourses that stereotype and oppress. As discussed in Chapter 3, these discourses shape what we think and feel and how we know ourselves and can distort how we view clients and supervisees. Activities such as those noted earlier provide an opportunity to bring these internalized messages into the open for personal reflection, accountability, and growth. Start by assuming you have internalized sexism, racism, classism, etc. Write responses to questions that generate self-examination (see Stone & ChenFeng, 2020). For instance, Émilie Ellis and Maria Bermúdez (2021) detailed questions that identify four aspects of internalized sexism: self-objectification, self-silencing, passive acceptance of gender roles, and internalized misogyny. Sample questions include:

- What does it stir in me when other women do not value culturally idealized beauty standards (i.e., thinness, femininity)?
- How do I limit my own self-expression and to benefit whom? How do I silence other women through labeling them (i.e., calling them "crazy")?
- How do I judge other women for not silencing themselves?
- What are three words I would use to describe what I believe women are most skilled at or are most naturally capable of?

While Ellis and Bermúdez directed these questions specifically to those who identify as female, they are relevant to everyone. For example, when Max asked himself these questions, he found that despite his feminist and progressive ideologies, he tends to judge women who conform to societal ideals of beauty as less smart and assumes that women are naturally more caring than others. When women (friends, family, teachers, employers, clients) do not demonstrate stereotypical caring behavior, he feels irritated and judgmental of them in ways he does not with men. Anna is becoming aware of the tension she feels around mixed sociocultural messages that she should excel in academic and work pursuits, while also silencing her opinions and hiding her intelligence.

Relational Activities to Generate Socio-Emotional Awareness

To stimulate contextual emotional awareness and encourage openness to new perspectives, group work is valuable. How you structure these experiences is important. You need to facilitate dialogue rather than debate (Becker et al., 1995) and create an atmosphere that encourages participants to listen from positions of curiosity, interest in complexity, openness to uncertainty, and willingness to question and change (Anderson, 2022). Drawing on lessons from the Public Conversations Project (Herzig & Chasin, n.d.) and the narrative practice of witnessing (White, 2007), I use the following principles to guide relational activities to promote socio-emotional awareness:

- Begin with personal stories—this engages emotion and experience rather than ideology
- Structure how speaking and listening happen—this makes space for usually silenced voices and prioritizes listening and reflection
- Ask about uncertainties and new questions—this enables new awareness to emerge
- Invite witnesses to share the personal impact of another's story on them—this validates experience and promotes connections across differences
- Lead with curiosity and step back from judgments, advice, and opinions—this creates safety to explore emergent awareness

Following are two relational activities I use regularly to promote socio-emotional awareness of self and others.

Socio-Emotional Dialogue Groups

This format may be used with a variety of socially charged topics. The example here is around race. What follows are the directions I give participants. Groups of five or six are ideal.

- Select one person to ask the questions. This person should also take a turn in answering the questions. Have each person respond to the first question, then move on to the next question. Don't always have the same person begin.
- For each question, each person may speak for up to two minutes. Select a timekeeper and respectfully enforce this rule.
- Listen to each person's reflections. Do not verbally respond. Do not engage in debate or discussion. Be aware of your own internal reactions.
- If you find yourself thinking about what you will say when it is your turn, gently return your thoughts to the speaker.
- If someone begins to respond to another group member, the facilitator should ask that person to simply listen.
- Speakers may pass and be returned to at the end of a round; no one is required to speak.

1. When thinking about the role of race in your life, what personal experience is especially meaningful to you? Share a story.
2. When thinking what your race means to others, what comes to mind? Share a story.
3. When you consider the impact of race in your life and interactions with others, what aspects are uncertain, confusing, or unclear to you?
4. As you listened and took in the experience of others in your group, what emotion was triggered for you? Give an example of why it is meaningful.
5. What new awareness and/or questions are raised for you as a result of this activity?

I use this format to challenge taken-for-granted thinking while honoring each person's perspective. It is especially helpful when people do not know each other well, but can be useful at any time. It is also a good structure for questions that help members of a group reflect on their experience with each other (how they engage, what they are learning about themselves, where they are struggling, etc.). You can be creative about the topic, keeping in mind that the order and focus of questions are important—move from personal story to uncertainties, then to what responses and new questions listening to others has stimulated. Sometimes after the small groups, I invite each person to share with the larger group one thing they are sitting with or reflecting on as a result of their experience. Naming the impact of relational experience and having it witnessed by others contribute to the emotional salience of the emerging contextual awareness.

Life Map Presentations

Life map presentations build on prior contextual awareness activities. They ask participants to examine key events in their lives through a contextual lens that considers not only what happened but also how social forces influenced their and their families' responses to these events. Creating the life map itself is an evocative symbolic activity that generates a new level of reflection. Sharing it with a group of witnesses and being witness to the life maps of others add emotional and relational meaning. Written reflection on the map and presentation helps bring the experiential to consciousness. Following are directions for this activity:

A) Create a life map. A life map is one way of expressing our histories—where we came from, where we are now, and where we are headed. Symbols, pictures, and drawings are used to represent important events, transitions, learning moments, and so on that stand out along your life path. You may use a large piece of paper (or other medium) and any materials you like—pictures from magazines, colored pens, photos, computer-generated graphics—to show your socio-contextual story. This personal presentation is NOT appropriate as a PowerPoint presentation (which tends to be more disembodied). However, you may use video, music, or other art forms to support/enhance presentation of your life map.

B) Include (a) how gender, class, race, sexual orientation, spirituality/religion, nation of origin, migration, physical and mental abilities, and other social and contextual issues intersect in your life; (b) specific and concrete ways these intersecting social locations afforded you privilege as well as lack of privilege or oppression in your day-to-day life; (c) how these sociocultural contexts framed significant events in your life and the resources/strengths that helped you overcome difficult times; and (d) the impact of these sociocultural contexts on your role as a therapist.

C) Share your life map with the class/group (15–20 minutes). The group will have approximately 10 minutes to share their reflections on how your life map impacted them (the thoughts or feelings they experienced). Only reflections that communicate human connection and are non-judgmental may be shared.

Presenter guidelines:

- Share your story in as open and reflective a way as possible
- Your goal is to experience the process of telling your story and having it received by interested others
- Be aware of your own internal responses
- Accept the genuine interest and curiosity of your witnesses

Witness guidelines:

- Open yourself to taking in the experience of another
- Engage from a position of curiosity
- If you find yourself making internal interpretations or judgments, stop to consider what these ideas say about you and what you may be curious to know or understand
- Reflect what moved you as you listened to the presenter's experience (speak from your experience)

I was moved when you said . . .
As you spoke of . . . I wondered . . .
As I listened to you, I couldn't help but think about times that . . .

- Do not attempt to interpret or explain

Confidentiality

- Treat everything shared in the life story as confidential
- Do not discuss any aspect of another person's story with anyone outside this room, including other class/group members

---

Comments by Anna and Slade after participating in the life map presentations illustrate increased socio-emotional awareness as a result of touching each other in this personal way.

Anna: I am so honored to have witnessed each of your stories. Honestly, I am still trying to take in how different each of your lives are from mine . . . I am aware of my privilege in having so much family support, and yet how little they actually know me. I have never felt so listened to—I felt uncomfortable, at first, being the center of attention, like I broke a cultural or gender rule.

Shade: With everything I've been through, I've done a lot of self-examination. But I felt a bit like you, Anna—uncomfortable being the center of attention. I realized my queer experience makes it hard for me to trust that others outside my group will understand. How could you? But today I'm feeling your interest and support. I think I'll be able to let my internalized guard down a little [smiles] and not have to depend on myself to have all the answers.

In written reflections afterward, participants are able to more fully draw the connections between their life experiences, social positions, and how they approach life and their work as therapists.

Max: My privilege stands out in ways I never saw before. In seventh grade, I had a hard time. Some kids at school picked on me because I was small for my age and liked "girly" things. And I was the only Jewish kid in my class. All the adults in my life supported me. My parents could afford for me to see a therapist, and they arranged for me to go to an expensive summer camp in another state where most of the other kids were also Jewish. That was the only time in my life when I felt different or targeted. Since then, I've been in situations that validated my academic achievements and skills in tennis and golf—thanks to extra coaching at my family's club. I have social capital almost everywhere, even here; since my mom is a clinical social worker, I've been hearing about therapy and meeting therapists all my life.

Charles: I've been a practicing psychologist for almost ten years. One of the things that struck me as I prepared this life map is how alone I've felt all my life. I didn't come out until college and mostly avoided confronting my racial identity. In some ways being a therapist is a safe space behind closed doors. Most of my clients are LGBTQI⁺. We talk a lot about social discourses regarding gender and sexuality. It's important, satisfying work, but I'm thinking now about ways it also keeps me in a bubble where I don't have to be so vulnerable.

Embody a Socioculturally Attuned Contextual Lens

Most of us do not automatically connect awareness to practice. Just as clients need focused, evocative experience to embody and enact the new ways of thinking generated in therapy, socially responsible practice requires systematically examining clinical work. This is best done with others—either through formal supervision or with a group of peers committed to shared growth and holding each other responsible.

Our action research included analyses of how we learned to apply a sociocultural framework. Participant researcher-therapists identified the importance of a supportive but challenging learning community. The outcome was an internalized lens they automatically applied in session. Next, I briefly summarize two of these studies.

Developing a Contextual Clinical Lens

The first study (Esmiol et al., 2012) analyzed the experience of 18 socioculturally diverse interns in four different quarters of an 11-week MFT doctoral practicum. Each practicum was structured as a participatory action project in which issues such as culture, power, race, class, gender, and sexuality were foregrounded in group discussions, weekly writing assignments, and video reviews of their interventions with clients. "Participants kept a weekly journal in which they (a) described the new [clinical/learning] actions they took, (b) reflected on their experience, (c) evaluated the outcome, and (d) reported what actions they would take next" (p. 576). Coding was a group process as members discussed their experience and reflections in the practicum class. For example:

> when a student said, "I was feeling anxious about raising culture as a relational issue, but when I did I was surprised by how engaged my clients got," this was discussed and coded by the group as "experienced positive client response."
>
> (p. 576)

Elisabeth Esmiol, Sarah Delgado, and I followed this initial open coding with focused coding to synthesize the data and organize it into grounded theory that explained the collective experience. This learning model is diagrammed in Figure 12.1. Although the authors emphasized that the experience was more recursive than the "stages" appear, growth began because I, as the instructor/supervisor, centered the issue. They found themselves needing to question practice as usual. Developing a personal contextual lens involved experimentation and reflection within

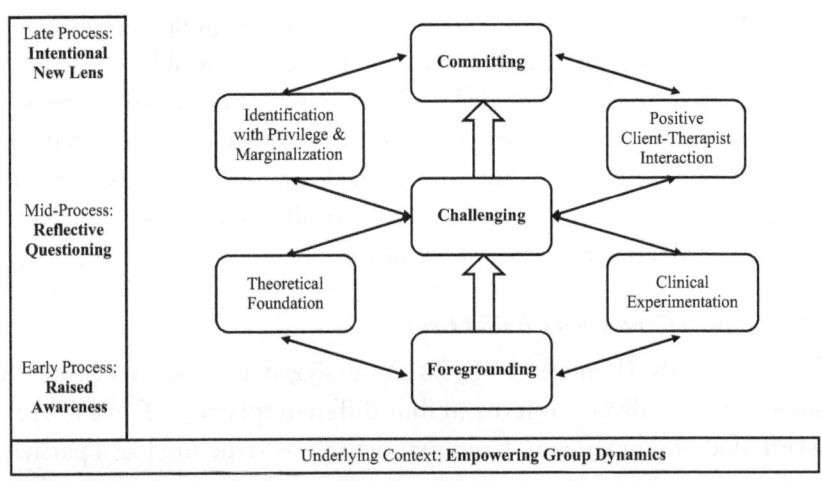

Figure 12.1 Model of Developing Contextual Consciousness

Source: Esmiol, E. E., Knudson-Martin, C., & Delgado, S. (2012). Developing a contextual consciousness: Learning to address gender, societal power, and culture in clinical practice. *Journal of Marital and Family Therapy, 38,* p. 577. (Used with permission).

"productive discomfort" (p. 579). Challenging, at the center of the diagram, is supported by a collaborative community. Esmiol et al. (2012) drew on quotes from final journals to explain:

> "Overall, I felt like I had nothing to prove. I felt like each person in the group knew where I was at in my program and I wasn't overly anxious to perform academically as I have in previous classes" [third author, four months later]. This sense of being accepted as mutual participants in an action research project helped cement the underlying safety that fueled our development. Furthermore, an "air of sincere humility and teachability reigned in the class" [third author, four months later]. By accepting the influence of each other and treating each other as equals, we were able to collaborate together and with our professor as equal participants. In addition, students felt free to question and challenge each other regarding their diverse cultural, racial, sexual, and religious perspectives.
>
> (p. 584)

Learning was both active and personal:

> We felt personally changed as we took ownership of our responsibility to address contextual issues in our own lives and the lives of our clients . . . consistently experiencing positive interactions with our clients [when we addressed contextual issues] was one of the strongest proponents for our adopting a contextual lens in therapy. . . . At some point, the distinction blurred between consciously integrating a contextual lens and automatically viewing clients through this new lens.
>
> (p. 582)

The reported collaborative learning experience mirrors the principles of equity, mutual support, and the Circle of Care foundational to SERT, as well as adoption of third order thinking.

Embodying a Relational Power Lens

A later study (Morrison et al., 2022) expanded on how researcher-participants learned to understand and recognize relational power and embody this lens in their clinical work. While in their MFT master's program, Tori Morrison, Midori Ferris-Wayne, Tahlia Harrison, and Emily Palmgren volunteered to help study markers of power processes in videos of couple therapy sessions and how what therapists did (or did not do) affected the flow of power. In this case, they were not watching their own videos, but rather videos of prior interns who had been supervised from a socioculturally attuned/SERT lens. Some of the sessions were also conducted by Lana Kim or me. The student researchers started the coding before seeing their first clients and continued as they began their internships.

Tori, Midori, Tahlia, and Emily each watched and individually coded the same video session, then we met to discuss their coding and organize the codes into categories that helped us understand what was happening in the sessions. To study *their* learning process during this research, we recorded our discussions. Grounded theory depicting their experience was based on coding transcripts of these conversations. Findings emphasized the value of watching actual therapy sessions with focused attention on the flow of power, that the process of coding involved a deeper-level engagement than is possible in classes or even in supervision of their own cases in which so many factors needed to be discussed. In addition to observing seasoned SERT clinicians, watching therapists in training was valuable, as it required more "work" and "creativity" (p. 414) to recognize power processes and imagine what could have been done. Viewing and coding these videos helped them bring a "critical observer" (p. 414) to their own in-session work.

As a result, they developed awareness of the relational nature of power and its presence in the clinical moment:

> We noticed that when themes including trust, communication, control and influence, vulnerability, or attunement were present in the therapy room, there was often some flow of power occurring in the moment.
>
> (Morrison et al., 2022, p. 412)

Observations made the flow of power real:

> Through our observations, the notion that power is not stagnant as relational systems and society continue to evolve and change became real to us.
>
> (p. 413)

The participant-researchers began to "feel" power and apply this awareness in their own practice, "Because of this study, I have this felt sense. I feel it in my body when something inequitable is happening in the room" (p. 414). They could no longer not see power:

> Once we became aware of the always-present nature of power, we could no longer not see it, regardless of what model or intervention was in use. In one conversation, the second author shared, "This is not . . . a lens that I take on and off at specific strategic moments in therapy; this has become something much more integrated into who I am . . . it's become part of my identity."
>
> (p. 416)

They experienced personal transformation, i.e., embodiment. Like the Esmiol et al. (2012) study, the group process was central:

> There's something that happens when you say it out loud [in this group], like I have this particular reaction when I see male partners using the language of emotional vulnerability in a way to manipulate the conversation . . . I feel it in my body, and it really is hard for me to sit with sometimes, but now that I've said it out loud, I have to address it and work to understand [my reaction].
>
> (p. 415)

Taken together, these studies reinforce that learning to see the workings of societal context and power processes benefits from systematic examination of actual therapy sessions and that such work—especially in relationship with others—is both personal and transformative. This sets the foundation for using your socio-emotional self in practice.

Use Contextual Self-of-the-Therapist in Session

Therapist use of contextual self is at the heart of socioculturally attuned practice. This reciprocal, interactive process of engagement with clients was a key finding of one of the first SERT studies. Melissa Wells, a co-researcher/therapist on our initial SERT team, took nearly verbatim notes of our discussions of what we did and why and where to go next. Julie Estrella, Veronica Kuhn, Cassidy Freitas, and Melissa studied these transcripts to identify what was involved in developing interventions that address the larger context (Estrella et al., 2015). Their findings highlighted that the therapists and the observing/consulting SERT team consistently drew on their personal experience and awareness of sociocultural context, as well as awareness of clients' emotional responses to context, to understand and respond to the clinical moment.

Contextual Emotional Awareness Gives Direction

Conversations revealed that when therapists felt confused or disconnected from clients' responses, they wanted to understand—to know what their clients were experiencing. To do so, they applied a contextual lens to both themselves and their clients, and this enabled them to move toward clients with more compassion *and* devise interventions that interrupted the flow of power. This use of contextual emotional awareness was demonstrated in therapists' descriptions of their in-session experience, as well as in consultations with the observing team. Consultations were especially helpful as "SERT therapists looked to one another to make sure they were not being [blocked] by their own experiences of larger societal discourses" (p. 59). For example, one therapist's emotional response reflected the common gender discourse that the woman should do something to make the relationship work,

> I feel so sad for her. It really feels like she has to do something different—he's not. I'm angry. How can you not be? He seems to be taking over the session and rationalizing everything.
>
> (p. 59)

Emotional awareness of unfairness and anger helped the team devise an alternative response that put the responsibility for change on the male partner:

> We're asking him to hold onto that hot wire and he's jiggling from the shock. We need to help him be grounded . . . coaching him through it by saying "This is important; stretch for her. She needs to know that you know what she's feeling. Try it again."
>
> (p. 59)

Study author Julie reported learning to "use my own experience as an emotional thermometer and . . . connect their experiences to one another's shared experience or to larger societal discourse" (p. 62). In other words, Julie learned to use herself as a socio-emotional bridge.

Sociocultural Attunement as Emotional Resonance

Another study focused specifically on how SERT therapists practice sociocultural attunement (Pandit et al., 2015). Live observers coded what they saw that told them therapists had attained sociocultural attunement, and after the session the therapists responded to "how did you know?" Findings illustrated a reciprocal process of connection as therapists' inner dialogue listened for social discourses, linked emotions and behaviors to discourses and power, and used awareness of their personal experience to inform their clinical actions. Therapists were highly attentive to how clients resonated with their feedback and to their own emotional responses. The authors concluded:

> We knew we demonstrated SCA [sociocultural attunement], not only when we were linking emotions and behaviors to discourse and power, but also from the reaction we felt toward our clients, a profoundly visceral sense of attunement . . . we resonated and sensed connection when clients seemed to feel "felt" (Siegel, 2007) and our sense of SCA included an emotional as well as physiological component . . . a [visceral] feeling of connection.
>
> (p. 73)

Participants in this study described sociocultural attunement as a cyclic relational process of using internal dialogue to "name emotions, experiences, and processes that are influenced by sociocultural context" (p. 74) and sensory awareness of connection with clients and client responses that demonstrate resonance. According to study author Jessica Chen-Feng, this experience of mutual resonance is like tuning a guitar:

> When tuning a guitar, if the tuning isn't right on pitch, then it's not tuned. Both the guitar and the tuning fork must be on the same note. In the same way, both the therapist and the clients must mutually resonate.
>
> (p. 74)

Learning to tune into and use your socio-emotional responses and those of your clients serves as relational glue to cement a therapist-client(s) alliance with the potential for third order change.

Tips for Using Your Socio-Emotional Awareness

Just as in our earlier example in which sharing her life story made Anna feel uncomfortable, as though she had broken a cultural or gender rule, moving toward your contextual experience in session with clients or in supervision/reflection afterward can raise a sense of trepidation, especially when power processes are involved. You may even feel like you're breaking professional rules of "neutral" emotional detachment and objectivity (Hardy, 2022). It can take courage to engage the potent confluence of power, emotion, and societal context (Knudson-Martin et al., 2015); socialization may tell you to step back. The following suggestions will help:

Ten tips for effective contextual use of self:

- Attune to your own sociocultural vulnerability
- Trust that your body and emotional reactions provide helpful feedback
- Use your socio-contextual lens to interpret/reflect upon your and your clients' emotional responses
- Use your wondering or confusion as a basis for questions—and to make sure you really understand
- Note your judgments and consider what values and interests they represent
- Be transparent about what you are seeing or experiencing
- Create a back-and-forth process of shared understanding based on resonance
- Own your role as an instrument of change
- Make interventions based on your attunement to sociocultural emotion
- Use supervision and peers as a sounding board

When Anna first started seeing clients, she was kind and understanding but had difficulty structuring a session and providing leadership that inspired change. In her personal life, Anna had always been good at apprehending another's felt experience; however, her socialized responses as an Asian American female are to accommodate that experience rather than question it. To be an effective instrument of change (Minuchin, 2017, see Chapter 1), Anna needs to be curious about her clients' reactions; rather than assuming she understands, she needs to ask questions informed by her sociocultural awareness and curiosity. Sometimes she has to name what she thinks the client may be experiencing and give voice to it. Doing so raises anxiety and takes courage; but when Anna does, clients respond positively.

For example, while working with the mother of a "misbehaving" young child, the mother was always attentive and open to suggestion. Anna resonates with her client's compliant behavior. Viewing her own and her client's experience through a contextual lens makes her wonder what else the mother may experience but not feel entitled to express. Anna is moved toward that curiosity in developing her attuned response:

Anna: Being a good mother is important to you. I can see that, feel it in how faithfully you work to help [child]. [client nods] I'm wondering what else is going on for you inside. It must be hard to feel loving toward [the child] all the time.

This response is hard for Anna to make. She senses social prohibition to speak of mothers as anything but loving. Yet using her own internal response and contextual awareness to guide how she questions and relates to the mother opens discussion of the mother's fear of the anger she sometimes feels toward her child and related feelings of helplessness and self-loathing that are important to address but had not previously been revealed. This lesson, and others like it, helps Anna value her own experience and voice in applying her clinical role.

Shade's lessons about use of contextual self in therapy are different. After living as a socially marginalized person for many years, Shade has a well-developed antenna for the presence of power inequities and skilled strategies for enacting personal autonomy despite the forces against them; they do not give the pain of ostracization space to control their life. When clients' life stories and struggles include the consequences of social inequities (as so many do), Shade readily intuits the power and larger context issues and can summarize and name them and identify potential resources. But taking in painful experiences so that clients "feel felt" is challenging for them because it involves accessing their own sociocultural vulnerabilities. While it is easier to move toward enacting change, they need to first stay emotionally *with* their clients and form a more collaborative process.

For example, Slade often tries to engage a powerful male partner in attuning to his spouse without first seeking to apprehend the man's socio-emotional experience and then is frustrated when he "resists." To attune to him (and his partner), Slade has to trust that the vulnerability they feel in the face of the client's enactments of power is an important indicator and respond by seeking to better know and resonate with the emotional underpinnings that maintain the client's power position. Then Slade is able to engage him in shifting the flow of power in his relationship.

Accountability Across the Professional Lifespan

Using self to engage with power and the consequences of power is challenging for nearly everyone, regardless of career stage. The goal is not for your emotional sensitivity to go away; it is to develop awareness of its contextual meaning and to use this information to effectively guide your clinical responses. Charles, who has been practicing for almost ten years, is getting better and better in recognizing when his sociocultural vulnerability presents as "protective pleasantness," especially with heterosexual White men. Now when he feels this, he is reminded to go toward his clients' sociocultural experience and get to know them. Charles regularly meets with a peer consultation group to process challenging cases, and as he does, he becomes ever more aware of his responses to the racial, gender, sexual, and socioeconomic nuances of his socio-emotional self, not only in his clinical practice but also in his personal life and social environment.

As a family therapy doctoral student, Max also participates in a clinical practicum and supervision, even though he is already licensed. Like Charles, he appreciates the accountability and "productive discomfort" these developmental activities provide. As a feminist, socially progressive, White, Jewish man, Max is exploring how he tends to respond to power imbalances by trying to protect or rescue those in less powerful positions. He's chagrined to discover how easily his responses can actually reinforce societal power processes. His supervisor and practicum group are helping him recognize these paternal emotions in session and channel it toward curiosity about his client's relational goals and strengths and work collaboratively to envision more equitable relationships.

All of the activities and practices described in this chapter are relevant across the professional lifespan. They apply to teaching, training, and supervisory roles, as well as clinical practice. Use the Circle of Care as a guide to your professional as well as personal relationships.

Therapist Checklist: Engaging Contextual Self

- ☐ Develop contextual awareness through reflection, shared interaction, and witnessing
- ☐ Pay attention to and value sensory, felt awareness
- ☐ Bring internalized messages about "normal," self, and others into the open
- ☐ Facilitate dialogue rather than debate
- ☐ Listen from a position of curiosity, complexity, uncertainty, and willingness to be emotionally impacted
- ☐ Engage through a reciprocal process of cyclic resonance
- ☐ Serve as a socio-emotional bridge between client and context
- ☐ Devise clinical responses based on contextual emotional awareness

13

STUDY CLINICAL PRACTICE

Like therapy, the answers research elicits depend on who you study, the questions you ask, and what you focus on. To know what is involved in creating a particular clinical outcome, you need to study practice. Socio-Emotional Relationship Therapy evolved out of action research directed toward learning how to better address gender, power, and other larger context issues in our clinical practice (see Chapter 1). Through practice-based research over more than 15 years, my colleagues, students, and I learned from our work and that of others to delineate the socially responsible approach to practice illustrated in this book. This ongoing linkage of research and day-to-day practice is both unusual and necessary (Simon, 2018; St. George et al., 2015).

◊ *You can and should research your practice*

In this chapter you will learn about the value of practice-based research and some of the principles involved. I will share the methods the SERT team used to research our clinical work and highlight key findings. The good news is that practice-based research is flexible; you can develop a method that works for you. You can integrate research into your practice, even without external funding. Practice-based research prioritizes discovery (Greenberg, 1991); it encourages and learns from creativity. I hope

DOI: 10.4324/9781003270232-13

this overview of the SERT research process inspires you to apply third order thinking to create research that helps you and others expand the potentialities that can be activated within therapeutic encounters.

What Is Practice-Based Research?

The field of systems/relational therapy emerged as practitioners reflected on, discussed, demonstrated, taught, and wrote about their work—often with teams observing "behind the mirror" (Hoffman, 2002). Though they published virtually no research on the processes or outcomes involved (Hardy et al., 2020), their tradition of reflecting on and questioning their work generated innovative, transformational clinical models.

When practitioners do not methodically reflect on their practices and share their findings, much important clinical knowledge is lost. Methods for conducting practice-based research vary from regular meetings to discuss and modify practice (perhaps similar to the founders of systems/relational therapy) to rigorous application of qualitative methodologies (e.g., grounded theory, discourse analysis, thematic analyses) and a variety of quantitative and mixed methods approaches (Johnson et al., 2020). What matters is that you identify a particular question and take a systematic approach to studying it.

The following principles guide practice-based research:

- Knowledge is not separate from how it is produced
- Inquiry is guided by intentional focus and goals
- Focus is on processes of change leading to desired outcomes
- There is access to personal voice and experience
- Emphasis is on discovery rather than verification
- Engagement in research improves practice

There are many questions to ask that will extend what we know about the *how* of practice. What you ask depends on the models you are working from and the particular issues that concern you. What you want to know, your context, and who your audience is shape the method you use (Daly, 2007). In other words, in practice-based research you are studying what you already know a lot about. Your research lens focuses you toward seeing and understanding what you would otherwise miss. According to Daly (2007), like family therapy, you take a stance of "not-knowing . . .

[which] does not mean, however that the therapist (or the researcher!) knows nothing or asks nothing" (p. 5). It means respect and openness to newness. According to Daly, this requires:

> learning how to observe, how to situate ourselves in order to see most effectively, and commitment to return again and again to our observations in order to build confidence in our understanding.
>
> (p. 4)

When developing a clinical model, as our team did with SERT, it is important that the researchers' observations and analyses work within the conceptual foundations of the model (Greenberg, 2007). You also need to be able to identify instances of the phenomenon of interest. Our SERT team needed a definition of power to guide our observations and interpretations. To detect power imbalances, we began with Anne Mahoney's and my previously published (Mahoney & Knudson-Martin, 2009) questions for assessing power in relationships based on relative status, attention to other, accommodation patterns, and well-being (see Chapter 4, Figure 4.1). Since our research emphasized discovery, our understanding of and ability to recognize power processes evolved over time. For example, a major outcome of participating in SERT practice research was learning to see inherent relational power processes when trust, communication, control and influence, vulnerability, or attunement were present in session (Morrison et al., 2022).

◊ *Practice-based research involves learning to see more clearly*

Similarly, researching the "how" of therapy means observing, distinguishing, and understanding different kinds of clinical circumstances/actions/responses on the part of therapists and clients and their impact on what happens next and the outcomes of interest. An important research focus for the SERT team was recognizing when sociocultural discourses were present, how therapists did (or did not) respond, and the impact of these actions on power and therapeutic goals, both in the short term and over the course of therapy. It was useful that at least some of the researchers had first-hand knowledge of the cases.

The intent is not to be "disinterested" observers, but rather observers open to discovery and intentional about exploring through multiple perspectives. As Sally St. George, Dan Wulff, and Karl Tomm reported about their experience doing practice-based research, the shared focus and commitment expand clinical learning and knowledge from an individual to a community endeavor and improve practice while also contributing to the collective clinical knowledge base (St. George et al., 2015).

SERT Action Research

We characterized our SERT inquiry as action research (Coghlan & Brannick, 2010). Action research involves planned actions to create "real-time change" (p. 15), while also making sense of what happened and developing useable knowledge or theory from this analysis. Action researchers draw on a variety of methods to gather and analyze data. Rather than being separate from these data, the researchers are connected to it; they engage in an ongoing cycle of taking action, evaluating action, constructing understanding, and planning new action.

The SERT team began with live observations of therapy sessions and analyses focused on developing a set of clinical competencies that informed subsequent clinical actions. Over the years, some members left the team and others joined, while the focus and methods evolved to address new questions, as described in this chapter. In all, over 60 researcher-clinicians have been part of the SERT team to date, representing a diverse range of social locations and perspectives.

Identifying SERT Competencies

The SERT clinical competencies emerged through a process similar to the consensual qualitative approach (Hill et al., 1997) "in which consensus is used to examine individual experiences, process multiple perspectives, and arrive at shared judgments about the meaning of the data" (Knudson-Martin et al., 2015, p. 207). At Loma Linda University, with institutional review board (IRB) approval, our clinical research team met weekly for six years. Some team members conducted live therapy while the rest watched and made notes about what happened; then we discussed our observations and experiences and refined our clinical actions.

While similar to live group supervision in some ways, our research process was more focused and systematic. The first year, team member Melissa Wells made transcriptions of our conversations. Douglas Huenergardt, Ketsia LaFontant, and I met between team meetings to identify themes in these notes, which we brought back to the group. Each team member responded to the themes until everyone's perspective was taken into account. From these themes we evolved a preliminary set of competencies, which we then used to guide our observations of the therapy sessions and raise new questions, as well as simultaneously inform therapists' subsequent work on the cases.

Our conversations involved a back and forth between detailed explorations of specific moments in the case at hand—the meaning of the contextual issues in the clients' experience, how therapists and clients responded, what worked and what interfered—and fine-tuning our practice-based clarification of the related clinical competencies. To implement these competencies, we discovered that therapists first had to develop contextual awareness, then needed to track the relational impact, followed by leadership in addressing the issue in session, and facilitating client empowerment (i.e., third order change).

We formulated a scale to help us both evaluate skill development and further determine what is involved in each competency. For example, Table 13.1 shows how we delineated levels of proficiency for competency 1, the ability to identify enactments of cultural discourse. This iterative process resulted in a set of seven clinical competencies for addressing gender, power, and societal context, along with the skills needed to implement them (Appendix I; Knudson-Martin et al., 2015). These initial seven competencies provided a foundation for further study and the development of SERT.

Developing a Map for Practice

Grounded theory methods are especially well-suited to describe or explain interpersonal processes (Charmaz, 2014). To get another perspective on what the early SERT team talked about and how we developed interventions to address the impacts of societal power, Julie Estrella, Veronica Kuhn, Cassidy Freitas, and Melissa Wells used grounded theory analysis to model our deliberative process (Estrella et al., 2015). According to

Table 13.1 Identify Enactments of Cultural Discourse

1–Limited	2–Aware	3–Tracks Process	4–Leads	5–Empowers
Therapist is aware that clients belong to a particular cultural context but is uncertain about how they are organized by culture or their relationship to it.	Therapist expands awareness of cultural context to include intersections with gender, class, race, religion, and other significant personal contexts such as prison experience and work environment.	Therapist identifies cultural markers in the conversation but does not explore how they uniquely link to personal experience or consider other discourses that might be involved.	Therapist extends conversations regarding cultural discourse— and alternative discourses— that influence personal experience and clients' patterns of relating.	Therapist guides clients to see their relationships as part of social patterns larger than themselves.

Kathy Charmaz (2014), researchers begin with curiosity and theoretical sensitivity to the topic, but with no predetermined categories or variables. They first use open coding of the transcript or observations to name what is happening through the perspective of the research lens. This organizes the data into conceptual bits that can then be formulated into larger categories. Theory is developed as researchers explore the dimensions of each category (focused coding) and how changes in one category relate to changes in another (selective coding). Julie's team used this process to analyze nearly verbatim transcripts of the SERT team's 2009 conversations and create a conceptual map of what guided the initial therapy/research team as we developed contextually informed interventions.

◊ *Sociocultural attunement and transforming power are connected*

This analysis captured a more personal component of the SERT team's practice (see Chapter 12), with discussions about identifying, disrupting, and transforming power at the center surrounded by awareness of their own and the clients' sociocultural experience and a contextual lens (Estrella et al., 2015). It became clear that sociocultural attunement and transforming power were interconnected and often difficult to sort out. The three-phase clinical process described in this book began to emerge as we grappled with how attention to power and sociocultural attunement promote relational alternatives based on equity and mutual support. Douglas Huenergardt and I summarized what we were learning (Knudson-Martin & Huenergardt, 2015):

> [Phase I] The challenge is to validate and support each partner without inadvertently organizing therapy around the dominant partner's view and to explore client goals in context of mutual support. (p. 9)
>
> [Phase II] We found that identifying power issues does not create change in and of itself. Before other significant progress can be made, therapists need to provide leadership that interrupts the flow of power so that partners can begin relating from more equitable positions. (p. 9–10)
>
> [Phase III] It is also not enough to identify and interrupt the flow of power. Therapists need to provide leadership in facilitating alternative experience.
>
> (p. 10)

Studying Clinical Actions

With an initial set of SERT competencies and general clinical sequence to work from, our ongoing weekly team meetings identified new questions and areas of focus as we worked with new cases. To augment our observing team, we collected transcripts of couple therapy contributed by marriage and family therapy (MFT) doctoral students and faculty. With support from the team as a whole, subgroups carried out grounded theory studies on specific issues.

The first of these studies was by Jessica ChenFeng and Aimee Galick early in their involvement in the SERT team (ChenFeng & Galick, 2015). They started coding transcripts of 23 couple therapy sessions through a focus on how societal discourses were present in session. When they found gender to be the most evident discourses, they narrowed their focus:

> When we began the grounded theory analysis, we had no idea what we would find because between us we knew very little about the dominant gender discourses that influence heterosexual couple

interactions. It is one thing to read about how gender organizes families and couples and another to be able to see it happening in moment-to-moment therapeutic processes.

(pp. 42–43)

Jessica and Aimee found that therapists regularly (a) reinforced male privilege by validating men while minimizing women's experiences, (b) expected women to accommodate by asking them to change, and (c) protected men from shame by reinforcing the idea that women are responsible for relationships.

Jessica and Aimee, and our team, did not anticipate that therapists (members of our early team and our colleagues) so frequently perpetuated male power. The study helped us see the interconnections between social discourse and norms and gendered power. It also identified exceptions that worked to interrupt gendered power, for instance, when therapists gave voice to and acknowledged alternative discourses such as validating relational needs, especially for men. The research identified the importance of making the implicit explicit, for example, by naming the discourse of female responsibility and highlighting examples of mutually supportive behavior. This study, together with a similar one conducted by Avigail Ward (Ward & Knudson-Martin, 2012), helped our team be more intentional and accountable for our clinical actions in each phase of therapy.

Recognizing Our Clinical Roles

Our team realized that identifying societal discourses and attuning to sociocultural emotion were preliminary to helping clients transform power imbalances and surprisingly elusive. Mia Pandit, Jessica ChenFeng, and Young Joo Kang took the lead in a grounded theory study of our team's experience of practicing sociocultural attunement (see Chapter 12). Behind the mirror observers focused specifically on what therapists did that suggested they were socioculturally attuned. Immediately afterward, in-session therapists wrote responses to how they knew they were socioculturally attuned (Pandit et al., 2014).

The team discussed our written responses, then Mia, Young Joo, and Jessica used grounded theory coding to develop a model of what constituted the practice of sociocultural attunement. Three aspects of the therapist's role stood out: (a) using a sociocultural lens to guide overall clinical focus; (b) interpretations of clinical process that link emotion and behavior to social discourse and were visible in questions asked, validation of emotion, and naming of sociocultural influence; and (c) attention to client resonance, i.e., evidence of a reciprocal feeling of connection. Their grounded theory model of sociocultural attunement highlighted the interconnections between each aspect of these skills.

◊ *Need for a strong leadership role*

Kirstee Williams (Williams et al., 2013) took understanding of what is required to create clinical change a step further with a task analysis of heterosexual cases involving infidelity. In a task analysis, researchers first identify clinical segments in which the desired change was accomplished and then ascertain the tasks involved in getting from the event marker (beginning of the change sequence) to positive resolution (Greenberg, 2007). Using the SERT team as experts to verify, Kirstee and Aimee Galick identified 13 successful change events and 7 unsuccessful ones, each beginning when therapists directed the focus of therapeutic conversation on the relationship between the couple.

> Change events are best examples of creating the desired change. Therefore, in watching videotapes, we looked for moments in which we thought the four components of mutual support (mutual attunement, mutual influence, shared vulnerability, and shared relational responsibility) were occurring between the partners.
> (Williams et al., p. 287)

Findings indicated four necessary tasks: (a) creating an equitable foundation for healing, (b) creating space for alternative gender discourse, (c) pursuing relational responsibility of the powerful partner, and (d) new experience of mutual support. The authors emphasized the need for therapists to take an active leadership role in creating space for an alternative gender discourse:

> Successful resolution required persistent efforts by the therapist to engage the powerful partner and support the less powerful

partner. Techniques ranged from helping the couple stay on task to structuring the session to initially engage the powerful partner in therapy, as well as therapist willingness to challenge power positions.

(p. 289)

Creating and Sustaining Change

Since relational engagement of the powerful partner proved significant to change that reflects mutual support (Williams et al., 2013), Sarah Samman analyzed 28 videos of couple therapy sessions (including 11 couples and 9 therapists) in which couples "reported high levels of distress as well as male partner relational disengagement" (Samman & Knudson-Martin, 2015, p. 82). Our purpose was "to develop a grounded theory about how therapeutic interventions can invite and sustain male relational engagement based on observations of therapists utilizing the SERT model" (p. 82). Rather than looking at specific change events, this study examined two or three sessions with each couple in their entirety.

◊ *Relationally engaging powerful partners must include both relational intent and impact*

We found five therapist interventions that consistently worked to relationally engage powerful male partners, as illustrated in Figure 13.1. Therapists had to use *all* of them. Importantly, naming and validating their relational intent needed to be immediately followed by highlighting the relational impact on his partner:

> Male validation without also highlighting the behavioral impact on his partner tended to reinforce the one-down position of the female partner. The most successful interventions were when men experienced personal and relational validation while also being able to recognize and take accountability for the impact of their behaviors on their partners. When these happened together, this effectively encouraged shared relational responsibility without reinforcing male privilege in session.

(p. 88)

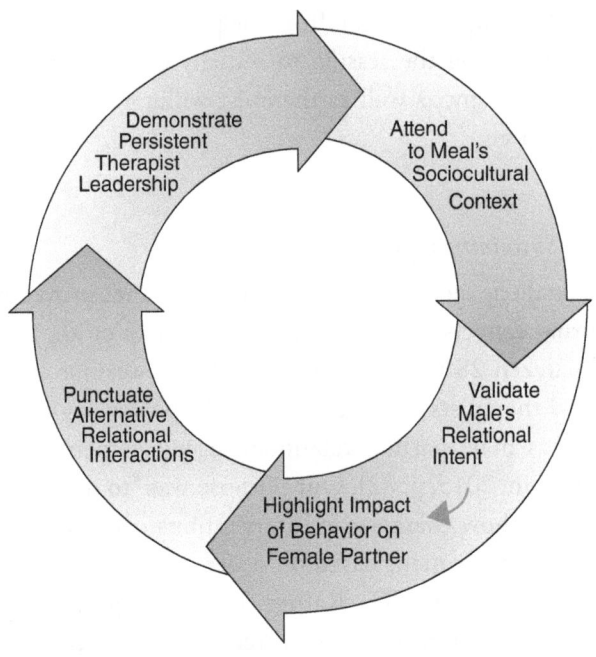

Figure 13.1 Relationally engaging heterosexual men in couple therapy

Source: Samman, S., & Knudson-Martin, C. (2015). Relational engagement in heterosexual couple therapy: Helping men move from "I" to "we." In C. Knudson-Martin, M. A. Wells, & S. K. Samman (Eds.), *Socio-emotional relationship therapy: Bridging emotion, societal context, and couple interaction* (pp. 79–91). AFTA Springer Briefs in Family Therapy. Springer. (used with permission).

Overall, the male partners moved from an individualistic mindset that kept them disengaged from their partners and focused on their own needs and interests to relational engagement that shared responsibility for the relationship and demonstrated attunement to her well-being. The study helped to clarify the importance of focusing on both relational desires and relational accountability.

◊ *Relational safety involves mutual vulnerability*

As we evolved SERT, it became clear that interrupting power imbalances was necessary to creating relational safety. It was more complicated in some cases than in others, particularly when one or both partners had histories of childhood abuse. Melissa Wells took the lead in an in-depth study of SERT therapy over time with four such heterosexual couples (Wells et al., 2017). Multiple team members completed line by line, constant comparison coding of 40 transcripts—10 sessions randomly selected across time with each couple. Focused and selective coding followed, together with analytic memos and regular meetings to compare codes and raise new questions that resulted in a grounded theory model of the key clinical processes involved in developing relational safety (Charmaz, 2014). To test the credibility of the model, Melissa conduced posttherapy interviews with two of the couples and applied the findings to current cases to confirm applicability of the model beyond the original studied couples.

◊ *The power context drives emotion and safety*

As the analysis (Wells et al., 2017) began to come together, it became clear that male emotion was driving the process in these heterosexual childhood survivor couples. To understand this interaction, the research team had to understand the sociocultural context of their emotion. The men in this study held a "dark view of themselves in the world," (p. 129) with corresponding nihilistic feelings of powerlessness relating to their experience of abuse. This linked with socialized male expectations that their needs be primary. From this position of "disentitled power," and compounded by other forms of social marginalization, the male partners appeared to protect themselves from vulnerability by acting harshly/dismissively toward their partners. Female partners responded with "reactive power . . . a defense against her fear of being vulnerable when she feels powerless and unsafe with her intimate partner" (p. 130). Clinical change followed men's shifts in use of power:

> As it became safer to be more vulnerable with each other, the men moved away from the automatic use of disentitled power, and the women reciprocally engaged more frequently through relational power. In the course of becoming mutually supportive, the partners demonstrated more trusting responses.
>
> (p. 132)

◊ *Sociocultural attunement to emotion is crucial*

The emphasis on shared vulnerability as the path to shifting from a power position to mutuality based on trust stood out to us as new information.

Facilitating this process included heightened attention to the sociocultural context of emotion:

> In order to help the couple build mutuality, they first had to experience safety. The therapists facilitated this by socio-emotionally attuning to the gendered context of each partner's protective responses. . . . The therapists worked to help the partners identify how their emotions were linked to disentitled and reactive power exchanges.
>
> (p. 133)

The findings detailed what is involved in mutual vulnerability: "being in touch with one's own emotions and their effect on the other partner; the capacity for self-reflection; recognizing one's positive relational intentions; accepting the partner's feedback; and desiring to tend to the partner's needs" (p. 136). As described in Chapter 5, these capacities tend to be gendered. When not mutual, they create and reinforce power imbalances. The Wells et al. (2017) analysis charted a detailed and nuanced understanding of how to work with the sociocultural connections between power, emotion, and vulnerability.

Teaching and Advancing SERT

When I moved to Lewis & Clark College in the fall of 2014, Socio-Emotional Relationship Therapy was well established, with in-press publications detailing the SERT competencies (Knudson-Martin et al., 2015; Knudson-Martin & Huenergardt, 2015). At Lewis & Clark, I was working with master's students just learning to do family therapy. My colleagues and I were interested in continuing to advance the development of SERT through teaching and action research. My Lewis & Clark IRB application listed the following initial goals:

(1) To advance development of an observational coding tool to guide training and research in Socio-Emotional Relationship therapy (SERT)

(2) To better articulate the clinical processes involved in practicing SERT

Toward this end, students interested in working from the SERT model invited clients to allow videos of their couple therapy sessions to become part of a SERT video bank and analyzed for research focused on "what works." Concurrently, I met regularly with a team of faculty colleagues at other master's-level MFT training programs to examine our experiences teaching and supervising SERT, using the evolving coding tool, and applying SERT across cultural contexts.

Recognizing Enactments of SERT Competencies

We introduced the development of SERT competencies scale (Appendix I; Knudson-Martin et al., 2015) to MFT trainees and engaged them in coding video of therapy sessions by identifying enactments of the competencies and noting the relevant time interval and level of competency, including missed opportunities. The trainee/researchers independently coded selected therapy sessions, then met biweekly with Lana Kim and me to discuss their coding. The goals were to see if the observers could recognize and agree on demonstrations of the competencies and to explore what is involved in enacting them.

Conversation regarding rationales for their codes was useful in deepening understanding of the complexities of applying the SERT competencies and contributed substantially to the observers' learning (O'Halloran et al., 2017; Morrison et al., 2022; Robillard et al., 2018). However, the competencies were hard to reliably distinguish because they tended to work together, and demonstrating them involved both conceptual and intervention skills.

◊ *Coding sessions overall achieved consensus*

As we continued to experiment with various coding formats, we learned that coders were able to distinguish sessions that adhered to the SERT model overall and that once they learned SERT concepts and the Circle of Care (Appendix A), even students who had not yet begun to see clients could recognize power imbalances in whose interests were the focus of attention, who attuned to and accommodated whom, and who focused on the relationship and their partner and who did not. Coders could also describe what therapists did or did not do in response and how clients responded. Recognizing societal discourses and sociocultural attunement was more challenging. We also learned that interrupting power did not work well if therapists did not connect power processes to the sociocultural context. These two dimensions—attention to power and sociocultural attunement—intersected in successful applications of SERT.

- *Attention to power and sociocultural attunement emerged as core dimensions*

Overall session ratings on (a) therapist adherence, (b) transforming the power imbalance, (c) sociocultural attunement, and (d) client responsiveness were the most reliable measures for identifying the application of SERT, as illustrated in Figure 13.2. An expanded session coding tool that includes more descriptors of the observation criteria is presented in Appendix H. We found that coding for specific clinical sequence competencies over time intervals in the session helps observers focus and assess the case. A version of the overall session coding tool with ten-minute intervals is in Appendix G. While overall ratings do *not* include a quantitative summary of the interval ratings, the process of coding competencies throughout the session enables coders to make good judgments

Therapist Adherence ("sticking to model")

0	1	2	3
Almost never	a little bit	tries, but let's go	persistent

Comments:

Transforming the Power Imbalance

0	1	2	3
Reinforces imbalance	maintains imbalance	creates opening for shift	enacts shift to mutuality

Comments:

Sociocultural Attunement

0	1	2	3
Colonizes	no curiosity/unpacking	connects to some	connects with SC Emotion

Comments:

Client Responsiveness (Clients connect to mutual ideals and/or SERT interventions)

0	1	2	3
not at all	a little	somewhat	a lot

Comments:

Overall Observations regarding session:

Figure 13.2 SERT Coding Tool

of the session overall. Coding competencies at time intervals also helps raise new questions about the case and SERT practice and is useful for detailed qualitative analysis or supervision. Appendix E includes an evaluation format for each competency.

From a Linear to Circular Clinical Sequence

Lana Kim, Lindsey Nice, Elisabeth Esmiol Wilson, and I met regularly to evaluate our experiences teaching and researching the SERT clinical sequence and competencies. Following our practice-based evidence that the SERT competencies work together and reinforce each other, we shifted the clinical sequence from a linear one (Knudson-Martin & Huenergardt, 2015) to a circular one (Appendix C). We renamed the phases with active, readily recognizable terms that capture the essence of SERT (position, interrupt, and practice) and reorganized competencies that had been difficult to distinguish. Since prior research and our ongoing analysis pointed to the importance of validating relational work and making relational consequences visible, we modified competency 1b and added competency 2a. Phase 3 was also reworked to clarify the skills involved in making change "stick."

Applying Socio-Emotional Awareness

Studying SERT heightened personal awareness of the socio-emotional aspects of our own clinical and supervisory roles. For example, Lana Kim, Jessica ChenFeng, Elisabeth Esmiol Wilson, and I set out to clarify how we practice sociocultural attunement to emotion in supervision (Kim et al., 2017). Using a consensual iterative method similar to the original SERT research team (which we all were part of), we determined that:

> Applying sociocultural attunement to supervision represents a significant departure from supervision as an instructional, supportive process focused primarily on modalities/theories, and case conceptualization. Instead . . . we assume a value stance that attunement to emotion as a sociocultural experience is at the heart of relationship building and is critical for the change process—for both client and supervisee.
>
> (p. 57)

We concluded supervision is isomorphic to therapy, that "change happens through the experience of feeling another person attuned to one's own SCE [sociocultural emotion]" (p. 65) and involves the following supervisory skills:

- Use a sociocultural framework
- Socially locate oneself
- Validate one's own sociocultural emotion
- Tolerate discomfort
- Pursue sociocultural emotion
- Demonstrate supervisory leadership
- Practice psychological resonance

We came to understand supervision as a reflexive process in which the supervisee experiences the supervisor as "someone who is open to learning and growing with [them] in their shared supervisory relationship" (p. 67). We expanded our awareness of socially responsible practice, concluding that "the supervisory relationship is a place where cultural equity is lived out" (p. 69).

Similarly, our growing socio-emotional awareness led Jessica Chen-Feng, Lana Kim, and I, together with international Chinese student Yuwei Wu, to examine our cases involving couples of Asian American heritages (ChenFeng et al., 2017). We met regularly to hold ourselves accountable to attuning to our clients, not through our lenses, but to see them within their own worlds. We focused on understanding their internal lived and felt reality and identified three themes that helped us make sense of our clients' experience—intangible loss, quiet fortitude/not burdening others, and duty to the family. Rather than stepping back in an attempt to be culturally sensitive, we had to socioculturally engage, understanding the Circle of Care and the flow of power through this felt awareness:

> to empower clients requires a proactive engagement and willingness to recognize and interrupt power imbalances. This work is inherently curious and appreciative. It involves a willingness to

acculturate ourselves to clients' multiple cultural worlds, while bringing an awareness of our own multiple cultural worlds and challenging rigid internalizations of cultural discourses.

(p. 570)

By centering socio-emotional engagement, we countered the stereotype of Asians as "not emotional" and instead oriented ourselves (and our clients) toward a culturally nuanced awareness of felt emotion.

Highlighting Sociocultural Attunement to Vulnerability

As you read our process of SERT discovery involving multiple projects and methods, you may have noticed our increasing awareness of what it means to work with emotion and the importance of vulnerability. Our study, *Sociocultural Attunement to Vulnerability in Couple Therapy: Fulcrum for Changing Power Processes* (Knudson-Martin et al., 2021), represented significant clarity regarding how sociocultural attunement and interrupting power processes work together.

We had learned from previous research that efforts to interrupt power did not seem to work when therapists interrupted by asking powerful persons to be vulnerable or attune to their partners without also bringing contextual meaning to power processes. In this study, we zeroed in on how this happens when therapy appears to successfully shift power imbalances. Beginning with 139 sessions in the SERT data bank, Emily Gibbs and Raquel Harmon identified 72 sessions with heterosexual couples with clearly distinguishable power disparities between partners, good audio quality, and access to multiple sessions over time, including nine couples and 12 therapists.

◊ *Success in transforming power involves attuning to sociocultural vulnerability*

Emily and Raquel began open coding by watching multiple videos of each couple and making notes about what was happening line by line, using the SERT lens as a theoretical guide. Lana Kim and I met regularly with them to discuss the codes and reflect on which seemed most salient and to decide which segments to return to for further analysis.

> A key analytic turn occurred when we found that shifts in power seemed to occur when therapists were able to use sociocultural awareness to engage less relationally attuned partners around their vulnerability. As a result, we tightened the analytic focus to explore sociocultural processes involved when working with vulnerability and transcribed specific video segments that informed this question.
>
> (p. 1157)

Subsequent coding identified different ways clients express sociocultural vulnerabilities. These were introduced in Chapter 2. The grounded theory analysis found that working with the connections to sociocultural vulnerability and power distinguished successful interventions and this involved *all* three of the following clinical actions:

(a) Identifying the power context of vulnerability
(b) Using responsive persistence to shift power inequities
(c) Facilitating mutual sociocultural attunement to vulnerability

A key take-away was that when power inequities persist, it is important to return to sociocultural attunement to vulnerability.

◊ *When power persists, attune to sociocultural vulnerability*

The case examples in this book incorporate our cumulative SERT studies. And since findings from the "ground up" invite researchers to return to the theoretical literature to help explain them (Charmaz, 2014), the SERT framework offered here is the result of a circular process between our action research and integration of the works of others. As a result, SERT theory on the connections between emotion, societal discourse, power, and the process of change has also evolved, becoming clearer and more focused over time.

Future Evolution

When US Surgeon General Vivek Murthy embarked on a listening tour, he found a crisis of social disconnection (U.S. Surgeon General's Advisory on the Healing Effects of Social Connection and Community, 2023):

> People began to tell me they felt isolated, invisible, and insignificant. Even when they couldn't put their finger on the word "lonely," time and time again, people of all ages and socioeconomic backgrounds, from every corner of the country, would tell me, "I have to shoulder all of life's burdens by myself," or "if I disappear tomorrow, no one will even notice." It was a lightbulb moment for me: social disconnection was far more common than I had realized.
>
> (p. 4)

There is growing research regarding the deleterious effects of societal inequities and dominant discourses that limit relational connections and health (e.g., McDowell et al., 2023; Watson et al., 2020). The healing effects of connectedness and a felt sense of belonging at intimate, family, community, and larger societal levels are substantial. The US Surgeon General's Advisory Report (2023) is a call to action to create social structures and relationships that build and support a culture of connection. How family practitioners and psychotherapists practice our roles has the potential to interrupt societal discourses and power processes that marginalize relational values and the worth, value, and health of many and to promote transformative third order change based on more equitable and relational alternatives.

Theory regarding the need for socially responsible clinical practices that take into account the impact of the larger societal context is growing (e.g., Dumaresque et al., 2018; Lini & Bertrando, 2022; Murphy & Hecker, 2020). Clinicians need to examine the values and interests our work supports and move toward contextually conscious practice. The practice-based research on Socio-Emotional Relationship Therapy reported here details *how* to do equity-based work that connects the dots between individual and relational well-being, client concerns and symptoms, and societal power processes. There is a need for so much more.

Socially responsible clinician-researchers need to be clear about which outcomes we measure. The SERT research began with mutual support as a desired relational outcome and research-based awareness that societal power processes interfere with its accomplishment (see Chapter 1). With an operationalized definition of power as whose interests and needs are valued, noticed, and attended to in relationship patterns and in societal structures and discourses, observers can readily qualitatively identify power inequities.

Studying power quantitatively is more challenging because the nature of power means it tends to be invisible to those who hold it and may seem "natural" to observers. Power is thus difficult to self-report and requires a systemic assessment of the power balance. For example, when Tom Luttrell (2016) asked whether the Relationship Balance Assessment—a measure of power that incorporates elements of the Circle of Care—could predict satisfaction in heterosexual relationships, he found that averaging individual scores yielded limited predictability. However, calculations of couples' *differences* in the perception of power, especially the woman's perspective, correlated with relational, sexual, and life satisfaction.

The many studies that have comprised the SERT action research thus far constitute a substantial body of information regarding the clinical processes that facilitate equity and mutual support as desired outcomes. With training to identify power processes and the presence of societal discourses, coders can use the SERT overall session rating scale to rate adherence to the SERT model and whether the session overall reinforces power imbalances or represents a shift or movement toward mutuality and the extent to which therapists colonize or impose dominant social discourses or connect with sociocultural emotion, as well as how responsive clients are to ideals of mutuality and SERT interventions. This coding tool offers the potential for future research that links socially responsible clinical practices to outcomes that reflect social connection, mutually supportive relationships, and health based on equitable worth and value as human beings.

Such research focuses beyond alleviation of individual symptoms to targeting the relational and social systems that give rise to and maintain them, and employs research designs that capture systemic processes

(Bermúdez et al., 2016; Priest et al., 2019). As a foundation for such research, scholar-practitioners need research that examines the detail of clinical discourse to identify when and how dominant discourses are present in clinical work. The discourse analyses conducted by Olga Smoliak and colleagues (2022a, 2022b, 2023) are excellent examples.

What and how we research depends on what we notice and value and what the systems that support and/or constrain our work value (Bermúdez et al., 2016). The future evolution of SERT—and socially responsible practice more broadly—depends on people like you, working in different contexts and using a range of methodologies to build on, and go beyond, existing theory and research to evolve and validate clinical practices that place equity, relationality, and mutual support at the center.

Therapist Checklist: Study Clinical Practice

- ☐ Integrate research into your own practice
- ☐ Apply third order thinking to clinical research
- ☐ Focus on relationality, mutual support, and equity as valued outcomes
- ☐ Recognize when and how dominant societal discourses are present in clinical work and research methodologies
- ☐ Identify the clinical processes involved in attaining desired clinical outcomes
- ☐ Use research to improve and be accountable for your clinical roles
- ☐ Integrate your practice-based findings with the larger knowledge base

14

CO-CREATE THE FUTURE

Every clinical encounter contains possibility. As you reflect on how Socio-Emotional Relationship Therapy is relevant to your practice, consider Salvador Minuchin's (2017) call to be an instrument of change (see Chapter 1). What clinicians think, say, and do matters. Even a small shift in perspective can have major implications for the trajectories of our clients' lives (Winslade, 2009). How we enact our therapeutic roles can determine whether we reinforce inequities built into and perpetuated by dominant discourses and an inequitable status quo, or are part of a path toward third order change based on equity and relationality (McDowell et al., 2018, 2023).

When Douglas Huenergardt, our students, and I first began to conceptualize SERT (Knudson-Martin & Huenergardt, 2010), we were drawn by the idea that within every situation are multiple sociocultural potentials. We were inspired by Boszormenyi-Nagy and Krasner (1986) to focus forward: to help clients consider how next generations will live their legacies and to take into account the consequences of our work for the future. As a SERT practitioner, you can and must address the immediate issues entrusted to your care; *how* you do this and what it means to be a responsive and responsible clinician matter, not only in the short term but for posterity.

SERT aligns with the goal of creating a just, relationally responsive world, which at its heart is an ethical and political project that involves

                    DOI: 10.4324/9781003270232-14

noticing what we do together and how we relate (Bava, 2023). When practicing SERT, you mindfully orient toward just relationships and challenge many dominant culture notions of professionalism and individualism (Knudson-Martin & Kim, 2023). In so doing, you are being accountable for how what you do together in therapy opens possibilities that have consequences.

The principles and practices illustrated in this book are thus a guide to co-creating the future. You begin by expanding the lens to see social patterns, standards, and expectations often so taken for granted you (and your clients) could not previously see them. You engage, not as a distant "objective" neutral observer, but as a curious partner seeking to socioculturally attune to each client's unique felt identities and experience. This can feel emotionally risky as you step away from a clinical power position. You reflectively frame interventions with attention to their impact on the flow of power among family members/intimate partners and between them and the larger society, as well as with you. Your leadership focuses on facilitating equitable relational processes that mutually nurture and support each person and enable them to join together to envision and enact relational patterns that transform what is possible and create new options.

Your role in determining what is privileged in the therapeutic process is influential, and your responsibility for it—conscious or not—cannot be avoided (see Chapter 6). The following questions for reflection will help your next steps in an ongoing journey toward socially responsible practice that co-creates a future that supports well-being through reciprocally responsive relationships based on equity and an expanded awareness of what is possible and desired.

1. What do I need to do to attune to my own socio-emotional experience and that of my clients?
2. What stereotypes and societal ideas have I (and my clients) internalized that perpetuate inequitable power processes and structures?
3. What kind of future do I want to be part of co-creating? In my practice in general? In this particular case?
4. How do the way I think, talk, and name things position my work toward the future I/we envision? Or not?

5. What helps me stay focused on equitable, mutually supportive relational processes? What takes me off-track?

6. How do desires to feel comfortable or perfect get in the way of co-creating an equitable future? In general? In this particular case?

7. How are my ideas about professionalism evolving as I move toward responsible, relationally responsive practice?

Socially responsible practice takes courage. Examining our worlds, our work, and our places in them asks us to explore what has been masked or oblivious to us and to move *with* our clients toward what previously has been hidden, overlooked, diminished, or discounted. It inevitably integrates the personal with the professional (Aponte & Carlsen, 2009). I encourage you to experiment with whatever the next steps are for you and to find supportive friends and colleagues to sustain you. Together we are co-creating what it means to practice responsibly, ethically, and effectively—what it means to do good therapy.

REFERENCES

Almeida, R. V. (2018). *Liberation based healing practices.* Institute for Family Services.

Anderson, H. (2022). Collaborative-dialogic practice: Conceptual framework. In H. Anderson & D. Gehart (Eds.), *Collaborative-dialogic practice: Generative relationships and conversations across contexts and cultures* (pp. 3–18). Routledge.

Aponte, H. J., & Carlsen, J. C. (2009). An instrument for person-of-the therapist supervision. *Journal of Marital and Family Therapy, 35*(4), 3395–405.

Baber, K., & Allen, K. (1992). *Women in families: Feminist reconstructions.* Guildford.

Baima, T. R. (2022). Transformative love: An antidote to white domination disorder. In K. V. Hardy (Ed.), *The enduring, invisible, and ubiquitous centrality of whiteness* (pp. 555–580). Norton.

Baima, T. R., & Feldhousen, E. B. (2007). The heart of sexual trauma: Patriarchy as a centrally organizing principle for couple therapy. *Journal of Feminist Family Therapy, 19,* 13–36.

Ball, J., Cowan, P., & Cowen, C. (1995). Who's got the power? Gender differences in partner's perceptions of influence during marital problem-solving. *Family Process, 34,* 303–321.

Bateson, G. (1972). *Steps to an ecology of mind: Collected essays in anthropology, psychiatry, evolution, and epistemology.* Jason Aronson.

Bava, S. (2019). Hyperlinked identity: A generative resource in a divisive world. In M. McGoldrick & K. V. Hardy (Eds.), *Revisioning family therapy: Addressing diversity in clinical practice* (3rd ed., pp. 318–335). Guilford.

Bava, S. (2023). A relationally responsive world: The politics of collaborative-dialogic space and process for generativity. In H. Anderson & D. Gehart (Eds.), *Collaborative-dialogic practice: Generative relationships and conversations across contexts and cultures* (pp. 37–54). Routledge.

Bava, S., & McNamee, S. (2019). Imagining relationally crafted justice: A pluralist stance. *Contemporary Justice Review, 22*(3), 290–306.

Beaudoin, M., & MacLennan, R. (2021). Mindfulness and embodiment in family therapy: Overview, nuances, and clinical applications in poststructural practices. *Family Process, 60*(4), 1555–1567.

Becker, C., Chasin, L., Chasin, R., Herzig, M., & Roth, S. (1995). From stuck debate to new conversation on controversial issues: A report from the public conversations project. *Journal of Feminist Family Therapy, 7*(1–2), 143–163.

Belenky, M. F., Clinchy, B. M., Goldberger, N. R., & Tarule, J. M. (1986). *Women's ways of knowing: The development of self, voice, and mind.* Basic Books.

Berg, I. K., & DeJong, P. (1996). Solution-building conversations: Co-constructing a sense of competence with clients. *Families in Society, 77*(6), 376–391.

Bergeron, G., De La Cruz, N., Gould, L., Liu, S., & Seligson, A. (2020). Association between racial discrimination and health-related quality of life and the impact of social relationships. *Quality of Life Research, 29*, 2793–2805.

Bermúdez, J. M., Muruthi, B. A., & Jordan, L. S. (2016). Decolonizing research methods for family science: Creating space at the center. *Journal of Family Theory & Review, 8*(2), 192–206.

Bernard, J. (1973). *The future of marriage.* World.

Boszormenyi-Nagy, I., & Krasner, B. R. (1986). *Between give and take: A clinical guide to contextual therapy.* Brunner/Mazel.

Brown, L. S. (2008). *Cultural competence in trauma therapy: Beyond the flashback.* American Psychological Association.

Bucciarelli, V., Nasi, M., Bianco, F., Seferovic, J., Ivkovic, V., Gallina, S., & Mattioli, A. V. (2022). Depression pandemic and cardiovascular risk in the COVID-19 era and long COVID syndrome: Gender makes a difference. *Trends in Cardiovascular Medicine, 32*, 12–17.

Burger, J. M., Sanchez, J., Imberi, J. E., & Grande, L. R. (2009). The norm of reciprocity as an internalized social norm: Returning favors even when no one finds out. *Social Influence, 4*(1), 11–17.

Burkitt, I. (2014). *Emotions and social relations.* Sage.

Butler, D. S., & Moseley, G. L. (2013). *Explain pain* (2nd ed.). Noigroup Publications.

Carli, L. L. (2020). Women, gender equality and COVID-19. *Gender in Management: An International Journal, 35*, 647–655.

Charmaz, K. (2014). *Constructing grounded theory: A practical guide through qualitative analysis* (2nd ed.). Sage.

ChenFeng, J., & Galick, A. (2015). How gender discourses hijack couple therapy–and how to avoid it. In C. Knudson-Martin, M. A. Wells & S. K. Samman (Eds.), *Socio-emotional relationship therapy: Bridging emotion, societal context, and couple interaction* (pp. 41–52). AFTA Springer Briefs in Family Therapy, Springer.

ChenFeng, J., Kim, L., Knudson-Martin, C., & Wu, Y. (2017). Application of socio-emotional relationship therapy with couples of Asian heritage: Addressing issues of culture, gender, and power. *Family Process, 56*, 558–573.

Coghlan, D., & Brannick, T. (2010). *Doing action research in your own organization* (3rd ed.). Sage.

Combs, G., & Freedman, J. (2012). Narrative, poststructuralism, and social justice: Current practices in narrative therapy. *The Counseling Psychologist, 40*, 1033–1060.

Combs, G., & Freedman, J. (2016). Narrative therapy's relational understanding of identity. *Family Process, 55*, 211–224.

Cowdery, R. S., & Knudson-Martin, C. (2005). Motherhood: Tasks, relational connection, and gender equality. *Family Relations, 54*, 335–346.

Cowdery, R. S., Scarborough, N., Knudson-Martin, C., Lewis, M., Shesadri, G., & Mahoney, A. R. (2009). Gendered power in cultural contexts part II: Middle class African American heterosexual couples with young children. *Family Process, 48*, 25–39.

Cozolino, L. (2016). *Why therapy works: Using our minds to change our brains.* Norton.

Daly, K. J. (2007). *Qualitative methods for family studies and human development.* Sage.

D'Aniello, C., Nguyen, H., & Piercy, F. (2016). Cultural sensitivity as an MFT common factor. *American Journal of Family Therapy, 44,* 234–244.

D'Arrigo-Patrick, E., Samman, S. K., & Knudson-Martin, C. (2020). Moving from "I" to "we": A grounded theory analysis of couple therapy with liver patients and their partners. *Family Process, 59,* 1517–1529.

D'Arrigo-Patrick, J., D'Arrigo-Patrick, E., & Hoff, C. (2018). Colliding discourses: Families negotiating religion, sexuality, and identity. In E. Esmiol Wilson & L. Nice (Eds.), *Socially just religious and spiritual interventions: Ethical uses of therapeutic power* (pp. 37–49). AFTA Springer Briefs in Family Therapy.

D'Arrigo-Patrick, J., Hoff, C., Knudson-Martin, C., & Tuttle, A. R. (2017). Navigating critical theory and postmodernism: Social justice and therapist power in family therapy. *Family Process, 56,* 574–588.

Dean, L., Churchill, B., & Ruppanner, L. (2022). The mental load: Building a deeper theoretical understanding of how cognitive and emotional labor over load women and mothers. *Community, Work & Family, 25,* 13–29.

de Shazer, S. (1991). *Putting difference to work.* Norton.

Dickerson, V. C. (2010). Positioning oneself within an epistemology: Refining our thinking about integrative approaches. *Family Process, 49,* 349–368.

Dickerson, V. C. (2013). Patriarchy, power, and privilege: A narrative/poststructural view of work with couples. *Family Process, 52,* 102–114.

Dumaresque, R., Thornton, T., Glaser, D., & Lawrence, A. (2018). Politicized narrative therapy: A reckoning and a call to action. *Canadian Social Work Review, 35,* 109–129.

Durkheim, E. (2005). *Suicide: A study in sociology.* Routledge. (Original published in French in 1897).

Ellis, É., & Bermúdez, M. (2021). Funhouse mirror reflections: Resisting internalized sexism in family therapy and building a women-affirming practice. *Journal of Feminist Family Therapy, 33*(3), 223–243.

Englar-Carlson, M., & Kiselica, M. S. (2013). Affirming the strengths in men: A positive masculinity approach to assisting male clients. *Journal of Counseling & Development, 91*(4), 399–409.

Esmiol, E. E., Knudson-Martin, C., & Delgado, S. (2012). Developing a contextual consciousness: Learning to address gender, societal power, and culture in clinical practice. *Journal of Marital and Family Therapy, 38,* 573–588.

Esmiol Wilson, E. (2018). From assessment to activism: Utilizing a justice-informed framework to guide spiritual and religious clinical interventions. In E. Esmiol Wilson & L. Nice (Eds.), *Socially just religious and spiritual interventions: Ethical uses of therapeutic power* (pp. 1–14). AFTA Springer Briefs in Family Therapy, Springer.

Estrella, J., Kuhn, V. P., Freitas, C., & Wells, M. A. (2015). Expanding the lens: How SERT therapists develop interventions that address the larger context. In C. Knudson-Martin, M. A. Wells & S. K. Samman (Eds.), *Socio-emotional relationship therapy: Bridging emotion, societal context, and couple interaction* (pp. 53–65). AFTA Springer Briefs in Family Therapy, Springer.

Ewing, J., Estes, R., & Like, B. (2017). Narrative neurotherapy (NNT): Scaffolding identify states. In M Beaudoin & J. Duvall (Eds.), *Collaborative therapy and neurobiology: Evolving practice in action* (pp. 87–99). Routledge.

Falicov, C. J. (1995). Training to think culturally: A multidimensional comparative framework. *Family Process, 34*(4), 373–388.

Falicov, C. J. (2014). Psychotherapy and supervision as cultural encounters: The multidimensional ecological comparative approach framework. In C. A. Falender, E. P. Shafranske & C. J. Falicov (Eds.), *Multiculturalism and diversity in clinical supervision* (pp. 29–58). American Psychological Association.

Fishbane, M. D. (2007). Wired to connect: Neuroscience, relationships, and therapy. *Family Process, 46*, 395–412.

Fraenkel, P. (2023). *Last chance couple therapy: Bringing relationships back from the brink.* Norton.

Fricker, M. (2007). *Epistemic injustice: Power and the ethics of knowing.* Oxford University Press.

Galick, A., D'Arrigo-Patrick, E., & Knudson-Martin, C. (2015). Can anyone hear me? Does anyone see me? A qualitative meta-analysis of women's experiences of heart disease. *Qualitative Health Research, 25*(8), 1123–1138.

Gallagher, C. (2003). Color-blind privilege: The social and political functions of erasing the color line in post race America. *Race, Gender & Class, 10*(4), 22–37.

Garcia, M., Košutić, I., & McDowell, T. (2015). Peace on earth/war at home: The role of emotion regulation in social justice work. *Journal of Feminist Family Therapy, 27*(1), 1–20.

Garcia, M., & McDowell, T. (2010). Mapping social capital: A critical contextual approach for working with low-status families. *Journal of Marital and Family Therapy, 36*, 96–107.

George, J., & Stith, S. M. (2014). An updated feminist view of intimate partner violence. *Family Process, 53*, 179–193.

Gergen, K. J. (1997). *Realities and relationships: Soundings in social construction.* Harvard University Press.

Gergen, K. J. (2021). *The relational imperative: Resources for a world on edge.* Taos Institute Publications.

Gerhardt, S. (2004). *Why love matters: How affection shapes a baby's brain.* Brunner/Mazel.

Gerson, K. (2009). *The unfinished revolution: Coming of age in a new era of gender, work, and family.* Oxford University Press.

Gilligan, C. (1982). *In a different voice: Psychological theory and women's development.* Harvard University Press.

Glebova, T., & Knudson-Martin, C. (2023). *Sociocultural trauma and relational well-being in the Eastern European context.* AFTA Springer Briefs in Family Therapy.

Goldner, V. (1985). Feminism and family therapy. *Family Process, 24*, 31–47.

Goodrich, T. J. (Ed.). (1991). *Women and power: Perspectives for family therapy.* Norton.

Gottman, J. M. (2011). *The science of trust: Emotional attunement for couples.* Norton.

Gouldner, A. W. (1960). The norm of reciprocity: A preliminary statement. *American Sociological Review, 25*(2), 161–178.

Greenberg, L. S. (1991). Research on the process of change. *Psychotherapy Research, 1*, 3–16.

Greenberg, L. S. (2007). A guide to conducting a task analysis of psychotherapeutic change. *Psychotherapy Research, 17*, 15–30.

Greenberg, L. S., & Goldman, R. N. (2008). *Emotion-focused couples therapy: The dynamics of emotion, love, and power.* American Psychological Association.

Greene, M. (2018). *The little #METOO book for men.* ThinkPlay Partners.

Grunebaum, H. (2006). On wisdom. *Family Process, 45*, 117–132.

György, G. (2023). Identity, security, and belonging: Healing from collective sociocultural trauma in Romania. In T. Glebova & C. Knudson-Martin (Eds.), *Sociocultural trauma and well-being in Eastern European family therapy* (pp. 45–57). AFTA Springer Briefs in Family Therapy, Springer.

Hanna, S. (2014). *The transparent brain in couple and family therapy: Mindful integrations with neuroscience.* Routledge.

Hardy, K. V. (1989). The theoretical myth of sameness: A critical issue in family therapy training and treatment. *Journal of Psychotherapy and the Family, 6*, 17–33.

Hardy, K. V. (2022). The centrality of whiteness. In K. V. Hardy (Ed.), *The enduring, invisible, and ubiquitous centrality of whiteness* (pp. 3–33). Norton.

Hardy, K. V., & Laszloffy, T. A. (1995). The cultural genogram: Key to training culturally competent family therapists. *Journal of Marital and Family Therapy, 21*(3), 227–237.

Hardy, N. R., Sabey, A. K., & Anderson, S. R. (2020). The process of change in systemic family therapy. *The Handbook of Systemic Family Therapy, 1*, 171–204.

Hare-Mustin, R. (1978). A feminist approach to family therapy. *Family Process, 17,* 181–194.

Hargrave, T. D., & Houltberg, B. J. (2020). Transgenerational theories and how they evolved into current research and practice. In K. S. Wampler, R. B. Miller & R. B. Seedall (Eds.), *The handbook of systemic family therapy* (Vol. 1, pp. 317–338). Wiley.

Harré, R., Moghaddam, F. M., Cairnie, T. P., Rothbart, D., & Sabat, S. R. (2009). Recent advances in positioning theory. *Theory & Psychology, 19*(1), 5–31.

Hays, P. (2008). *Addressing cultural competencies in practice: Assessment, diagnosis and therapy* (2nd ed.). American Psychological Association.

Herman, J. L. (2015). *Trauma and recovery: The aftermath of violence—From domestic abuse to political terror.* Basic Books.

Herzig, M., & Chasin, L. (n.d.). A nuts and bolts guide from the Public Conversations Project Fostering Dialogue Across Divides. From the Public Conversations Project. publicconversationsproject.org. (Also see the PCP Dialogue Tool Box.).

Hill, C. E., Thompson, B. J., & Williams, E. N. (1997). A guide to conducting consensual Qualitative research. *The Counseling Psychologist, 25*, 517–572.

Hill, S. A. (2005). *Black intimacies: A gender perspective on families and relationships.* AltaMira Press.

Hoffman, L. (2002). *Family therapy: An intimate journey.* Norton.

Hurtado, A. (1996). Strategic suspensions: Feminists of color theorize the production of knowledge. In N. Goldberger, J. Tarule, B. Clinchy & M. Belenky (Eds.), *Knowledge, difference and power: Essays inspired by women's ways of knowing* (pp. 372–392). Basic Books.

Imber-Black, E. (1992). *Families and larger systems: A family therapist's guide through the labyrinth.* Guilford Press.

Jack, D. C. (1991). *Silencing the self: Women and depression.* HarperPerennial.

Johnson, L. N., Evans, L. M., Baucom, B. R., & Whiting, J. B. (2020). Process research: Methods for examining mechanisms of change in systemic family therapies. *The Handbook of Systemic Family Therapy, 1*, 467–489.

Johnson, S. M. (2004). *The practice of emotionally focused couple therapy* (2nd ed.). Brunner-Routledge.

Johnson, S. M. (2005). *Emotionally focused couple therapy with trauma survivors.* Guilford.

Johnson, S. M. (2019). *Attachment theory in practice: Emotionally Focused Therapy (EFT) with individuals, couples, and families.* Guilford.

Jonathan, N. (2009). Carrying equal weight: Relational responsibility and attunement among same-sex couples. In C. Knudson-Martin & A. R. Mahoney (Eds.), *Couples, gender and power: Creating change in intimate relationships* (pp. 79–103). Springer Publishing.

Jonathan, N., & Knudson-Martin, C. (2012). Building connection: Attunement and gender equality in heterosexual relationships. *Journal of Couple and Relationship Therapy, 11*, 95–111.

Jordan, J. V. (2004). Relational resilience. In J. V. Jordan, M. Walker & L. M. Hartling (Eds.), *The complexity of connection: Writings from the Stone Center's Jean Baker Miller training institute* (pp. 28–46). Guilford.

Jordan, J. V. (2010). *Relational-cultural therapy.* American Psychological Association.

Jordan, L. S., Grogan, C., Muruthi, B., & Bermúdez, J. M. (2017). Polyamory: Experiences of power from without, from within, and in between. *Journal of Couple & Relationship Therapy, 16*, 1–19.

Kelly, S. (2017). *Diversity in couple and family therapy: Ethnicities, sexualities, and socioeconomics.* Praeger.

Kelly, S., Jérémie-Brink, G., Chambers, A. L., & Smith-Bynum, M. A. (2020). The black lives matter movement: A call to action for couple and family therapists. *Family Process, 59*(4), 1374–1388.

Kiecolt-Glaser, J., Malarkey, W., Cacioppo, J., & Glaser, J. (1994). Stressful personal relationships: Immune and endocrine function. In R. Glaser & J. Kiecolt-Glaser (Eds.), *The handbook of human stress and immunity* (pp. 321–339). Academic Press.

Kim, L., ChenFeng, J., Esmiol Wilson, E., & Knudson-Martin, C. (2017). Towards safe and equitable relationships: Sociocultural emotional attunement in supervision. In R. Allan & S. Poulsen (Eds.), *Cultural safety in couple and family supervision and training* (pp. 57–70). AFTA Springer Briefs in Family Therapy, Springer.

Kim, L., Knudson-Martin, C., & Tuttle, A. (2019). Transmission of intergenerational migration legacies in Korean American families: Parenting the third generation. *Journal of Contemporary Family Therapy, 41*, 180–190.

Knudson-Martin, C. (1992). Balancing the ledger: The applications of Nagy's theories to the study of continuity and change among generations. *Contemporary Family Therapy, 14*(3), 241–258.

Knudson-Martin, C. (1994). The female voice: Applications to Bowen's family systems theory. *Journal of Marital and Family Therapy, 20*(1), 35–46.

Knudson-Martin, C. (1995). Constructing gender in marriage: Implications for counseling. *The Family Journal, 3*, 188–199.

Knudson-Martin, C. (1997). The politics of gender in family therapy. *Journal of Marital and Family Therapy, 23*, 431–447.

Knudson-Martin, C. (2009). An unequal burden: Gendered power in diabetes care. In C. Knudson-Martin & A. R. Mahoney (Eds.), *Couples, gender and power: Creating change in intimate relationships* (pp. 105–123). Springer Publishing.

Knudson-Martin, C. (2013). Why power matters: Creating a foundation of mutual support in couple relationships. *Family Process, 52*, 5–18.

Knudson-Martin, C., & Huenergardt, D. (2010). A socio-emotional approach to couple therapy: Linking social context and couple interaction. *Family Process, 49*, 369–386.

Knudson-Martin, C., & Huenergardt, D. (2015). Bridging emotion, societal discourse, and couple interaction in clinical practice. In C. Knudson-Martin, M. A. Wells & S. K. Samman (Eds.), *Socio-emotional relationship therapy: Bridging emotion, societal context, and couple interaction* (pp. 1–13). AFTA Springer Briefs in Family Therapy, Springer.

Knudson-Martin, C., Huenergardt, D., Lafontant, K., Bishop, L., Schaepper, J., & Wells, M. (2015). Competencies for addressing gender and power in couple therapy: A socio-emotional approach. *Journal of Marital and Family Therapy, 41*, 205–220.

Knudson-Martin, C., & Kim, L. (2023). Socioculturally attuned couple therapy: Socio-Emotional Relationship Therapy. In J. L. Lebow & D. K. Snyder (Eds.), *Clinical handbook of couple therapy* (6th ed., pp. 267–291). Guilford.

Knudson-Martin, C., Kim, L., Gibbs, E., & Harmon, R. (2021). Sociocultural attunement to vulnerability in couple therapy: Fulcrum for changing power processes. *Family Process, 60*, 1152–1169.

Knudson-Martin, C., & Mahoney, A. (1996). Gender dilemmas and myth in the construction of marital bargains. *Family Process, 35*, 137–153

Knudson-Martin, C., & Mahoney, A. (1998). Language and processes in the construction of marital equality in new marriages. *Family Relations, 47*, 81–91.

Knudson-Martin, C., & Mahoney, A. (1999). Beyond different worlds: A "post-gender" approach to relational development. *Family Process, 38*, 325–340.

Knudson-Martin, C., & Mahoney, A. (2005). Moving beyond gender: Processes that create relationship equality. *Journal of Marital and Family Therapy, 31*, 235–246.

Knudson-Martin, C., & Mahoney, A. (Eds.). (2009). *Couples, gender, and power: Creating change in intimate relationships.* Springer Publishing.

Knudson-Martin, C., McDowell, T., & Bermudez, M. (2020). Sociocultural attunement in systemic family therapy. In K. Wampler & R. Miller (Eds.), *Handbook of systemic therapies* (Vol. 1., pp. 619–637). Wiley.

Knudson-Martin, C., Wells, M., & Samman, S. (Eds.). (2015). *Socio-emotional relationship therapy: Bridging societal context, emotion, and power.* AFTA Springer Briefs in Family Therapy, Springer.

Kosutic, I., Garcia, M., Graves, T., Barnett, F., Hall, J., Haley, E., Rock, J., Bathon, A., & Kaiser, B. (2009). The critical genogram: A tool for promoting critical consciousness. *Journal of Feminist Family Therapy, 21*(3), 151–176.

Krolokke, C., & Sorensen, A. S. (2006). *Gender communication theories and analysis: From silence to performance.* Sage.

Laird, J. (1999). Culture and narrative as metaphors for clinical practice with families. In D. H. Demo, K. R. Allen & M. A. Fine (Eds.), *Handbook of family diversity* (pp. 338–358). Oxford University Press.

Lareau, A. (2011). *Unequal childhoods: Class, race, and family life.* University of California Press.

Larner, G. (2015). Ethical family therapy: Speaking the language of the other. *Australian & New Zealand Journal of Family Therapy, 36*, 434–449.

Larson, R., & Richards, M. H. (1994). *Divergent realities: The emotional lives of mothers, fathers, and adolescents.* Basic Books.

Lawson, L., Knudson-Martin, C., Hernandez, B. C., Lough, A., Benesh, S., & Douglas, A. (2017). Student healthcare clinicians' illness narratives: Professional identity development and relational practice. *The American Journal of Family Therapy, 45*(3), 149–162.

Leslie, L. A., & Southard, A. L. (2009). Thirty years of feminist family therapy: Moving into the mainstream. In S. A. Lloyd, A. L. Few & K. R. Allen (Eds.), *Handbook of feminist family studies* (pp. 328–339). Sage.

Lini, C., & Bertrando, P. (2020). Finding one's place: Emotions and positioning in systemic-dialogical therapy. *Journal of Family Therapy, 42*(2), 204–221.

Lini, C., & Bertrando, P. (2022). Positional responsibility in systemic-dialogical therapy. *Journal of Family Therapy, 44*, 339–350.

Loscocco, K., & Walzer, S. (2013). Gender and the culture of heterosexual marriage in the United States. *Journal of Family Theory & Review, 5*, 1–14.

Luttrell, T. B. (2016). *Exploring factors in the relationship balance assessment.* Loma Linda University.

Mahoney, A. R., & Knudson-Martin, C. (2009). Gender equality in intimate relationships. In C. Knudson-Martin & A. Mahoney (Eds.), *Couples, gender, and power: Creating change in intimate relationships* (pp. 3–16). Springer Publishing Company.

Malpas, J. (2011). Between pink and blue: A multidimensional family approach to gender nonconforming children and their families. *Family Process, 50, 4*, 453–470.

Matta, D., & Knudson-Martin, C. (2006). Couple processes in the co-construction of fatherhood. *Family Process, 45*, 19–37.

Mazanec, M. J., & Duck, S. (1999). Responding and relating: Response-ability to individuals, relating, and difference. In S. McNamee & K. J. Gergen (Eds.), *Relational responsibility: Resources for sustainable dialogue* (pp. 121–128). Sage.

McDowell, T. (2015). *Applying critical social theories to family therapy practice.* AFTA Springer Briefs in Family Therapy, Springer.

McDowell, T., Knudson-Martin, C., & Bermudez, M. (2018). *Socioculturally attuned family therapy: Toward equitable theory and practice.* Routledge.

McDowell, T., Knudson-Martin, C., & Bermudez, M. (2019). Toward third thinking in family therapy: Addressing social justice across family therapy practice. *Family Process, 58,* 9–22.

McDowell, T., Knudson-Martin, C., & Bermudez, M. (2023). *Socioculturally attuned family therapy: Toward equitable theory and practice* (2nd ed.). Routledge.

McGoldrick, M. (1998). Introduction: Re-visioning family therapy through a cultural lens. In M. McGoldrick (Ed.), *Re-visioning family therapy: Race, culture, and gender in clinical practice* (1st ed., pp. 3–19). Guilford.

McGoldrick, M. (2016). *The genogram casebook.* Norton.

McGoldrick, M., Anderson, C. M., & Walsh, F. (Eds.). (1989). *Women in families: A framework for family therapy.* Norton.

Mehl-Madrona, L. (2010). *Healing the mind through the power of story: The promise of narrative psychiatry.* Bear & Company.

Mehl-Madrona, L., & Mainguy, B. (2015). *Remapping your mind: The neuroscience of self-transformation through story.* Bear & Company.

Minuchin, S. (2017, January/February). The art of creating uncertainty. Psychotherapy Networker, pp. 37–38.

Minuchin, S., Reiter, M., & Borda, C. (2014). *The craft of family therapy: Challenging certainties.* Routledge.

Moghadam, S., & Knudson-Martin, C. (2009). Keeping the peace: Couple relationships in Iran. In C. Knudson-Martin & A. Mahoney (Eds.), *Couples, gender, and power: Creating change in intimate relationships* (pp. 255–274). Springer Publishing Co.

Morrison, T., Ferris-Wayne, M., Harrison, T., Palmgren, E., & Knudson-Martin, C. (2022). Learning to embody equitable couples therapy: A qualitative analysis. *Journal of Contemporary Family Therapy, 44*(4), 408–421.

Murphy, M. J., & Hecker, L. L. (2020). Ethical and legal issues unique to systemic family therapy. In K. S. Wampler, R. B. Miller & R. B. Seedall (Eds.), *Handbook of systemic family therapy* (Vol. 1, pp. 533–554). John Wiley & Sons.

O'Halloran, E., Dunford, K., Kim, L., & Knudson-Martin, C. (2017, June 2). Learning to apply social justice: Studying SERT. [Poster]. American Family Therapy Academy Annual Conference, Philadelphia, PA.

Oswald, R. F., Kuvalanka, K. A., Blume, L. B., & Berkowitz, D. (2009). Queering "the family". In S. A. Lloyd, A. L. Few & K. R. Allen (Eds.), *Handbook of feminist family studies* (pp. 43–55). Sage.

Pandit, M., ChenFeng, J., & Kang, Y. J. (2015). SERT therapists' experience of practicing sociocultural attunement. In C. Knudson-Martin, M. A. Wells & S. K. Samman (Eds.), *Socio-emotional relationship therapy: Bridging emotion, societal context, and couple interaction* (pp. 67–78). AFTA Springer Briefs in Family Therapy, Springer.

Pandit, M., Kang, Y. J., ChenFeng, J., Knudson-Martin, C., & Huenergardt, D. (2014). Practicing socio-cultural attunement: A study of couple therapists. *Journal of Contemporary Family Therapy, 36,* 518–528.

Paré, D. (1996). Culture and meaning: Expanding the metaphorical repertoire of family therapy. *Family Process, 35,* 21–42.

Pascoe, C. J. (2007). *Dude you're a fag: Masculinity and sexuality in high school.* University of California Press.

Piercy, F. P. (2020). The future of systemic family therapy: What needs nurturing and what does not. In K. S. Wampler, R. B. Miller & R. B. Seedall (Eds.), *Handbook of systemic family therapy* (Vol. 1, pp. 753–770). Wiley.

Porges, S. W. (2009). Reciprocal influences between body and brain in the perception and expression of affect. In D. Fosha, D. J. Siegel & M. F. Solomon (Eds.), *The healing power of emotion: Affective neuroscience, development & clinical practice* (pp. 27–54). Norton.

Priest, J. B., Roberson, P. N. E., & Woods, S. B. (2019). In our lives and under our skin: An investigation of specific psychobiological mediators linking family relationships and health using the biobehavioral family model. *Family Process*, *58*(1), 79–99.

Quek, K. M., & Knudson-Martin, C. (2006). A push towards equality: Processes among dual-income couples in a collectivist culture. *Journal of Marriage and Family*, *68*, 56–69.

Quek, K. M., & Knudson-Martin, C. (2008). Reshaping marital power: How dual career newlywed couples create equality in Singapore. *Journal of Social and Personal Relationships*, *25*, 513–534.

Rober, P. (2021). The dual process of intuitive responsivity and reflective self-supervision: About the therapist in family therapy practice. *Family Process*, *60*(3), 1033–1047.

Robillard, G., Dilley-Bucciarelli, G., Decker, A., Willis, V., Kim, L., & Knudson-Martin C. (2018, June 22). Learning to socioculturally attune from inside and out. [Brief presentation]. American Family Therapy Academy, Austin, TX.

Roesch, E., Amin, A., Gupta, J., & García-Moreno, C. (2020). Violence against women during covid-19 pandemic restrictions. *BMJ*, *369*, 1712.

Rusovick, R., & Knudson-Martin, C. (2009). Gender discourse in relationship stories of young American couples. In C. Knudson-Martin & A. Mahoney (Eds.), *Couples, gender, and power: Creating change in intimate relationships* (pp. 275–294). Springer Publishing Co.

Salmon, L. (2017). The four questions: A framework for integrating an understanding of oppression in clinical work and supervision. In R. A. Allan & S. S. Poulsen (Eds.), *Creating cultural safety in couple and family therapy supervision and training* (pp. 11–22). AFTA Springer Briefs in Family Therapy, Springer.

Samman, S., & Knudson-Martin, C. (2015). Relational engagement in heterosexual couple therapy: Helping men move from "I" to "We". In C. Knudson-Martin, M. A. Wells & S. K. Samman (Eds.), *Socio-emotional relationship therapy: Bridging emotion, societal context, and couple interaction* (pp. 79–91). AFTA Springer Briefs in Family Therapy, Springer.

Scheinkman, M., & Fishbane, M. (2004). The vulnerability cycle: Working with impasses in couple therapy. *Family Process*, *43*, 279–299.

Scher, S., & Kozowska, K. (2012). Thinking, doing and the ethics of family therapy. *American Journal of Family Therapy*, *40*(2), 97–114.

Schore, A. (2021). The interpersonal neurobiology of intersubjectivity. *Frontiers in Psychology*, *12*, 648616. http://doi.org/10.3389/fpsyg.2021.648616

Seedall, R. B., & Butler, M. H. (2006). The effect of proxy-voice intervention on couple softening in the context of enactments. *Journal of Marital and Family Therapy*, *32*(4), 421–437.

Seedall, R. B., Butler, M. H., Zamora, J. P., & Yang, C. (2016). Attachment change in the beginning stages of therapy: Examining change trajectories for avoidance and anxiety. *Journal of Marital and Family Therapy*, *42*(2), 217–230.

Siegel, D. J. (2007). *The mindful brain: Reflection and attunement in the cultivation of well-being*. Norton.

Siegel, D. J. (2012). *The developing mind: How relationships and the brain interact and shape who we are*. Guildford.

Siegel, D. J. (2019). The mind in psychotherapy: An interpersonal neurobiology framework for understanding and cultivating mental health. *Psychology and Psychotherapy*, *92*, 224–237.

Siegel, D. J., & Bryson, T. P. (2016). *No-drama discipline: The whole-brain way to calm the chaos and nurture your child's developing mind.* Bantam.

Silverstein, R., Bass, L. B., Tuttle, A., Knudson-Martin, C., Huenergardt, D. (2006). What does it mean to be relational? A framework for assessment and practice. *Family Process, 45*, 391–405.

Simon, G. (2018). Eight criteria for quality in systemic practitioner research. uobrep. openrepository.com

Smoliak, O., LaMarre, A., Rice, C., Tseliou, E., LeCouteur, A., Myers, M., Vesely, L., Briscoe, C., Addison, M., & Velikonja, L. (2022a). The politics of vulnerable masculinity in couple therapy. *Journal of Marital and Family Therapy, 48*, 427–446.

Smoliak, O., Rice, C., Knudson-Martin, C., Briscoe, C., LeCouteur, A., LaMarre, A., Tseliou, E., Velikonja, L., Myers, M., Addison, M., & Vesely, L. (2022b). Denials of responsibility in couple therapy. *Journal of Couple and Relationship Therapy, 21*, 344–365.

Smoliak, O., Rice, C., LaMarre, A., Tseliou, E., LeCouteur, A., & Davies, A. (2023). Gendering of care and care inequalities in couple therapy. *Family Process* (advanced on line publication). http://doi.org/10.1111/famp12804

Spencer, C. M., Keilholtz, B. M., & Stith, S. M. (2020). The association between attachment styles and physical intimate partner violence perpetration and victimization: A meta-analysis. *Family Process, 60*, 270–284.

St. George, S., & Wulff, D. (2014). Braiding socio-cultural interpersonal patterns into therapy. In K. Tomm, S. St. George, D. Wulff & T. Strong (Eds.), *Patterns in interpersonal interactions: Inviting relational understandings for therapeutic change* (pp. 124–142). Routledge.

St. George, S., Wulff, D., & Tomm, K. (2015). Research as daily practice. *Journal of Systemic Therapies, 34*(2), 3–14.

Stith, S. M., McCollum, E. E., & Rosen, K. H. (2011). *Couples therapy for domestic violence: Finding safe solutions.* American Psychological Association.

Stone, D. J., & ChenFeng, J. L. (2020). *Finding your voice as a beginning marriage and family therapist.* Routledge.

Strong, T. (2017). Neuroscience discourse and collaborative therapies? In M. Beaudoin & J. Duvall (Eds.), *Collaborative therapy and neurobiology: Evolving practice in action* (pp. 116–127). Routledge

Sullivan, O. (2005). *Changing gender relations, changing families; Tracing the pace of change over time.* Rowman & Littlefield.

Sutherland, O., Turner, J., & Dienhart, A. (2013). Responsive persistence Part I: Therapist influence in postmodern practice. *Journal of Marital and Family Therapy, 39*, 470–487.

Taylor, S. (2006). Tend and befriend: Biobehavioral bases of affiliation under stress. *Current Directions in Psychological Science, 15*(6), 273–277.

Tichenor, V. J. (2005). *Earning more and getting less: Why successful wives can't buy equality.* Rutgers University Press.

Thompson, E. (2016). Introduction to the revised edition. In F. J. Varela, E. Thompson & E. Rosch (Eds.), *The embodied mind: Cognitive science and human experience* (2nd ed., pp. xvii–xxix). The MIT Press.

Tuttle, A., Kim, L., & Knudson-Martin, C. (2012). Parenting as relationship: A framework for assessment and practice. *Family Process, 51*, 73–89.

U.S. Surgeon General's Advisory on the Healing Effects of Social Connection and Community (2023). Our epidemic of loneliness and isolation. www.hhs.gov/sites/default/files/surgeon-general-social-connection-advisory.pdf

van der Meiden J., Verduijn, Noordegraff, M., & van Ewijk, H. (2020). Strengthening connectedness in close relationships: A model for applying contextual therapy. *Family Process, 59*, 346–360.

Varela, F. J., Thompson, E., & Rosch, E. (2016). *The embodied mind: Cognitive science and human experience* (2nd ed.). The MIT Press.

Vargas, L., & Wilson, C. M. (2011). Managing worldview influences: Self-awareness and self-supervision in a crosscultural therapeutic relationship. *Journal of Family Psychotherapy, 22*(2), 97–113.

Walters, M., Carter, B., Papp, P., & Silverstein, O. (1991). *The invisible web: Gender patterns in family relationships.* Guilford Press.

Ward, A., & Knudson-Martin, C. (2012). The impact of therapist actions on the balance of power within the couple system: A Qualitative analysis of therapy sessions. *Journal of Couple and Relationship Therapy, 11*, 221–237.

Watson, M. F. (2013). *Facing the black shadow.* BookBaby.

Watson, M. F., Bacigalupe, G., Daneshpour, M., Han, W., & Parra-Cardona, R. (2020). Covid-19 interconnectedness: Health inequality, the climate crisis, and collective trauma. *Family Process, 59*, 832–846.

Wells M. A., & Kuhn, V. P. (2015). Couple therapy with adult survivors of child abuse: Gender, power, and trust. In C. Knudson-Martin, M. A. Wells & S. K. Samman (Eds.), *Socio-emotional relationship therapy: Bridging emotion, societal context, and couple interaction* (pp. 107–119). AFTA Springer Briefs in Family Therapy, Springer.

Wells, M. A., Lobo, E., Galick, A., Knudson-Martin, C., Huenergardt, D., & Schaepper, J. (2017). Fostering trust through relational safety: Applying SERT's focus on gender and power with adult-survivor couples. *Journal of Couple & Relationship Therapy, 16*, 122–145.

Wetherell, M. (2012). *Affect and emotion: A new social science understanding.* Sage.

White, M. (2007). *Maps of narrative practice.* Norton.

Williams, K., Galick, A., Knudson-Martin, C., & Huenergardt, D. (2013). Toward mutual support: A task analysis of the relational justice approach to infidelity. *Journal of Marital and Family Therapy, 39*, 285–298.

Williams, K., & Knudson-Martin, C. (2013). Do therapists address gender and power in infidelity? A feminist analysis of the treatment literature. *Journal of Marital and Family Therapy, 39*, 271–284.

Winslade, J. (2009). Tracing lines of flight: Implications of the work of Gilles Deleuze. *Family Process, 48*, 332–346.

Yancy, G. (2012). *Look, a white! Philosophical essays on whiteness.* Temple University Press.

Zimmerman, J. (2018). *Neuro-narrative therapy: New possibilities for emotion-filled conversations.* Norton.

Zimmerman, T. S., Haddock, S. A., Ziemba, S., & Rust, A. (2002). Family organizational labor: Who's calling the plays?. *Journal of Feminist Family Therapy, 13*(2–3), 65–90.

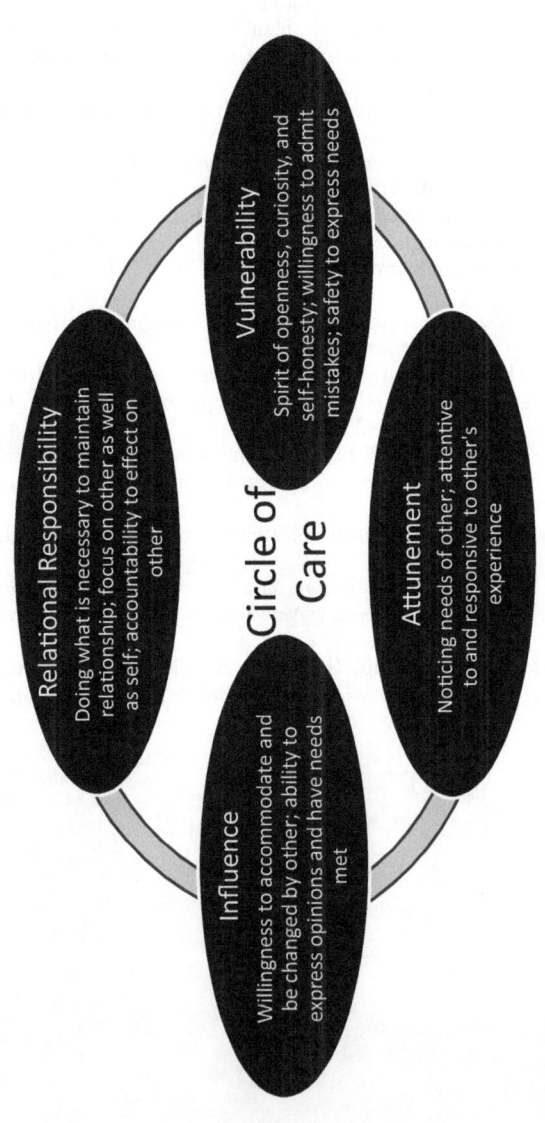

Figure BM2 Circle of Care

Source: Knudson-Martin, C. & Huenergardt, D. (2015). Bridging emotion, societal discourse, and couple interaction. In C. Knudson-Martin, M. E. Wells, & S. Samman (Eds.). *Socio-Emotional Relationship Therapy: Bridging emotion, societal context, and couple interaction* (p. 6). Springer. Used with permission.

APPENDIX B
TYPOLOGY OF RELATIONAL ORIENTATIONS

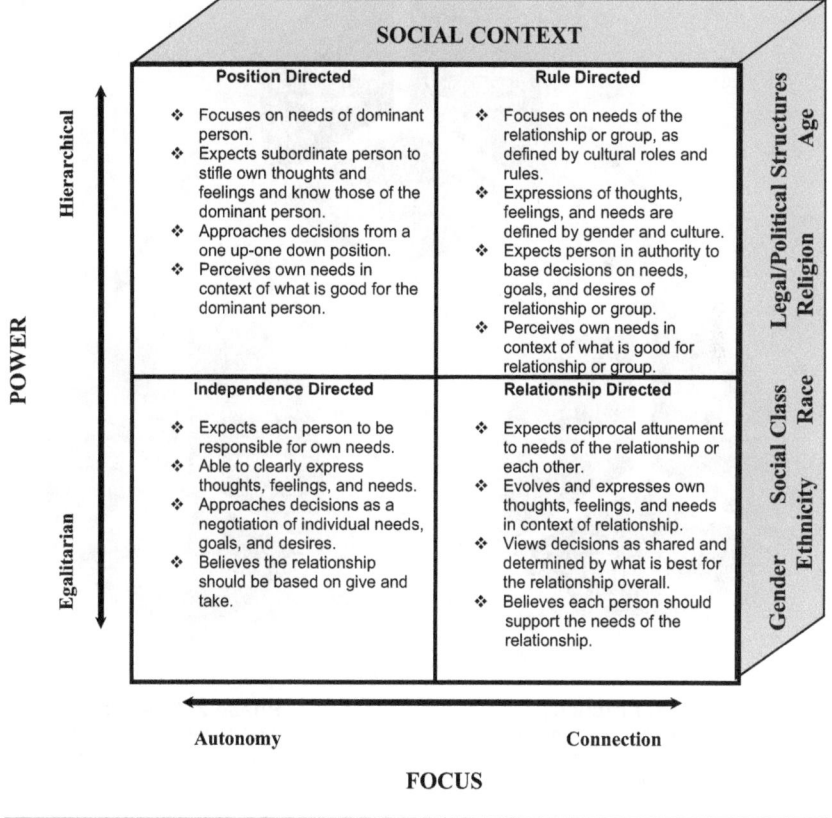

Figure BM3 Typology of Relational Orientations

Source: Silverstein, R., Bass, L. B., Tuttle, A., Knudson-Martin, C., & Huenergardt, D. (2006). What does it mean to be relational? A framework for assessment and practice. *Family Process, 45*, p. 399 (used with permission)

Appendix C
SERT Clinical Sequence

Phase 1: Position
Position therapy to counter inequities and orient toward relationality

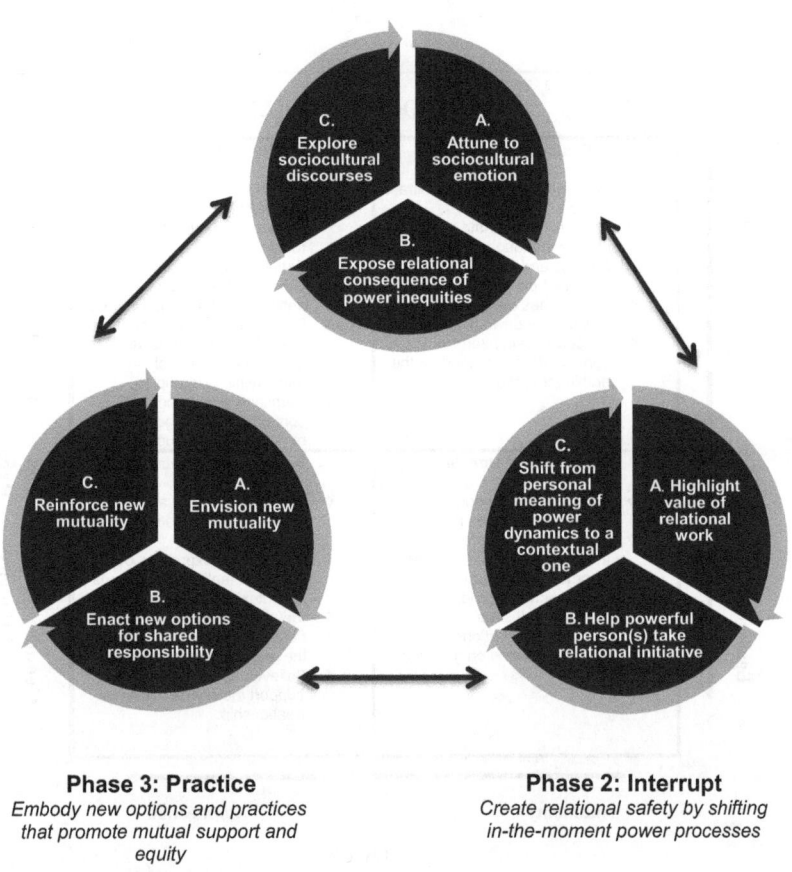

Phase 3: Practice
Embody new options and practices that promote mutual support and equity

Phase 2: Interrupt
Create relational safety by shifting in-the-moment power processes

Figure BM4 Circle of Care

Source: Knudson-Martin, C., & Kim, L. (2023). Socioculturally attuned couple therapy. In J. L. Lebow & D. K. Snyder (Eds.). *Clinical Handbook of Couple Therapy* (6th ed., p. 279). Guildford (used with permission)

APPENDIX D
SERT CLINICAL COMPETENCIES AND OUTCOMES

SERT CLINICAL COMPETENCIES

Phase 1. Position

Competencies	Steps involved	Outcomes
1a. Attune to sociocultural emotion	1. Know your place in the system 2. Identify emotionally salient words or actions 3. Engage emotionally to resonate with client's contextual situation 4. Mirror, sharpen, and focus felt contextual experience 5. Voice sociocultural context of relational hopes and fears	A. Clients feel felt, and the boundary between the personal and the societal begins to dissolve B. Powerful clients begin to be aware of their position and demonstrate openness to accountability for their impact on others and shared relational responsibility
1b. Expose relational consequences of power inequities	1. Consider power contexts of client issues 2. Track flow of power 3. Explore relational impact of the flow of power 4. Name consequences of power imbalance on relational goals	C. Clients begin to see themselves and their relationships from a new, sociocultural angle and open themselves to relational possibilities based on equity and mutual support
1c. Explore sociocultural discourses	1. Move from the personal to the contextual 2. Name the expectation/discourse 3. Explore the personal/relational effect of the discourse 4. Invite possibility of alternative or marginalized discourse	

(Continued)

Continued

Phase 2. Interrupt		
Competencies	**Steps involved**	**Outcomes**
2a. Highlight the value of relational work	1. Look for and uncover examples of unrecognized relational work 2. Detail what is involved in doing relational work 3. Identify the positive consequences of relational work for others	A. Relationally oriented persons, who are usually also in less powerful positions, experience validation B. Powerful persons experience the positive consequences of relational engagement; less powerful persons begin to feel safer and cared about C. Less powerful, more vulnerable persons are likely to be heard, and clients join together to resist negative societal effects
2b. Help more powerful persons take relational initiative	1. Consider the flow of power when inviting clients to express vulnerability or attune 2. Address accountability for the impact of a nonrelational position 3. Name the powerful person's relational interest in engaging in the Circle of Care 4. Support the powerful person in carrying out relational acts 5. Identify the positive consequences of the relational act	
2c. Connect interruptions in the flow of power to contextual meaning	1. Frame behaviors or conflicts in terms of social position and/or competing societal discourses 2. Identify personal meaning around the societal discourse 3. Explore consequences of enacting the societal discourse 4. Discuss choices and preferences regarding enactments of societal discourse	

Phase 3. Practice		
Competencies	**Steps involved**	**Outcomes**
3a. Envision new mutuality	1. Invite relational/equitable ideals to the foreground 2. Create a detailed image of mutual support/equity in this circumstance 3. Identify what is involved in enacting the ideal 4. Envision the meaning and consequences of the ideal in clients' lives	A. Clients use images of mutual support to describe and evaluate how they relate B. Clients incorporate images of mutual support into their felt identities C. Clients experience confidence that they can safely communicate on hard topics
3b. Enact new options for shared relational responsibility	1. Create the relational focus and goal 2. Clarify what clients will do 3. Coach behind the scenes 4. Process what happened and how 5. Carry learning forward	D. Clients are able to intentionally break from dominant discourse to consider and enact new options E. Clients demonstrate and embody new models of relating
3c. Reinforce new mutuality	1. Identify demonstrations of transformative action 2. Amplify what was involved 3. Reinforce positive relational outcomes 4. Encourage commitment to reflective action	

APPENDIX E
SERT COMPETENCIES EVALUATION FORM

SERT PHASE 1: Positioning Competencies			
Competency	Steps involved	Observed?	Notes
1a. Attune to socio-cultural emotion	1. Know your place in the system 2. Identify emotionally salient words or actions 3. Engage emotionally to resonate with client's contextual situation 4. Mirror, sharpen, and focus felt contextual experience 5. Voice sociocultural context of relational hopes and fears		
1b. Expose relational consequences of power inequities	1. Consider power contexts of client issues 2. Track flow of power 3. Explore relational impact of the flow of power 4. Name relational consequences of power imbalance		
1c. Explore sociocultural discourses	1. Move from the personal to the contextual 2. Name the expectation/discourse 3. Explore the personal/relational effect of the discourse 4. Invite possibility of alternative or marginalized discourse		
Phase 1 Client Outcomes			
Outcome		Observed?	Notes
1A. Clients feel felt, and the boundary between the personal and the societal begins to dissolve			
1B. Powerful clients begin to be aware of their position and demonstrate openness to accountability for their impact on others and shared relational responsibility			
1C. Clients begin to see themselves and their relationships from a new, sociocultural angle and open themselves to relational possibilities based on equity and mutual support			

SERT PHASE 2: Interrupting Competencies			
Competency	Steps involved	Observed?	Notes
2a. Highlight the value of relational work	1 Look for and uncover examples of unrecognized relational work 2. Detail what is involved in doing relational work 3. Identify the positive consequences of relational work for others		
2b. Help more powerful persons take relational initiative	1. Consider the flow of power when inviting clients to express vulnerability or attune 2. Address accountability for the impact of a nonrelational position 3. Name the powerful person's relational interest in engaging in the Circle of Care 4. Support the powerful person in carrying out relational acts 5. Identify the positive consequences of the relational act		
2c. Connect interruptions in the flow of power to contextual meaning	1. Frame behaviors or conflicts in terms of social position and/or competing societal discourses 2. Identify personal meaning around the societal discourse 3. Explore consequences of enacting the societal discourse 4. Discuss choices and preferences regarding enactments of societal discourse		

Phase 2 Client Outcomes		
Outcome	Observed?	Notes
2A. Relationally oriented persons, who are usually also in less powerful positions, experience validation		
2B. Powerful persons experience the positive consequences of relational engagement; less powerful persons begin to feel safer and cared about		
2C. Less powerful, more vulnerable persons are likely to be heard and clients join together to resist negative societal effects		

(Continued)

Continued

SERT PHASE 3: Practicing Competencies			
Competency	**Steps involved**	**Observed?**	**Notes**
3a. Envision new mutuality	1. Invite relational/equitable ideals to the fore-ground 2. Create a detailed image of mutual support/equity in this circumstance 3. Identify what is involved in enacting the ideal 4. Envision the meaning and consequences of the ideal in clients' lives		
3b. Enact new options for shared relational responsibility	1. Create the relational focus and goal 2. Clarify what clients will do 3. Coach behind the scenes 4. Process what happened and how 5. Carry learning forward		
3c. Reinforce new mutuality	1. Identify demonstrations of transformative action 2. Amplify what was involved 3. Reinforce positive relational outcomes 4. Encourage commitment to reflective action		
Phase 3 Client Outcomes			
Outcome		**Observed?**	**Notes**
3A. Clients use images of mutual support to describe and evaluate how they relate			
3B. Clients incorporate images of mutual support into their felt identities			
3C. Clients experience confidence that they can safely communicate on hard topics			
3D. Clients are able to intentionally break from dominant discourse to consider and enact new options			
3E. Clients demonstrate and embody new models of relating			

Appendix F

SERT Assessment
Guide (SAG)

Social Identities [Context and Discourses]

- In what kinds of societal contexts are clients embedded? How have these changed over time?
- What messages about gender, sexuality, and intimate relationships has each internalized?
- How do socioeconomic status and economic situation impact constructions of self, access to resources, and relationship patterns?
- How do social institutions (immigration, justice system, medical, health, social services, etc.) impact the client's sense of self and relationships with others?
- How do each person's religion, age, race, ethnicity, and disabilities impact constructions of self and experience in their relationships?
- How are the client's expressions of thoughts, feelings, and needs influenced by cultural, religious, or gender discourses?
- To what extent are the client's decisions determined by cultural, religious, or gender traditions?

Flow of Power

- How much personal, interpersonal, and institutional power does each client experience as a result of their societal positions?
- To what extent is each person equally able to express and attain personal interests/goals?
- To what extent do each expect to define what is "real"?
- To what extent does each person organize around what matters to the other(s)?
- Whose interests are most reflected in "shared" decisions?
- Whose interests and schedule organize daily schedules and routines?
- How are differences in opinion handled?
- Who is more likely to accommodate the other person(s)?
- Does accommodation often occur automatically without anything being said?
- Does one person's sense of competence, optimism, or well-being seem to come at the expense of the other's physical or emotional health?
- Does the relationship support the economic viability of each person?

(Continued)

Continued

Mutuality in the Circle of Care

Vulnerability

- How able is each to let down their guard to take in the other's experience?
- How willing is each to admit weakness, uncertainty, or mistakes in the other's presence?
- How safe does each feel to share innermost thoughts and feelings with partner(s)?
- How able are partners to seek relationship repair by expressing a feeling or concern? Who is more likely to do this?
- How are expressions of vulnerability related to social identity/norms and/or trauma and marginalized experience?

Attunement

- How interested is each person in knowing and understanding the other's experience and perspective?
- Who listens to the other(s)? About what? In what circumstances?
- To what extent does each notice and respond to the other's feelings and needs?
- How able is each to witness and respond to the other's negative emotions?
- To what extent is each attuned to what is good for the relationship overall, compared to what is good for the self?
- How are attunement processes related to social identity/norms and/or trauma and marginalized experience?

Influence

- How able is each person to engage the other(s) in addressing issues of concern?
- How free does each feel to directly express their opinions or make requests?
- Whose expectations define standards in the relationship?
- How open is each to being impacted by the other(s)?
- Whose interests determine daily routines?
- How are influence processes related to social identity/norms and/or trauma and marginalized experience?

Relational Responsibility

- To what extent does each focus on what is needed to maintain or improve the relationship(s)? How do they do this?
- Who keeps track of what needs to be done in the home? For the children? For the relationship(s)?
- Who does the emotional work in the relationship(s)? What does that look like?
- How aware are each of the emotional work each one does?
- How responsible does each feel for the relationship(s)? How is this experienced?
- How does responsibility shift from person to person? When?
- How is the balance of relational responsibility related to social identity/norms and/or trauma and marginalized experience?

Relational Ideals

- Do the clients seek relationships that mutually benefit and support each person?
- How valued is emotional work in the relationship?
- What relationship ideals and personal characteristics do clients endorse that support mutual engagement in the Circle of Care?

APPENDIX G

SERT SESSION RATING ACROSS INTERVALS

Therapist Adherence ("sticking to model")

0	1	2	3
Almost never	a little bit	tries, but let's go	persistent

Transforming the Power Imbalance

0	1	2	3
Reinforces imbalance	maintains imbalance	creates opening for shift	enacts shift to mutuality

Sociocultural Attunement

0	1	2	3
Colonizes	no curiosity/unpacking	connects to some	connects with SC Emotion

Client Responsiveness (Clients connect to mutual ideals and/or SERT interventions)

0	1	2	3
not at all	a little	somewhat	a lot

SERT OVERALL SESSION RATING

Session code_____   Rater_____

Date_____

Table BM9 SERT Overall Session Rating

Therapist Adherence ("sticking to model")			
0	1	2	3
Almost never	Some attempts without follow-through	Inconsistent; portions of session represent SERT, other portions do not	Consistent throughout session overall

Comments/explanation

Transforming the Power Imbalance			
0	1	2	3
Therapist actions reinforce power imbalance throughout most of session	Therapist does not intervene in power imbalance and thus maintains status quo	Therapist creates or builds upon opening for shift in power imbalance but either does not follow through or client(s) resist	Session outcome represents a shift or movement toward mutuality

Comments/explanation

Sociocultural Attunement			
0	1	2	3
Therapist colonizes and/or imposes dominant discourse	Limited curiosity or unpacking of societal discourse/context	Inconsistent; connects to some key societal discourses but misses others	Connects with sociocultural emotion

Comments/explanation

Client Responsiveness (clients connect to mutual ideals and/or SERT interventions)			
0	1	2	3
Not at all	A little, then is lost	Somewhat or mixed	A lot

Comments/explanation

APPENDIX I

COMPETENCIES FOR WORKING WITH GENDER AND POWER IN COUPLE RELATIONSHIPS (2015)

Awareness → Tracking Process → Providing Leadership → Empowerment

1. Identify Enactments of Cultural Discourse

1	2	3	4	5
Therapist is aware that clients belong to a particular cultural context but is uncertain about how they are organized by culture or their relationship to it	Therapist expands awareness of cultural context to include intersections with gender, class, race, religion, and other significant personal contexts such as prison experience and work environment	Therapist identifies cultural markers in the conversation but does not explore how they uniquely link to personal experience or consider other discourses that might be involved	Therapist extends conversations regarding cultural discourse—and other contradictory discourses—that influence personal experience and couples' patterns of relating	Therapist guides partners to see their relationship as part of social patterns larger than themselves

2. Attune to Underlying Sociocultural Emotion

1	2	3	4	5
Therapist processes client emotion at an individual level but does not probe underlying relational or socio-emotional contexts	Therapist processes relational context of client emotions but does not explore how they are part of larger sociocultural experience	Therapist identifies the origin of the emotion in the larger sociocultural discourse in an abstract way that is hard for clients to understand and is not connected to their relationship process	Therapist explores underlying sociocultural emotions and begins to link them to relationship patterns	Therapist reflects sociocultural attunement to clients that affectively engages them in the therapy and creates a new basis for addressing relationship processes

3. Identify Relational Power Dynamics

1	2	3	4	5
Therapist ignores or takes power issues at face value and validates complaints of the powerful person without attending to power imbalances in the relationship	Therapist identifies power issues but minimizes them by attributing them equally to the relationship system without addressing the nuances of individual socio-emotional experience	Therapist is attuned to underlying power processes and validates individual experiences such that client "feels felt," but alienates the partner	Therapist names underlying power issues in a way that both partners feel validated	Therapist names underlying power issues in a way that both partners feel validated and engages them to relate in ways that challenge

4. Facilitate Relational Safety

1	2	3	4	5
Therapist assumes an inherent equality between partners that ignores power and safety issues that encourages vulnerability when it is not safe to do so	Therapist's exploration of safety and vulnerability issues in the relationship is limited to concerns regarding physical safety and potential violence	Therapist begins to identify and name emotional as well as physical safety issues and takes a clear stance that encourages partners to be accountable for the safety of self and other	Therapist demonstrates ongoing tracking of safety and vulnerability issues as they relate to the couple's emotional and relational processes in and out of session	Therapist actively supports both partners in building a relational bond based on mutual accountability, emotional vulnerability, and safety.

5. Foster Mutual Attunement

1	2	3	4	5
Therapist reinforces gender stereotypical power differences by encouraging the more emotionally attuned person to focus on the less attuned	Therapist encourages both partners to tune into each other but does not address the underlying power differences	Therapist identifies gendered behaviors that influence each partner's ability to attune to the other but normalizes them instead of challenging them	Therapist asks less attuned person to stretch toward partner without putting this experience in a socio-emotional context	Therapist challenges gender stereotypes and empowers each partner to empathically imagine the other's experience such that they "feel felt" and are mutually changed by that resonance

(Continued)

Awareness → Tracking Process → Providing Leadership → Empowerment

6. Create a Relationship Model Based on Equality

1	2	3	4	5
Therapist uses language that collapses individual positions in the system and ignores how gendered power contributes to the relational issues	Therapist identifies unequal relationship patterns but doesn't know how to engage clients in further exploration of these issues	Therapist interrupts unequal relationship processes and introduces questions that begin to	Therapist clearly names invisible power processes and helps couple identify their options and goals regarding relationship equality	Therapist helps couple create a relationship model based on equality and works with their micro-processes to expand and develop their picture of equality

7. Facilitate Shared Relational Responsibility

1	2	3	4	5
Therapist actions allow stereotypical gender patterns to organize the session	Therapist points out stereotypical gender interactions but does not link them to shared responsibility and mutual accountability	Therapist names the gender patterns that limit mutual responsibility and begins to track their emotional and relational impact	Therapist asks the less responsible partner to initiate relationship change but does not support the couple in establishing a new relational pattern	Therapist facilitates a process that enables both partners to genuinely engage with difficult issues while maintaining concern for the other's well-being and for the relationship

Source: Knudson-Martin, C., Huenergardt, D., Lafontant, K., Bishop, L., Schaepper, J., & Wells, M. (2015). Competencies for addressing gender and power in couple therapy: A socio-emotional approach. *Journal of Marital and Family Therapy, 4*, p. 220 (used with permission)

APPENDIX J
RELATIONAL PRACTICES CHECKLIST

Rate yourself and your significant other (**usually, sometimes, seldom**) Where there is a discrepancy in your perceptions, discuss how your internalized social schemas may contribute to your differing perceptions.

Identify areas for discussion and practice in your therapy sessions

Relational Practices	Perception of Self	Perception of Other
Attunement to Other • How interested are you in knowing and understanding the other's experience and perspective? • Do you listen to your partner? Your children? About what? In what circumstances? • To what extent do you notice and respond to the other's feelings and needs?		
Openness to Vulnerability • How willing are you to show weakness, uncertainty, or mistakes in your partner's presence? • How safe and willing do you feel to share innermost thoughts and feelings with your partner? • How likely are you to seek relationship repair by expressing a feeling or concern?		
Accepting Influence • How able are you to engage the other in addressing issues that concern you? • How free do you feel to directly express opinions or make requests? • How readily do you accommodate your interests/schedule to fit your partner's/the family's needs and schedule?		

(Continued)

Continued

Relational Practices	Perception of Self	Perception of Other
Relational Responsibility • To what extent do you focus on what is needed to maintain or improve your relationship? • To what extent do you keep track of what needs to be done in the house? For the children? For the relationship? • How responsible are you for doing the emotional work in the relationship?		

Source: McDowell, T., Knudson-Martin, C., & Bermudez, J. M. (2023). Socioculturally Attuned Family Therapy: Toward Equitable Theory and Practice. Routledge, p. 224 (used with permission)

INDEX

Page numbers in *italics* indicate a figure and page numbers in **bold** indicate a table on the corresponding page.